MICHAEL J. STROBEL

Manual of
ARTHROSCOPIC
SURGERY

With 2352 Separate Color Illustrations

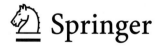

Michael J. Strobel, Professor Dr. med.
sporthopaedicum Straubing
Orthopädisch-chirurgische Gemeinschaftspraxis
Bahnhofplatz 8
D-94315 Straubing
Germany

Revised, updated, and enlarged translation
of the German edition.

Title of the German edition:

Strobel: Arthroskopische Chirurgie
© Springer-Verlag Berlin Heidelberg 1998
ISBN 3-540-63571-8

Translated by:

Terry C. Telger
6112 Waco Way
Fort Worth, TX 76133, USA

ISBN 978-3-540-85737-2

e-ISBN 978-3-540-87410-2

DOI 10.1007/978-3-540-87410-2

Library of Congress Control Number 2008933861

© 2008 Springer-Verlag Berlin Heidelberg

Cover design: eStudio Calamar Steinen, Barcelona
Illustrations: Th. Heller, Tübingen
Data conversion and layout: B. Wieland, Heidelberg
Printing and bookbinding: Stürtz GmbH, Würzburg

Printed on acid-free paper

9 8 7 6 5 4 3 2

springer.com

Acknowledgments

A book of this magnitude cannot reflect the work of a single individual. Rather, it is the result of years of collaboration among my surgical colleagues in Straubing, the illustrator, Springer Verlag, and the author.

I am grateful to the surgical staff at our clinic, especially Andrea Kienberger, Evi Schwarz, Agnes Albert, and Petra Baumann, for their valuable assistance and for putting so much time and effort into the digital documentation of interesting intraoperative findings. I thank Markus "Willi" Wild for his help in organizing the digital documentation and the many image files, and I thank Petra Broschinsky for her help with patient records. I also thank Karl-Heinz Semmelmann for scanning the many radiographs into the computer and setting up the digital data files.

Prof. Dr. Jörg Grünert (Erlangen) provided a wealth of technical advice and proofread the chapters on wrist arthroscopy and endoscopic carpal tunnel release. I am also grateful to Prof. Andre Gächter (St. Gallen, Switzerland), Dr. Andreas Weiler (Berlin), Scott Rodeo (New York), Prof. Peter Habermeyer (Heidelberg), and Dr. Kai-Uwe Jensen (Hamburg) for their many technical suggestions and for providing illustrations.

I thank my partner Dr. Hanns M. Fett (Straubing) for proofreading the manuscript and for supplying many helpful suggestions, illustrations, and additional materials for the chapter on shoulder arthroscopy. I thank Dr. Heinz-Jürgen Eichhorn for his support and technical input.

I extend special thanks to Petra Flechtner, who did most of the typing and almost all the revisions, and to Uli Schultes and Carola Urlinger.

I thank Thomas Heller (Tübingen) for the brilliant computer-rendered graphics, which reflect a precision and level of detail that I would not have thought possible. He has succeeded in combining exceptional esthetic value with an extremely high information content.

This book would not have been possible without the commitment of Springer-Verlag and its staff. I particularly acknowledge the efforts of my friend Dr. Udo Schiller, who regrettably is no longer with Springer-Verlag. He helped to plan the book and laid the groundwork for reproducing the illustrations in digitized form. I thank Gabriele Schröder for her support and for the many encouraging conversations involved in the sometimes difficult task of transforming my wishes into reality. I thank Mrs. Linde Prodehl for handling the copyediting, which was not always easy given the extensive subheadings in the manuscript.

I am particularly indebted to Bernd Wieland of Springer-Verlag, with whom I forged a friendship during the many months of the production process. Mr. Wieland took care of the proof arrangements and page layouts, processed the many digital image files, and handled technical problems and updates in a calm, efficient, and supportive manner. It is largely the result of his personal commitment that the book has achieved its present form and qualitative perfection.

In closing, I express thanks to my family and personal friends for their support and ask them to forgive me for neglecting them during the planning and production phases of this book.

Without all these friends and colleagues, it would not have been possible to create this book in its present form.

Michael J. Strobel

Preface to the English Edition

After the German book "Arthroskopische Chirurgie" proved to be such a success, both friends and visiting physicians as well as Springer-Verlag asked me to prepare an English edition. Compared to the numerous, well-known textbooks of arthroscopic surgery in the English-language literature, particularly in the US, this volume deliberately does not intend to present purely scientific treatises on the individual disease entities and surgical techniques. On the contrary, the goal of this book is to present and describe in detail those arthroscopic techniques which have proven to be clinically effective in hundreds and thousands of patients on a daily basis, and thus it does not aspire to meeting the demand of being "complete." In particular, the therapy and surgical techniques have been standardized and the operative steps are presented in a "how to do" format which is easy to follow. Particular importance has been attached to problems and pitfalls, which can affect the operative procedure considerably and in the worst-case scenario even cause the surgical treatment to fail.

With respect to the German edition, the chapters on lesions of the meniscus and on the anterior and posterior cruciate ligaments have been completely revised and expanded. The other chapters have been reworked and updated. Furthermore, many of the illustrations have been replaced and modified so that the visual presentation of arthroscopic findings and operative steps is even better. Hence, there are over 340 more illustrations than in the German edition. A superb visual presentation is essential, particularly in arthropscopic surgery, not only to be able to recognize and diagnose pathological conditions and to distinguish them from the large range of normal findings and normal variations, but also for intraoperative use in performing specific surgical procedures with care.

I would like to extend my thanks to Gabriele M. Schröder (Springer-Verlag, Heidelberg), who actively supported me in the conception and planning of the English edition of the book. Special thanks also go to Bernd Wieland (Springer-Verlag, Heidelberg), who – as for the German edition – not only designed the layout but also has produced the book cover and the illustrations to my utmost satisfaction. I thank my friend Andreas Weiler (Berlin) for the numerous histological figures and the corrections. Thanks also go to Dr. U. Horras (Giessen), who provided several histological and electron microscopic illustrations. Mr. Terry C. Telger (Fort Worth, Texas) in his reliable way provided a perfect translation of the book into English. For this, I owe him a genuine debt of gratitude. Thanks are extended once again to Petra Flechtner (Straubing), who spent a tremendous amount of time in typing and correcting the manuscript of this book, too. I would also like to thank my wife Patricia for the proof reading and at the same apologize to her for the "months of neglect" for the time it took to put this English edition together.

I do hope that the readers will find pleasure in this book and also that it helps them in their daily clinical work and furthers their enjoyment of the field of arthroscopy.

Michael J. Strobel
September 2001

Preface to the German Edition

Arthroscopic surgical procedures are no longer limited to the knee but are commonly performed on a variety of joints. While numerous books have been published on arthroscopic surgery, many deal with only a single joint or address various joints and surgical techniques in a somewhat haphazard fashion. As a result, many colleagues have approached me with the suggestion that I author a practice-oriented textbook on arthroscopic surgery.

This book is intended to cover the full spectrum of arthroscopic surgical procedures and endoscopically-assisted intraarticular operations in an up-do-date, practice-oriented "how to" format that takes into account current arthroscopic trends. The information is presented in a consistent, easy-to-use format that permits rapid referencing of specific topics of interest. The coverage of specific disorders is clear, practice-applicable, and detailed, with particular emphasis placed on arthroscopic findings, therapeutic management, and the surgical techniques that have proven most successful in the day-to-day practice of arthroscopic surgery at our institution.

A problem in all arthroscopic textbooks is how best to convey diagnostic findings and the various steps involved in surgical procedures. While schematic drawings are useful for describing operative procedures, they often convey only a vague impression of the actual practice of arthroscopic surgery. For this reason, I have chosen to illustrate the various types of joint pathology and their treatment in series of arthroscopic views that give a detailed, step-by-step visual account of the procedures. This approach requires exceptionally high-quality images in which even fine details can be appreciated. My initial plan was to use video prints as illustrations. But improvements in digital image technology caused me to reconsider, and almost all the arthroscopic views presented in this book consist of digitized video images. This accounts for their exceptionally fine quality.

It is hoped that this surgical textbook will motivate the reader to delve more deeply into arthroscopic techniques, their indications, and the differentiated management of arthroscopically treatable disorders in various joints. May the book serve as a reference tool and perhaps even a manual for arthroscopic practitioners, enabling them to plan and conduct arthroscopic surgical procedures more efficiently and successfully for the benefit of their patients.

Straubing, May, 1998
Michael J. Strobel

Contents

VOLUME 1

VOLUME 2

Ankle Joint

Ankle Joint – General Part

The ankle joint (talocrural joint) ranks third after the knee and shoulder joints in terms of the frequency of arthroscopic interventions (1036 were performed at our institution from 1992 to 2000).

3.1 Historical Development

Bircher (1921) limited arthroscopy to the knee joint. As early as 1931, however, the American surgeon Michael Burman found that the wrist and ankle joint were suitable for arthroscopy. But it was not until the late 1970s that ankle arthroscopy was practiced clinically. Chen (1976) was the first author to report on a large clinical series. He was followed by Johnson (1978), Plank (1978), and Parisien (1981).

Since then, ankle arthroscopy has become established as a standard procedure.

3.2 Instrumentation (Arthroscopy System)

Basically the same instruments are used as in knee arthroscopy (see Sect. 1.2). However, the use of a long scope in the small ankle joint would be cumbersome and would place the surgeon's hands too far from the joint. It is better to use a short-barreled scope, therefore (Fig. 3.2-1). The examiner can maneuver this scope with greater accuracy and position it more accurately within the joint. Accuracy is further improved by bracing the hand against the patient's foot.

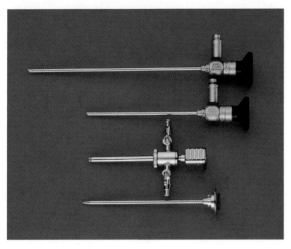

Fig. 3.2-1. Short-barrel scope (diameter 4 mm) for arthroscopy of the ankle and elbow joints. The working length is 14 cm, which is considerably shorter than a standard scope (*above*) (Karl Storz, Tuttlingen, Germany)

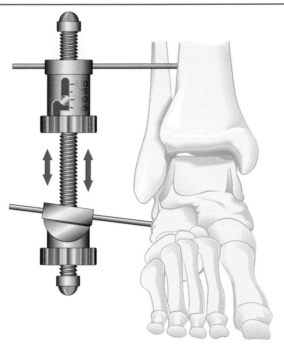

Fig. 3.5-1. Invasive distraction of the ankle joint using an external frame

3.3 Video System

The video system is identical to that used in knee arthroscopy (see Sect. 1.3).

3.4 Probe

The probing hook is used for precision palpation. We recommend using a shorter probe than in the knee joint, as this permits greater accuracy and causes less trauma.

A curved mirror is useful for selected indications (see Sect. 1.5). For example, multiple intraarticular loose bodies may slip beneath the sheath where they cannot be seen. They can be visualized by passing a mirror through the instrument portal opposite to the scope (see Fig. 8.3-4).

3.5 Distraction

The talocrural joint space is very narrow if the fibular capsule and ligaments are intact and not hyperlax. The joint space can be expanded by manual traction or with a mechanical distractor.

Some manufacturers offer special distractors that are similar in design to a single-rod external fixation device, with one pin placed in the calcaneus and the other in the tibia (Fig. 3.5-1). This is an invasive technique, however. Distractor fixation in the talus has been described, but this is hazardous due to the potential for vascular injury.

▶ **Caution:** Avascular necrosis of the talus.

To date, we have not had to use invasive distraction for ankle arthroscopy. We prefer manual distraction by an assistant or surgical nurse. Arthroscopic arthrodesis is the only procedure that requires a mechanical distractor.

▶ **Note:** Complete muscular relaxation greatly facilitates manual distraction.

3.6 Operating Instruments

The same mechanical, motor-driven, and electrosurgical instruments are used as in the knee joint (see Sect. 1.6). Smaller instruments of the type used in wrist arthroscopy (small joint set, see Sect. 5.6) should also be available. Loose bodies or detached osteophytes may occur in tight, hard-to-reach joint areas that are not accessible to larger instruments. Motorized instruments must be handled carefully when used to remove synovium or scar tissue from the anterior capsule, due to the proximity of the anterior tibial artery and other essential structures.

Following osteophyte removal, an endoscopic laser can be used to smooth the resection site and control bleeding (Fig. 3.6-1). A deep zone of necrosis should be produced to inhibit the regrowth of osteophytes following laser ablation.

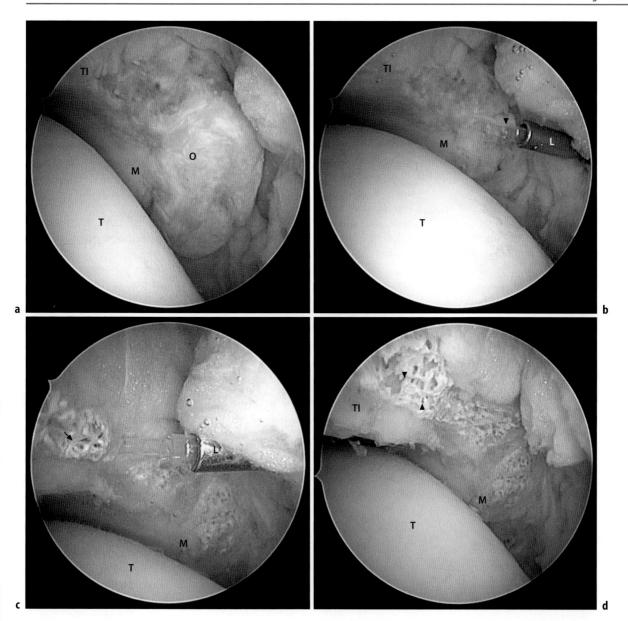

Fig. 3.6-1 a–d. Arthroscopic laser use. **a** Inspection reveals an osteophyte (*O*) on the anterior border of the medial malleolus (*M*) (*T* talus, *TI* tibia). **b** The laser handpiece (*L*) protects the laser fiber (*arrowhead*). **c** Removal of the osteophyte exposes cancellous bone. The central red beam (*arrow*) indicates the site of laser ablation. **d** Appearance of the treated area following osteophyte removal (*arrowheads* opened cancellous bone areas)

3.7 Anesthesia

General anesthesia, spinal block, or epidural anesthesia can be used for arthroscopic surgery (see Sect. 1.7). General anesthesia is preferred, as it allows for precise control of relaxation. Since most ankle procedures are done on an outpatient basis, short-acting agents are used (see Sect. 1.7).

3.8 Positioning

The patient is positioned supine with the foot 15–20 cm past the end of the operating table. A side post of the kind used in knee arthroscopy is mounted lateral to the lower leg. A special leg holder is not required.

This position is advantageous, as it affords access to the ankle from all sides and permits the use of posterior portals.

3.9 Tourniquet

A tourniquet is used for all arthroscopic procedures. Exsanguination is preferred for more complex procedures such as the reattachment of osteochondral fragments, the retrograde cancellous bone grafting of osteochondral lesions (osteochondritis dissecans), arthroscopic fracture treatment, and arthroscopic arthrodesis (thigh cuff inflated to 450 mm Hg).

3.10 Draping

Since arthroscopy is performed in a fluid medium, watertight draping of the operative field is required. Disposable materials are used. After the tourniquet has been placed and/or the limb wrapped for exsanguination, the operative limb is aseptically prepared. The contralateral leg is draped first. Then a sterile surgical glove is pulled onto the operative foot to cover the toes. Next the foot is passed through the aperture in the waterproof extremity sheet (fenestrated drape), and the sheet is secured about 15 cm proximal to the ankle with a small, sterile piece of tape. The glove on the foot is also fixed with sterile tape to prevent slipping (Fig. 3.10-1).

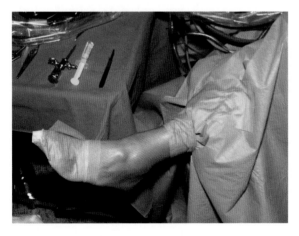

Fig. 3.10-1. Draping for ankle arthroscopy

3.11 Distention Medium

Since electrosurgical instruments will be used, the joint should be distended with a nonelectrolytic solution (e.g., Purisole, Fresenius). Adequate distention pressure is maintained with a gravity-flow system. The pressure is adjusted by raising or lowering the level of the reservoir bag. Because the joint capsule is very thin at certain sites, a high distention pressure should be avoided.

▶ **Caution:** Capsular rupture.

3.12 Setup and Preparations for Arthroscopy

The equipment setup is the same as for knee arthroscopy. The scrub nurse stands next to the instrument table on the operative side at the level of the patient's lower leg. The surgeon sits slightly lateral to, or in line with, the foot on the operative side.

3.13 Portal Placement

Ankle arthroscopy makes use of anterior, posterior, transmalleolar, and transtalar access portals.

3.13.1 Gross Anatomy

First the bony structures about the ankle are palpated to establish orientation. The malleoli are key landmarks that are palpable in every patient. The tip of the lateral malleolus is approximately 1.5 cm distal and slightly posterior to the medial malleolus. The anterior joint space is located approximately 2 cm proximal to the medial malleolus, i.e., about 3–4 cm proximal to the tip of the lateral malleolus.

Anterior Ankle Region

Anterior structures of the ankle region include cutaneous nerves and veins in the subcutaneous tissue, extensor tendons, and the neurovascular bundle. The extensor tendons are easily identified during active dorsiflexion of the foot. Prior to the induction of anesthesia, the surgeon should always palpate and identify the extensor hallucis longus tendon, the tibialis anterior tendon medially, and the extensor digitorum longus tendons laterally.

Simultaneous supination and plantar flexion displace the tendons medially, allowing the examiner to palpate the anterolateral trochlear surface of the talus and the anterior joint space. The saphenous nerve runs with the long saphenous vein over the anterior border of the medial malleolus and then passes to the medial side of the extensor hallucis longus tendon.

Coursing between the extensor tendons are the dorsal pedal artery with its accompanying veins and the deep peroneal nerve. This region should not be violated during portal placement. The superficial peroneal nerve runs lateral to the extensor digitorum longus tendon and peroneus brevis muscle.

Posterior Ankle Region

The central landmark is the Achilles tendon. Descending medial to the Achilles tendon are the posterior tibial artery with its accompanying veins, the tibial nerve, and the sensory nerve fibers for the heel. Lateral to the Achilles tendon, the sural nerve and the venous plexus of the short saphenous vein run posterior to the lateral malleolus. The peroneal tendon group is also on the lateral side.

The talocrural joint space is considerably closer to the skin anteriorly than posteriorly. The long flexor tendons (flexor digitorum longus, flexor hallucis longus, tibialis posterior) cross the joint space posteromedially. These tendons are almost immobile, being held in place by tendon sheaths and retinacula. Vessels and tendons on the medial side contraindicate a posteromedial approach to the ankle joint. The posterolateral portal is placed between the flexor hallucis longus tendon and the peroneal tendons; this area is not traversed by essential structures.

Central Region

The anterior articular border of the lower tibia runs horizontally except for a notch at its junction with the medial malleolus. Proximal to the distal tibiofibular joint, the fibula is bound to the tibia by strong interosseous ligaments (syndesmosis). A small synovial fold extends about 5 mm proximally from that level and can cause intermittent catching.

The talar dome, or trochlear surface, is broader anteriorly than posteriorly. It is convex in the sagittal plane and concave in the coronal plane. This geometry makes it difficult to advance an arthroscope posteriorly. The raised medial and lateral margins of the talar dome contribute to the relatively high incidence of osteochondral fractures in this region.

The lateral malleolus gives attachment to the anterior and posterior fibulotalar ligaments, the fibulocalcaneal ligament, and the posterior and posterior inferior tibiofibular ligaments. The lowermost fibers of the latter ligament form the transverse tibiofibular joint, which augments the posterior tibial flange. It deepens the tib-

ial plafond, preventing posterior displacement of the talus during sudden landing on the forefoot.

Although anatomic atlases portray these ligaments as separate structures, they combine with the joint capsule to form components of a multilayered capsuloligamentous restraint system. Deliberate dissection is often necessary to display the ligaments as separate structures in anatomic specimens.

3.13.2 Anterior Portals

Generally it is sufficient to establish two anterior portals, although accessory anterolateral and anteromedial portals may be created. An anterocentral portal is also described (Figs. 3.13-1 and 3.13-2).

Anteromedial Portal

This portal is located medial to the tibialis anterior tendon. It is useful for evaluating the anterolateral joint structures and is frequently recommended. The long saphenous vein and saphenous nerve are at risk during creation of this portal.

Anterolateral Portal

This portal is placed lateral to the extensor digitorum longus tendon or peroneus tertius muscle (if present). At risk are the short saphenous vein and superficial cutaneous branches of the superficial peroneal nerve.

The anterolateral portal is always the first portal to be established (arthroscope portal).

Anterocentral Portal

An anterocentral portal is very often described, as it reportedly gives better access to the medial and lateral portions of the joint. Placed lateral to the extensor hallucis longus tendon, it has been particularly recommended for evaluating posterior joint areas in patients with capsuloligamentous instability or hyperlax ligaments. The anterocentral portal has significant disadvantages, however. An arthroscope in this portal can pass only a very short distance into the joint and can easily slip out of the joint space. Also, placement of the portal can injure the anterior tibial artery if that vessel takes an anomalous course. This portal cannot be recommend, therefore. To date, we have had no need for an anterocentral portal in our arthroscopic ankle operations. By using anteromedial and anterolateral portals and switching the arthroscope and instrument portals as required, we can obtain complete visualization of the

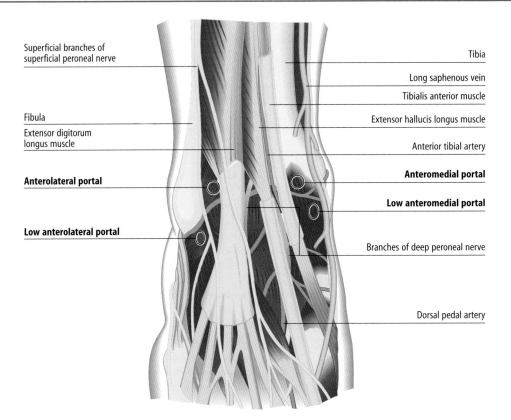

Fig. 3.13-1. Relationship of the anterior portals to anatomic structures about the ankle. (Modified from Ferkel 1996)

anterior joint space. The posterior joint space can also be viewed when distraction is applied to a joint with lax ligaments or chronic lateral instability.

Low Anterolateral Portal

This portal serves as an accessory portal on the lateral side. It is placed several millimeters proximal and about 1 cm anterior to the tip of the fibula. The low anterolateral portal gives access to the tip of the fibula and more distal structures such as fixed intraarticular bodies.

Low Anteromedial Portal

The low anteromedial portal can be a useful adjunct to the standard anteromedial portal. It is placed approximately 1 cm in front of the anterior border of the medial malleolus.

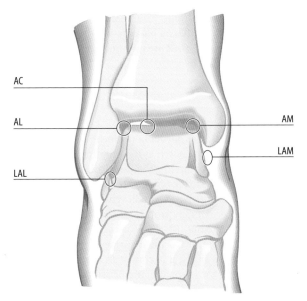

Fig. 3.13-2. Relationship of the anterior portals to the bony structures about the ankle (*AM* anteromedial, *AL* anterolateral, *AC* anterocentral, *LAM* low anteromedial, *LAL* low anterolateral). (Modified from Ferkel 1996)

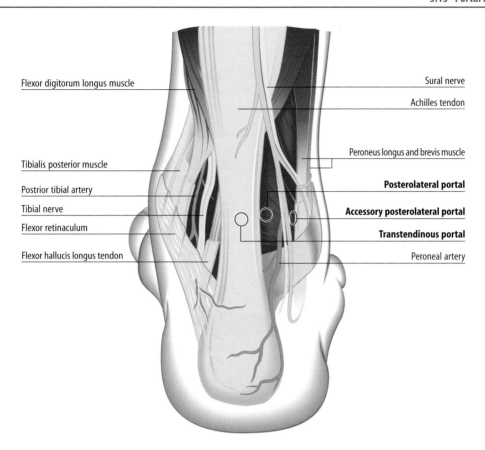

Flexor digitorum longus muscle

Tibialis posterior muscle

Postrior tibial artery

Tibial nerve

Flexor retinaculum

Flexor hallucis longus tendon

Sural nerve

Achilles tendon

Peroneus longus and brevis muscle

Posterolateral portal

Accessory posterolateral portal

Transtendinous portal

Peroneal artery

Fig. 3.13-3. Relationship of the posterior portals to anatomic structures about the ankle. (Modified from Ferkel 1996)

3.13.3 Posterior Portals

Posterior portals are necessary for accessing the posterior joint space (Figs. 3.13-3 and 3.13-4).

Posterolateral Portal

Placed lateral to the Achilles tendon, this is the standard posterior portal for the ankle joint. It can be used to inspect the posterior portion of the ankle mortise and the posterior aspect of the talar dome. Structures at risk during portal placement are the sural nerve and short saphenous vein.

Transtendinous Portal

Surgical procedures on the posterior part of the ankle joint may necessitate a second portal placed through the Achilles tendon. It is analogous to the Gillquist portal placed through the patellar tendon in knee arthroscopy. There is no risk to essential anatomic structures.

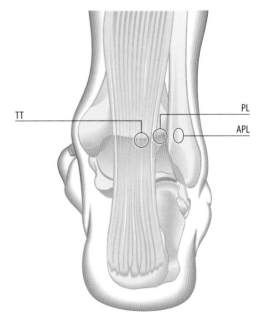

TT

PL

APL

Fig. 3.13-4. Relationship of the posterior portals to the bony structures about the ankle (*TT* transtendinous, *PL* posterolateral, *APL* accessory posterolateral). (Modified from Ferkel 1996)

Posteromedial Portal

The posteromedial portal is placed medial to the Achilles tendon. This portal is not recommended due to the high risk of injury to the posterior tibial artery and posterior tibial nerve.

▶ **Note:** The posteromedial portal is obsolete.

Accessory Posterolateral Portal

An accessory posterolateral portal can be established about 1 cm anterior to the posterolateral portal, just posterior to the peroneus tendons.

3.13.4 Transmalleolar Portals

There are some situations (e. g., an osteochondral lesion or severe cartilage damage on the middle third of the talus) in which a portal can be established through the lateral or medial malleolus (Fig. 3.13-5). This is indicated if the lesion cannot be reached through the anteromedial or anterolateral portal despite maximum plantar flexion.

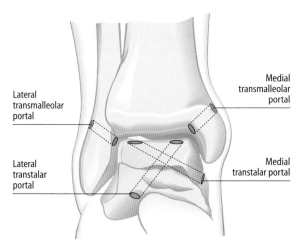

Fig. 3.13-5. Transmalleolar and transtalar portals for ankle arthroscopy. (Modified from Ferkel 1996)

Medial Transmalleolar Portal

This portal is placed about 15 mm proximal to the joint space on an imaginary vertical line through the center of the medial malleolus. A 6- to 10-mm skin incision is made, and the skin and subcutaneous tissue are spread longitudinally with a small clamp to the level of the periosteum. Then the periosteum is elevated from the

malleolus. Portal placement can be facilitated by using a drill guide or by locating the portal site with a thin Kirschner wire drilled through the malleolus. When the desired area of the talus has been reached, the definitive portal can be made by drilling back and forth with the Kirschner wire and changing the flexion angle. Otherwise the portal can be accurately modified with a parallel drill sleeve. If an osteochondral fragment requires fixation with Ethipins or small-fragment screws, the fragment is fixed initially with an optimally placed Kirschner wire. This wire is removed and exchanged for a collared wire, which is overdrilled with a coring reamer (5 or 6 mm diameter). The bone plug from the reamer can be replaced in the portal at the end of the operation.

Lateral Transmalleolar Portal

The technique is the same as for the medial portal. The Kirschner wire should not be overdrilled with a large-bore reamer, however, due to the risk of fibular fracture.

3.13.5 Transtalar Portals

Osteochondral lesions can be bone-grafted through a medial or lateral transtalar approach (see Fig. 3.13-5). A drill guide is used in placing these portals, which are rarely indicated. Although transtalar portals have been described in the literature (Ferkel 1996), we have not used them in our patients due to the precarious blood supply of the talus.

3.13.6 Placement of the Arthroscope Portal

The anterolateral portal has become the standard primary arthroscope portal. Sheath insertion is performed in a well-defined sequence of steps:

1. **Palpation of the joint line.** The joint line is located about 3 cm proximal to the tip of the lateral malleolus. It is palpated while the ankle is flexed and extended. Supination is helpful for palpating the anterolateral joint line.

2. **Needle test** (Fig. 3.13-6). First an ordinary hypodermic needle is inserted into the joint. The needle is held by the hub, without an attached syringe, to improve tactile feedback. The needle is moved laterally and medially to confirm that it has entered the joint.

3. **Joint distention** (Fig. 3.13-7). With intraarticular needle placement confirmed, the syringe is attached and

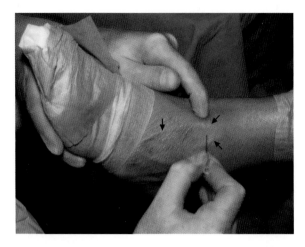

Fig. 3.13-6. Needle test. The superficial veins (*arrows*) should be preserved

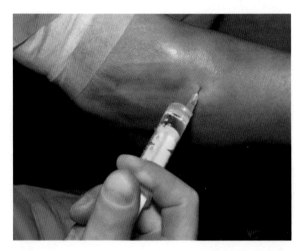

Fig. 3.13-7. The joint is distended with irrigating fluid

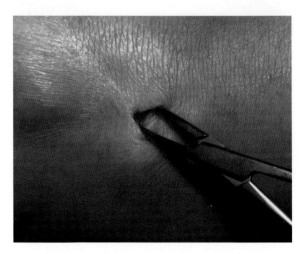

Fig. 3.13-8. The subcutaneous tissue is spread with a blunt clamp

the joint distended with irrigating fluid. Normally up to 15 mL can be instilled.

Resistance to further injection after the first 1–2 mL can have two possible causes:

- **The needle tip is in the capsule or outside the joint.** In the latter case a soft resistance is felt due to subcutaneous tissue distention, which is detectable visually and by palpation.

- **Massive intraarticular adhesions.** If the joint is lined with scar tissue, only a few milliliters of fluid can be injected intraarticularly. This diagnosis may be suggested preoperatively by the history (trauma, surgery, infection) and clinical findings (severe motion loss, feeling of anterior joint tightness).

  After 5 mL has been injected, the syringe is removed and joint entry confirmed by fluid backflow from the needle. If the needle tip is within the joint, the injection is continued. As the fluid is instilled, the ankle dorsiflexes slightly. The tense joint capsule is palpable medially, laterally, and anteriorly. Local retracted sites that may signify adhesions are sometimes detected by visual inspection.

  When the joint has been adequately distended, the needle is withdrawn while pressure is maintained on the plunger. Intraarticular placement can be reconfirmed by disconnecting the syringe and noting backflow from the needle, but this will compromise joint distention and make the arthroscope more difficult to insert.

4. **Skin incision.** A 3- to 4-mm skin incision is made, making certain that the knife cuts only the skin. Cutting into the subcutaneous tissue or to the joint capsule is avoided, as this risks injury to tendons and nerve branches.

5. **Spreading the subcutaneous tissue** (Fig. 3.13-8). The subcutaneous tissue is spread longitudinally and transversely with a blunt clamp. The joint capsule is not yet perforated, as this would cause fluid extravasation and collapse the capsule, making it difficult to insert the sheath.

6. **Inserting the sheath** (Fig. 3.13-9). The sheath with blunt obturator is inserted medially with a gentle twisting motion. Fluid backflow through the open spigot confirms that the sheath has entered the joint. The blunt obturator is exchanged for the scope, and arthroscopy is begun. A short scope (Fig. 3.2-1) is advantageous, as it has a shorter extraarticular lever arm than a standard scope, which facilitates handling (Fig. 3.13-9 b, c).

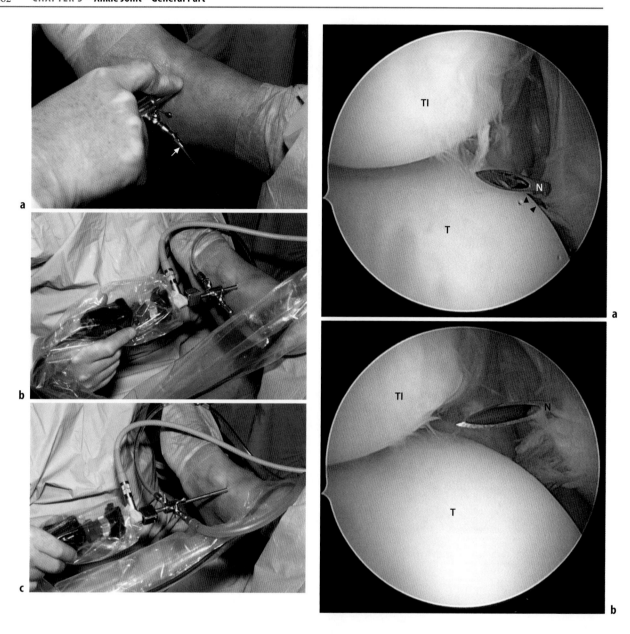

Fig. 3.13-9 a–c. The sheath with blunt obturator is inserted. **a** The spigot is open to permit fluid outflow (*arrows*) from the joint. **b, c** Comparison of the short scope (**b**) and long scope (**c**)

Fig. 3.13-10 a, b. Locating the medial instrument portal site. **a** A trial needle (*N*) is used to determine the level of the portal. If the portal is placed too far distally, the needle and subsequent operating instruments will be deflected by the medial border of the talus (*arrowheads*) (*T* talus, *TI* anterior tibial border). **b** The portal is placed just proximal to the medial border of the talus

3.13.7 Placement of the Anteromedial Portal

The instrument portal, like the arthroscope portal, is created in a series of steps:

1. **Transillumination.** The medial part of the joint is visualized. The light spot from the scope defines the location of anteromedial blood vessels by transillumination.

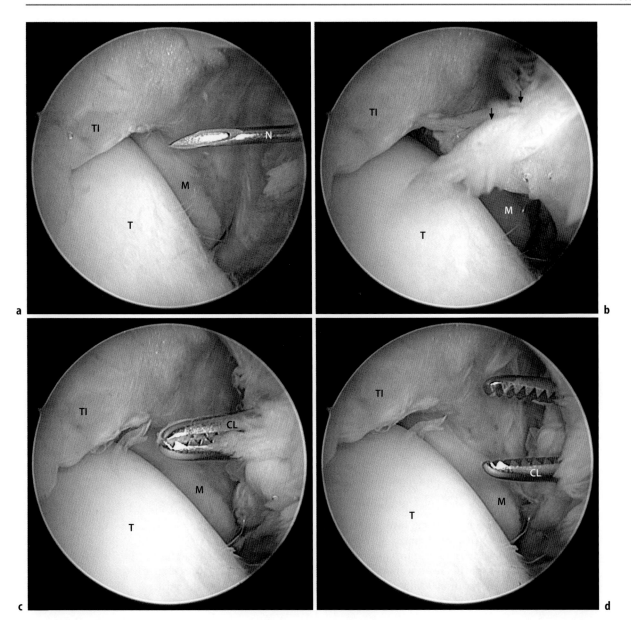

Fig. 3.13-11 a–d. Creating the anteromedial portal. **a** The portal site is determined with a needle (*N*) (*M* medial malleolus, *T* talus, *TI* anterior tibial border). **b** A small clamp with jaws closed is passed into the portal, raising a soft-tissue bulge (*arrows*). **c** When the clamp (*CL*) has passed through the synovium, **d** the jaws are opened to spread the tissues and create a capsular opening

2. **Determining portal location** (Fig. 3.13-10). The portal site is located by inserting a percutaneous needle and noting its relation to the joint space. If the medial portal is placed too low, subsequent inspection of the lateral joint structures will be difficult. The portal should be placed at the level of the joint line, therefore. It is better to reposition the needle than perform arthroscopy through an unfavorably placed anteromedial portal.

3. **Skin incision.** A skin incision 3–4 mm long is made at the needle insertion site. Only the skin should be incised to avoid injury to subcutaneous nerve branches.

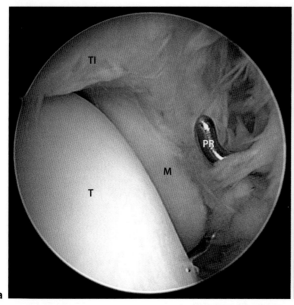 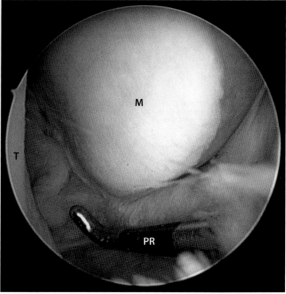

a   b

4. **Spreading the subcutaneous tissue and joint capsule** (Fig. 3.13-11). The subcutaneous tissue is carefully spread in the longitudinal and transverse directions with a blunt clamp. Then the clamp, with jaws closed, is advanced toward the joint space, creating a bulge in the joint capsule that can be seen with the arthroscope. Sometimes vision is obscured by synovitis. The closed clamp is further advanced to perforate the joint capsule, and the jaws are spread to widen the capsular opening.

5. **Inserting the probe and operating instruments** (Fig. 3.13-12). In the absence of pronounced synovitis, the probing hook is inserted and used to palpate the cartilage surfaces. If synovitis is present, a partial synovectomy should be performed with a small synovial resector to improve visualization.

3.13.8 Placement of the Posterolateral Portal

With the arthroscope in an anterior portal, an inflow cannula is placed in the other portal to prevent loss of joint distention during the rest of the procedure. The joint can be safely distended through the inflow cannula, which eliminates the risk of accidentally distending the subcutaneous tissue by attempting to reinject the joint with a needle and syringe.

1. **Determining portal location** (Fig. 3.13-13 a, b). A percutaneous needle is inserted at the posterolateral portal site next to the Achilles tendon. Fluid backflow from the hub confirms posterior joint entry. In patients

Fig. 3.13-12 a, b. Insertion of the probe. **a** The probe (*PR*) is used to palpate the medial malleolus (*M*), the medial portion of the talus (*T*), and the anterior tibial border (*TI*). **b** The probe is moved distally to palpate the tip of the medial malleolus

with a lax joint or posttraumatic instability, joint distraction may be sufficient to allow inspection of the insertion site from the anterior side (Fig. 3.13-13 c).

2. **Skin incision.** A skin incision 3–4 mm long is made at the needle site, again taking care to cut only the skin.

3. **Spreading the subcutaneous tissue.** The subcutaneous tissue is spread with a blunt clamp. The closed clamp is advanced into the posterior joint space, and the posterior capsule is spread open.

4. **Inserting the switching rod.** A switching rod is inserted into the posterolateral portal (Fig. 3.13-13 d). A gush of fluid alongside the switching rod confirms entry into the joint.

5. **Inserting the sheath.** The arthroscope is removed from the front of the joint, leaving the inflow cannula in place. The sheath is inserted over the switching stick into the posterior joint space, the switching stick is withdrawn, and the arthroscope is inserted.

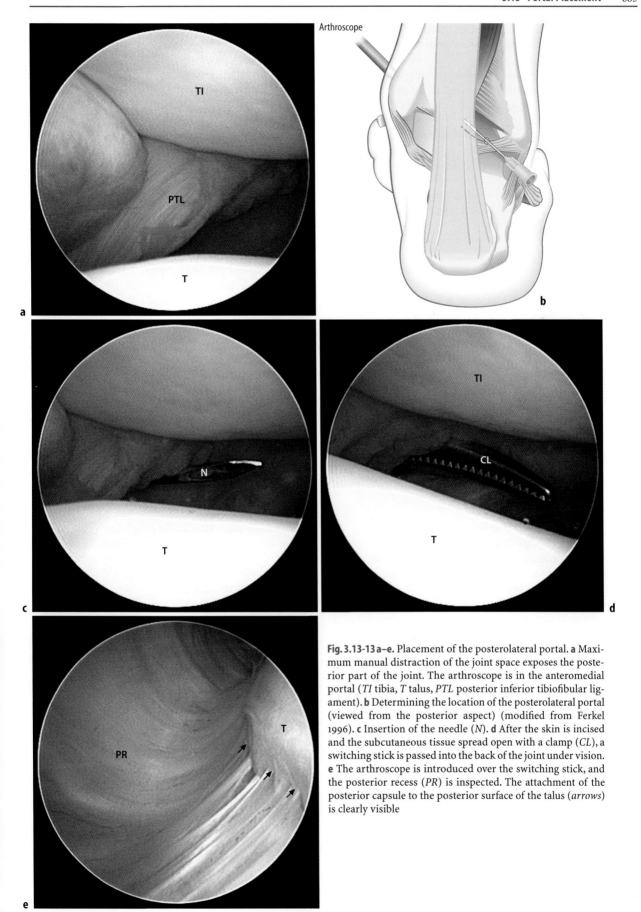

Fig. 3.13-13 a–e. Placement of the posterolateral portal. **a** Maximum manual distraction of the joint space exposes the posterior part of the joint. The arthroscope is in the anteromedial portal (*TI* tibia, *T* talus, *PTL* posterior inferior tibiofibular ligament). **b** Determining the location of the posterolateral portal (viewed from the posterior aspect) (modified from Ferkel 1996). **c** Insertion of the needle (*N*). **d** After the skin is incised and the subcutaneous tissue spread open with a clamp (*CL*), a switching stick is passed into the back of the joint under vision. **e** The arthroscope is introduced over the switching stick, and the posterior recess (*PR*) is inspected. The attachment of the posterior capsule to the posterior surface of the talus (*arrows*) is clearly visible

3.13.9 Switching the Arthroscope and Instrument Portals

The portals in ankle arthroscopy are always used in an alternating fashion for viewing and for instrumentation. The medial part of the joint can be inspected from the anterolateral arthroscope portal, and the anterolateral part of the joint can be viewed through the anteromedial portal.

A switching rod should always be used for portal changes to avoid perforation of the joint capsule, predisposing to synovial fistulae. The technique is the same as in the knee joint (see Sect. 1.13.6).

3.14 Examination Sequence

The ankle joint consists of an anterior and posterior joint space, each of which is subdivided into three compartments:

Anterior Joint Space

- Anterior compartment
- Anterolateral compartment
- Anteromedial compartment

Posterior Joint Space

- Posterior compartment
- Posterolateral compartment
- Posteromedial compartment

In more than 90% of ankle arthroscopies, surgery is confined to the anterior joint space. After the anterolateral arthroscope portal has been created (see above) and intraarticular orientation has been established, arthroscopic evaluation proceeds as follows:

1. **Anterior compartment.** The medial half of the anterior compartment is inspected (anterior tibial border and talar trochlear surface), and the scope is advanced medially.

2. **Anteromedial compartment.** This area starts medial to the medial margin of the talus. The adjacent medial malleolus, the medial aspect of the talus, and sometimes the distal end of the medial malleolus can be seen in the absence of synovitis (see Fig. 3.13-12 b).

3. **Anterior capsule.** The arthroscope is retracted to inspect the anterior joint capsule and the talar insertion of the capsule.

4. **Switching portals.** The arthroscope is moved to the anteromedial portal.

5. **Anterior compartment.** The lateral part of the anterior compartment, with the talus and anterior tibial surface, is inspected.

6. **Anterolateral compartment.** The lateral aspect of the talus and the anterior part of the lateral malleolus are inspected. Sometimes more of the lateral malleolus can be visualized. Inspection is often hampered by scar tissue and adhesions.

7. **Posterior joint space.** The posterior joint space is inspected through the posterolateral portal, starting with the posteromedial compartment (Fig. 3.14-1). The scope is then retracted to inspect the posterior and posterolateral compartments. The posterolateral compartment can be viewed more clearly through a transtendinous approach.

3.15 Complications

Varying complication rates have been reported in the literature. Small (1988) found a complication rate in the range of 0.5% to 0.6% in his retrospective analysis of 146 ankle arthroscopies. Guhl (1993) described an initial complication rate of 11.1%, but this decreased to 2.9% as more experience was gained. Schiessler et al. (1991) had a high complication rate of 15.1% in their patients, but their series did not include any serious complications.

3.15.1 Intraoperative Local Complications

Vascular injury. Injury to the dorsal pedal artery and an aneurysm of that vessel (Morgan 1993) have been described.

If surgery is performed in a bloodless field (thigh tourniquet or exsanguination), significant bleeding cannot be diagnosed intraoperatively.

Nerve injury. Nerve lesions have repeatedly been described. Most involve injury to superficial branches of the peroneal or saphenous nerve. Some transient paresthesias have been reported.

Cartilage injury. The most frequent intraoperative complication is cartilage injury. Presumably a large percentage of these lesions go undetected. The use of standard portals and small, short instruments is essential for minimizing these complications.

Portal placement problems. A nonstandard technique of portal placement can cause unnecessary perforations of

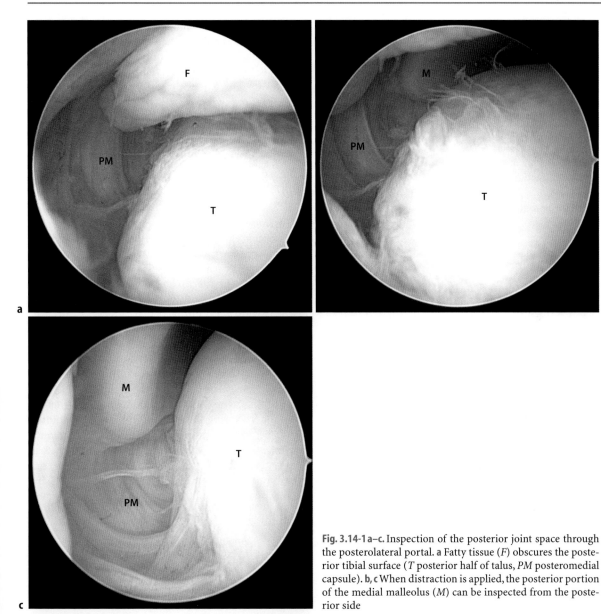

Fig. 3.14-1 a–c. Inspection of the posterior joint space through the posterolateral portal. **a** Fatty tissue (*F*) obscures the posterior tibial surface (*T* posterior half of talus, *PM* posteromedial capsule). **b, c** When distraction is applied, the posterior portion of the medial malleolus (*M*) can be inspected from the posterior side

the synovium or joint capsule, allowing fluid extravasation into the subcutaneous tissue. This subcutaneous distention can cause significant constriction of the joint cavity.

Ligament and tendon injuries. The overaggressive resection of scar tissue can cause the undesired resection of capsuloligamentous tissue. The surgeon should proceed very carefully, therefore, when significant adhesions are present.

3.15.2 Postoperative Local Complications

Synovial fistula. Synovial fistulae have been known to develop at anterior portal sites. Typical cases are marked by delayed healing and the localized collection of sterile synovial fluid. Guhl (1988) found 4 synovial fistulae in 172 arthroscopies, Gächter (1991) reported only 1 fistula in 217 arthroscopies, and Schiessler et al. (1991) found 1 fistula in 31 arthroscopies. Among our patients (n = 1036), we have seen only two cases of delayed healing at the instrument portal, and this was not associated with drainage of synovial fluid.

Hemarthrosis (rare).

Infection. This is still the most dreaded complication of arthroscopic procedures (see Sections 1.15.7 and 2.18 for the management of intraarticular infections).

Compartment syndrome (rare).

Reflex sympathetic dystrophy. Staging and diagnosis are reviewed in Sect. 1.15.14.

3.15.3 Distraction-Related Complications

Various complications can result from the use of mechanical ankle distractors:

- Pin fracture
- Pin site infection
- Traction injury to tendons, ligaments, nerves, and vessels
- Stress fracture

In summary, it may be said that the precise, atraumatic placement of arthroscopic portals is the most important safety factor in ensuring a low complication rate.

3.16 Documentation

Documentation in ankle arthroscopy should fulfill the same requirements as in any arthroscopic procedure (see Sect. 1.16).

All data and findings can be recorded on a special documentation sheet similar to that used in knee arthroscopy (see p. 87). Routine photographic documentation (video print) is obtained to document the initial findings and the result of the arthroscopic procedure.

3.17 Outpatient Arthroscopy

Outpatient ankle arthroscopy should meet the same requirements as in other joints. More than 95% of the arthroscopic procedures performed at our institution (n = 1036) have been done on an ambulatory basis.

3.18 Indications

Since numerous arthroscopic surgical techniques are known, the spectrum of indications has expanded considerably in recent years. It is still common in the literature for authors to draw a distinction between diagnostic and operative arthroscopy. We deliberately omit this distinction, because the goal in every patient is to provide definitive arthroscopic treatment. Purely diagnos-

tic arthroscopy no longer has a significant role to play in modern arthroscopic surgery and, in the ankle joint, should be the absolute exception.

Very often a detailed clinical examination that includes imaging studies (radiographs, MRI) will suggest a presumptive diagnosis that justifies proceeding with arthroscopy. However, the surgeon must be able to provide effective arthroscopic treatment for the anticipated lesion. In the ankle as in other joints, no arthroscopist has ever cured a patient by furnishing a diagnosis.

3.18.1 Unexplained Pain

Pain of unknown cause is a frequent indication for arthroscopy. The pain may result from chronic degenerative changes (osteoarthritis), various forms of synovitis, bony or soft-tissue impingement (e.g., lateral meniscoid syndrome), intraarticular adhesions, or pronounced capsular fibrosis.

Patients often describe persistent anterior ankle pain after conservatively or operatively treated fractures and after sprains. Years of "reassurance" are not uncommon in these cases. Unfortunately, the radiograph is very often considered the essential diagnostic tool. When X-rays are unrevealing, patients are often told that nothing

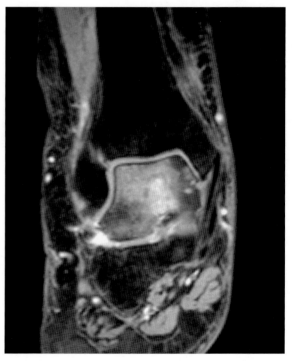

Fig. 3.18-1. Chronic ankle pain in a 47-year-old woman 6 weeks after jumping from a height of 1 meter. MRI demonstrates bone edema throughout the talus

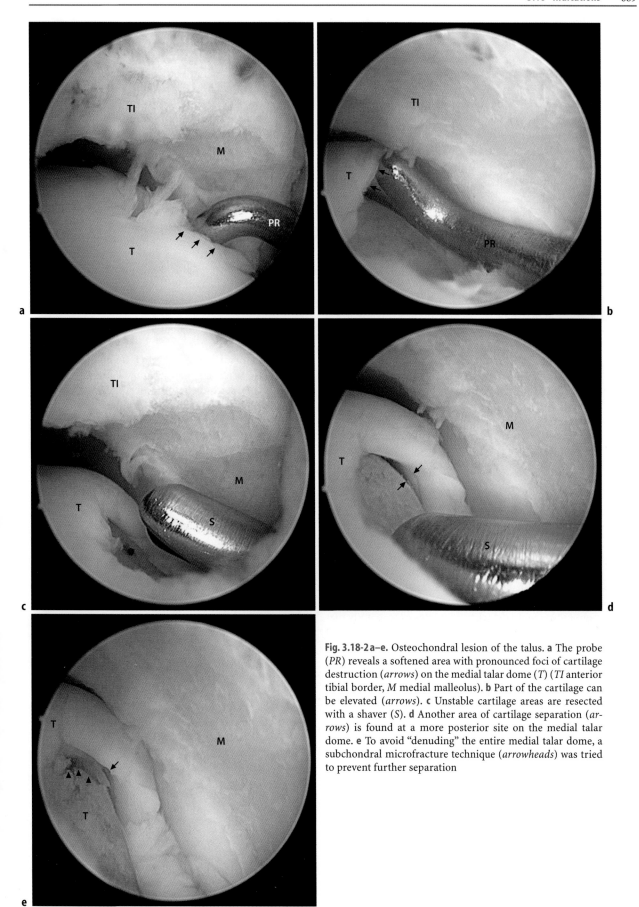

Fig. 3.18-2a–e. Osteochondral lesion of the talus. **a** The probe (*PR*) reveals a softened area with pronounced foci of cartilage destruction (*arrows*) on the medial talar dome (*T*) (*TI* anterior tibial border, *M* medial malleolus). **b** Part of the cartilage can be elevated (*arrows*). **c** Unstable cartilage areas are resected with a shaver (*S*). **d** Another area of cartilage separation (*arrows*) is found at a more posterior site on the medial talar dome. **e** To avoid "denuding" the entire medial talar dome, a subchondral microfracture technique (*arrowheads*) was tried to prevent further separation

is causing the pain or that it is an acceptable outcome. MRI can provide valuable clues in some cases (Fig. 3.18-1). The arthroscopic era has shown that there are many potential intraarticular changes that can underlie chronic, refractory pain.

A local anesthetic test is helpful in determining whether joint pain has an intraarticular or extraarticular cause. If intraarticular injection of the anesthetic relieves the pain, it may be assumed that the cause is intraarticular. If the pain persists, it is unlikely that arthroscopic treatment will be of substantial benefit. Nevertheless, arthroscopy may be the last available recourse in many cases.

3.18.2 Locking

The differential diagnosis of intermittent locking includes loose bodies, scarring, synovial villi, adhesive bands, and fixed intraarticular bodies. Frequently a loose body is not visible on radiographs. The presumptive diagnosis of a loose body is expressed more often than it can be confirmed at arthroscopy.

Rounded calcifications in the lateral capsule and ligaments or in the medial ligaments are usually intraligamentous even if they appear on radiographs as intraarticular loose bodies.

By contrast, calcifications seen in the anterior part of the joint (lateral radiograph) are more likely to be true intraarticular loose bodies.

3.18.3 Osteochondral Lesions (Osteochondritis Dissecans)

The clinical symptoms of osteochondral lesions are diverse, ranging from a complete absence of complaints or intermittent exertion-related pain to severe, persistent complaints with joint swelling (Fig. 3.18-2). If the fragment becomes detached, it creates a loose body that can cause intermittent locking. Arthroscopy is indicated for staging and definitive treatment.

Arthroscopy should be performed in patients with a known or suspected, acute or chronic osteochondral fracture. The osteochondral fragment can be evaluated arthroscopically to determine whether reattachment is feasible. The bed, which may be located on the lateral or medial margin of the talus, can also be identified and treated (abrasion, fibrocartilage induction, reattachment).

3.18.4 Unexplained Effusion

Joint effusion can have various causes that include rheumatoid disease, hyperuricemia, and pigmented villonodular synovitis. Arthroscopy is useful for establishing the diagnosis (synovial biopsy) and performing a partial or complete synovectomy.

3.18.5 Bony Impingement

It is common to find osteophytes on the anterior tibia, the talus, or both (Fig. 3.18-3). Particularly common in athletes, these spurs can cause limitation of motion and painful, refractory irritation of the anterior joint capsule. The lesion usually appears more significant at arthroscopy than on radiographs.

3.18.6 Ligament Impingement Syndromes

Intraarticular scars may develop following a lateral ankle sprain or direct ankle trauma. Patients complain of persistent anteromedial or anterolateral ankle pain. This may be accompanied by intermittent locking or by a "snap" or "click." Anterolateral impingement syndrome (synonym: lateral meniscoid syndrome) is a common finding after lateral capsuloligamentous injuries.

3.18.7 Cartilage Lesions

Various stages of traumatic and degenerative cartilage lesions may be found, especially on the talus. Complaints range from intermittent pain and locking to unremitting pain.

3.18.8 Chronic Lateral Instability

Before a ligament reconstruction is performed to stabilize the lateral capsule and ligaments, it is recommended that arthroscopy be performed so that intraarticular pathology such as severe cartilage damage or scar tissue can be diagnosed and treated. This has an important bearing on prognosis. Among our own patients, we have seen several cases in which the clearing of intraarticular lesions (lysis of adhesions) so improved subjective instability that the patient no longer desired a stabilizing operation.

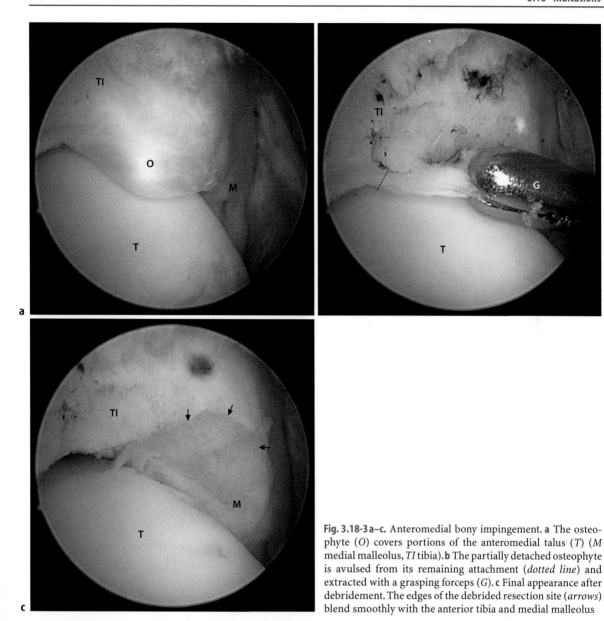

Fig. 3.18-3 a–c. Anteromedial bony impingement. **a** The osteophyte (*O*) covers portions of the anteromedial talus (*T*) (*M* medial malleolus, *TI* tibia). **b** The partially detached osteophyte is avulsed from its remaining attachment (*dotted line*) and extracted with a grasping forceps (*G*). **c** Final appearance after debridement. The edges of the debrided resection site (*arrows*) blend smoothly with the anterior tibia and medial malleolus

3.18.9 Arthrodesis

Advanced degenerative changes with pain unresponsive to conservative therapy may be an indication for arthrodesis. Tibiotalar fusion can be performed as an arthroscopically assisted procedure.

3.18.10 Infection

If infection results from an injection, needle aspiration, or prior arthroscopy, arthroscopic eradication of the infection is an option.

3.18.11 Fractures

Fractures with articular involvement, such as a medial malleolar fracture or a Weber type A or B fracture, are amenable to arthroscopically assisted treatment. These techniques are still at an early stage of development, and large clinical series are not yet available for review.

3.18.12 Tumors

Rarely, tumors are encountered that are suitable for arthroscopic removal.

3.19 Contraindications

Besides the general contraindications to arthroscopy (see Sect. 1.19), advanced degenerative changes in the ankle joint are considered a relative contraindication unless arthrodesis is planned. Acute injuries with massive soft-tissue swelling are another relative contraindication. Edema involving the lower leg or ankle region and advanced stages of arteriovenous occlusive disease also contraindicate arthroscopy. The first priority in these cases is to treat the underlying disease.

Ankle Joint – Special Part

4.1 Synovitis

Cause

Synovitic reactions can have various causes (see Sect. 2.3).

Symptoms

Pain is the most common symptom and may be accompanied by swelling, warmth, and catching. The catching of synovial villi between the articular surfaces is much more common than in other joints (see below, Therapeutic Management).

Clinical Diagnosis

On clinical examination, external manual pressure will elicit pain over the affected joint area. An intraarticular effusion is sometimes palpable.

Range of motion is compared with the opposite side. Angular deformity and capsuloligamentous instabilities are excluded as potential causes of joint irritation.

Radiographs

It is not uncommon to find osteophytic spurs on the anterior talus and/or the anterior tibial border. Contour irregularities of the talus, calcifications, or intraarticular loose bodies are sometimes revealed. In many cases radiographs findings are normal.

MRI

MRI can verify a radiographic suspicion of intraosseous changes. The articular cartilage can also be evaluated.

Arthroscopic Findings

General aspects of arthroscopic synovial evaluation are reviewed in Sect. 2.3. Synovial changes in the ankle joint are commonly found in the anterior joint space. They may be localized to the anteromedial or anterolateral compartment or may involve the joint diffusely. In most cases, accompanying lesions such as cartilage damage, osteophytes, etc. can be identified as the cause.

Therapeutic Management

Synovitis can cause pain as well as catching. This may seem curious at first but is explained by the anatomy and motion characteristics of the ankle joint.

In its normal state, the synovial membrane is thin and lines all of the joint cavity except for the cartilaginous surfaces. If the synovium becomes thickened, individual synovial villi or even portions of the synovial membrane may become caught in the tibiotalar joint space during plantar flexion (Fig. 4.1-1). This exerts traction on the synovial membrane, which has a sensory nerve supply, and on the anterior capsule, resulting in pain. This "traction effect" is reduced by synovectomy.

Given the rich sensory innervation of the anterior capsule, lesions such as capsular fibrosis, scarring, or adhesive capsulitis (see Sections 4.2 and 4.6) can cause severe clinical symptoms.

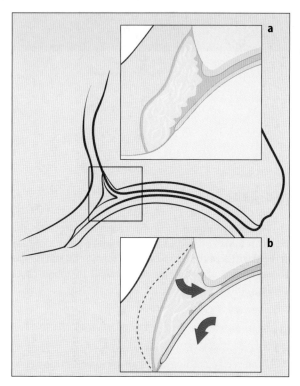

Fig. 4.1-1. a Thickening of the synovium in the anterior joint space. **b** On plantar flexion, synovial villi become entrapped in the tibiotalar joint space. (Modified from Lundeen 1992)

The pathogenic mechanism described for synovial "entrapment" and the resulting capsular tension are partly responsible for the complaints that develop in impingement syndromes (see Sect. 4.2).

Whenever chronic pain and degenerative changes are present, one should always consider that an accompanying synovitis can produce clinical symptoms either directly or through traction on the capsule. As a result, a great many cases can benefit from synovectomy, especially if the synovitis is accompanied by scarring, loose bodies, or osteophytes. Partial synovectomy is usually a necessary first step at arthroscopy so that these lesions can be accurately located and evaluated (Fig. 4.1-2).

The changes found in rheumatoid synovitis are the same as in the knee joint (see Sect. 2.3). Also as in the knee, the ankle synovium tends to encroach upon the articular cartilage and overgrow the cartilage margins. These types of synovitis as well as synovial chondromatosis are an indication for complete arthroscopic synovectomy, which should include the posterior compartments.

Operative Technique

Partial Synovectomy
(Figs. 4.1-2 and 4.1-3)

1. **Inspection and probing.** First the extent of the synovitis is assessed by inspection. Then the synovium is probed to determine whether the tissue is soft or whether tough adhesive bands have form over the affected synovium.

2. **Synovectomy.** A partial synovectomy is performed in the affected joint area with a motorized shaver (see Figs. 4.1-2 and 4.2-3). If synovitis is found in the anterolateral recess, the shaver is introduced through the anterolateral compartment. For synovitis on the anteromedial side, the shaver is introduced through the anteromedial compartment.
   Synovectomy involving the anterior capsule requires a very careful technique using the small-lumen synovial resector from the small joint set. An aggressive synovectomy of the anterior capsule using a large instrument can easily resect portions of the anterior capsule. The anterior tibial artery runs just anterior to the very thin joint capsule.

3. **Additional measures.** Most cases require additional measures such as the removal of scar tissue, the resection of impingement tissue, osteophyte removal, or cartilage shaving. These measures determine the rest of the procedure and the postoperative protocol.

Complete Synovectomy
(Fig. 4.1-4)

1. **Inspection and probing.** The extent of the synovectomy is determined by inspection. The joint is then probed for pathologic structures such as adhesive bands and loose bodies. Vision is often markedly reduced if generalized synovitis is present.

2. **Synovial biopsy.** Whenever generalized synovitis is found, a synovial biopsy should be taken with a small ronguer or grasping forceps.

3. **Synovectomy.** First the anteromedial compartment is synovectomized with a synovial resector to improve vision. If the lower part of the anteromedial compartment cannot be reached through the anteromedial instrument portal, an accessory low anteromedial portal may be needed. A small synovial resector (small joint set) can be passed through this portal to continue the synovectomy at a more caudal level.
   After the portals have been interchanged (arthroscope portal anteromedial, instrument portal anterolateral), the synovectomy is continued in the lateral

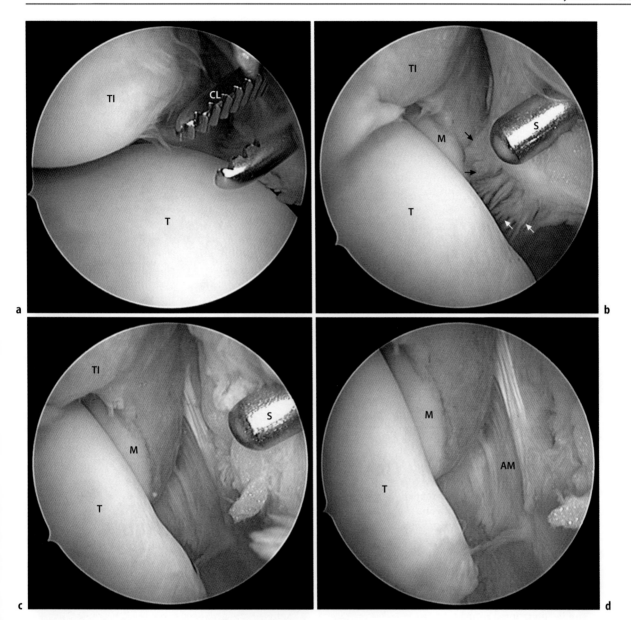

Fig. 4.1-2 a–d. Anteromedial synovitis. **a** The portal site is determined, and the puncture hole in the anteromedial capsule is widened with a clamp (*CL*) (*T* talus, *TI* tibia). **b, c** Synovial villi (*arrows*) are resected with a shaver (*S*). **d** The medial malleolus (*M*) and anteromedial capsule (*AM*) can be evaluated

part of the anterior compartment and the anteromedial compartment. Access to the inferior part of the anteromedial compartment may require an accessory portal.

4. **Posterior synovectomy.** If generalized (e.g., rheumatoid) synovitis is present, a posterior synovectomy is always performed. First the posterolateral portal is established (see Sect. 3.13.8). An inflow cannula is left in the anterior joint space. After the posterior joint space has been inspected, a transtendinous portal is created through the Achilles tendon, and a shaver (small synovial resector) is passed through the portal to synovectomize the posterior part of the joint. An accessory posterolateral portal may prove necessary

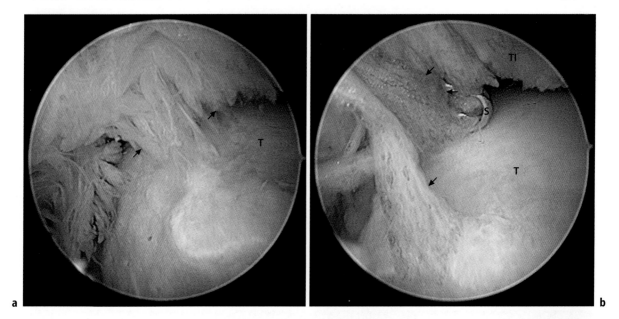

Fig. 4.1-3 a, b. Synovitis in the anterior joint space. **a** The tibia and talus (*T*) are obscured by synovitis (*arrows*). **b** Following synovectomy with a shaver (*S*), the anterior tibial border (*TI*) can be seen

if problems arise. The arthroscope and instrument portals are switched (arthroscope portal transtendinous, instrument portal posterolateral) to complete the synovectomy in the posterolateral compartment.

5. **Completing the operation.** An intraarticular drain is rarely needed because the ankle joint is not prone to postoperative effusion. The portals are closed with simple interrupted sutures.

▶ **Tip:** Make certain that the sutures encompass the skin only. Deeper suture passes risk injury to subcutaneous nerve branches.

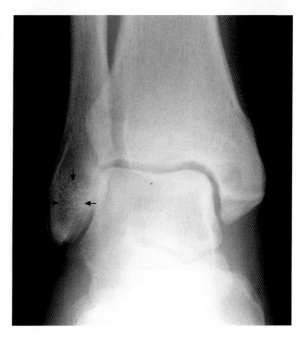

Fig. 4.1-4 a (Legend see next page)

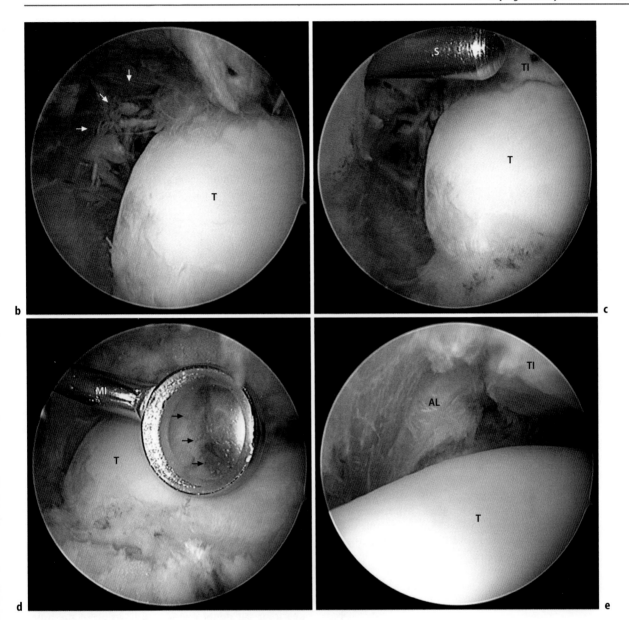

Fig. 4.1-4a–e. Pigmented villonodular synovitis. **a** Radiograph shows a small, localized lucency in the distal fibula (*arrows*). **b** A dark-brown area of pigmented synovitis (*arrows*) is visible on the anterior capsule. The lateral malleolus and anterior tibial border cannot be seen (*T* talus). **c** Anterolateral synovectomy is performed with a shaver (*S*) (*TI* anterior tibial border). **d** The mirror (*MI*) reveals additional areas of dark brown synovitis on the anterior capsule (*arrows*). **e** After the synovectomy is completed, the anteromedial capsule (*AL*) and anterior tibial border can be evaluated

4.2 Impingement Syndromes

Impingement syndromes are among the most common intraarticular lesions. Soft-tissue impingement is distinguished from bony impingement, in which osteophytes and degenerative changes are present. This section deals only with soft-tissue impingement syndromes (Fig. 4.2-1).

These lesions were unknown during the "prearthroscopic" era, because the complaints were very often classified as idiopathic or as an endpoint. Exploratory arthrotomy was generally withheld, especially since radiographs were usually unrevealing. If arthrotomy was performed, either the lesions were not found or were tran-

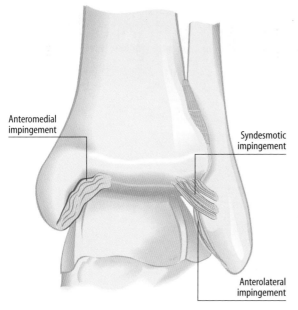

Anteromedial
impingement

Syndesmotic
impingement

Anterolateral
impingement

Fig. 4.2-1. Sites of occurrence of medial and lateral impingement syndromes (soft-tissue impingement)

sected when the joint was entered. When new scar tissue formed after the arthrotomy, the "unexplained" complaints remained unchanged or became even worse.

4.2.1 Lateral Impingement Syndrome

Synonyms are lateral meniscoid syndrome, lateral meniscoid type lesion, synovial impingement, and lateral impingement. We prefer the term lateral impingement syndrome or lateral meniscoid syndrome.

Cause

The most frequent cause is a disruption of the lateral capsule and ligaments. Soft-tissue impingement can also result from direct trauma such as surgery, fracture, or a direct blow to the ankle during sports.

Symptoms

Patients describe persistent anterior joint pain that is often localized to the anterolateral compartment. Some patients notice catching or may display a "snap" or "click" on forcible dorsiflexion of the ankle.

Clinical Diagnosis

Clinical examination typically elicits tenderness in the anterolateral compartment and anterior to the lateral malleolus. Terminal dorsiflexion may be limited or painful. The pain is aggravated by forced dorsiflexion or plantar flexion while pressure is placed on the anterolateral capsule.

Clinical examination shows tenderness in the area of the syndesmosis, the anterior fibulotalar ligament, and possibly the fibulocalcaneal ligament.

Other causes of pain should be considered in the differential diagnosis:

- Adhesions
- Osteochondral lesion of the talus
- Calcifications involving the medial or lateral malleolus
- Peroneal tendon tear
- Peroneal tendon subluxation
- Degenerative joint changes
- Nerve lesions
- Fractures (talus or calcaneus)
- Subtalar joint irritation
- Sinus tarsi syndrome
- Chronic lateral instability
- Syndesmotic injury

Radiographs

Radiographs in typical soft-tissue impingement are unrevealing unless the impingement has been caused by a fracture.

Local calcifications or small, detached bone fragments result from lateral ankle sprains. The examiner should always note the radiographic distance between the fibula and tibia in the area of the syndesmosis. Widening of the diastasis at this level suggests a previous injury. If doubt exists, a radiograph of the uninvolved side can help to detect syndesmosis widening.

MRI

Soft-tissue impingement cannot be confidently diagnosed on MR images, and therefore MRI is not indicated for this type of lesion. MRI can help evaluate the ankle for associated lesions that must be excluded in differential diagnosis.

Arthroscopic Findings

In typical cases, arthroscopy initially shows local synovitis in the anterolateral compartment of the ankle

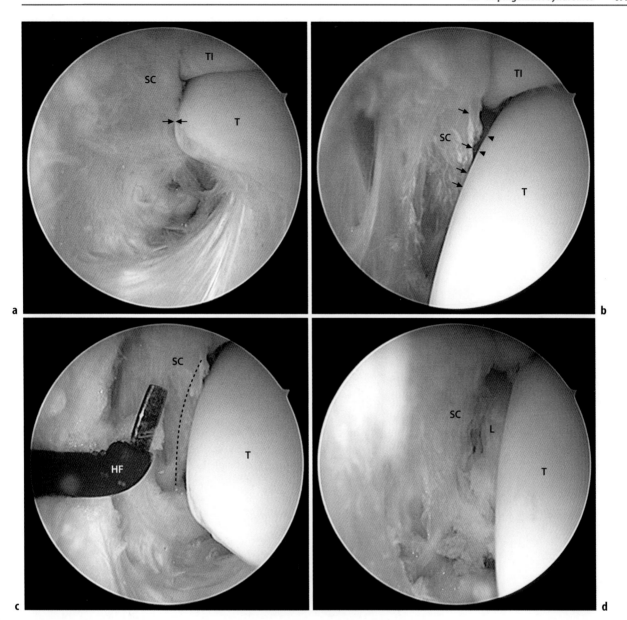

Fig. 4.2-2 a–d. Anterolateral impingement syndrome. The patient, a 26-year-old man, presented with chronic pain 7 months after a lateral ankle sprain. **a** Anterolaterally, the fibula is obscured by scar tissue (*SC*) abutting the lateral talar dome (*arrows*) (*T* talus, *TI* tibia). **b** A small space has been developed between the scar tissue (*arrows*) and lateral talar dome (*arrowheads*) with a shaver. **c, d** The scar tissue is partially resected (*dashed line*) with a cautery knife (*HF*), exposing a portion of the lateral malleolus (*L*)

joint. Soft-tissue changes are most commonly found at the inferior margin of the anterior fibulotalar ligament, in the anterolateral compartment, and on the anterior fibulotalar ligament.

The status of the impingement tissues can be evaluated by flexion-extension and by probing under arthroscopic control. Tough, ligament-like fibrous bands are found in addition to very soft, synovial-like tissue. Dorsiflexion and plantar flexion can demonstrate contact of the impinging structures on the talus. The lateral talar margin should be scrutinized for cartilage damage and erosions caused by the chronic pressure.

▶ **Tip:** When evaluating the joint, always consider that the joint is in a distended condition during arthroscopy.

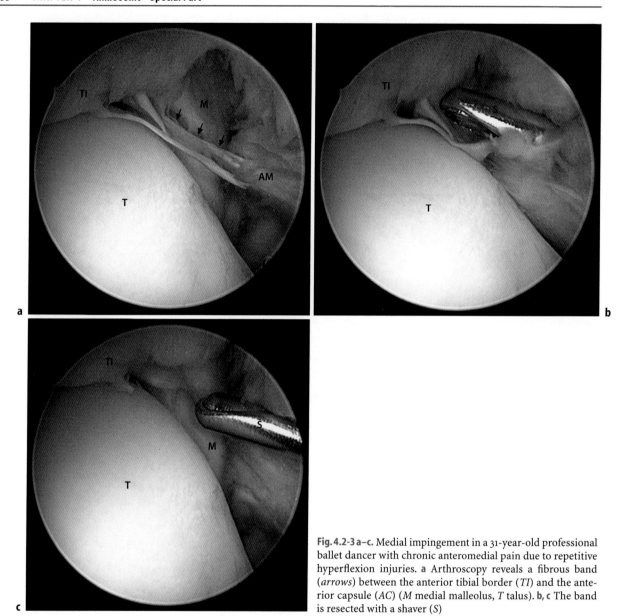

Fig. 4.2-3 a–c. Medial impingement in a 31-year-old professional ballet dancer with chronic anteromedial pain due to repetitive hyperflexion injuries. **a** Arthroscopy reveals a fibrous band (*arrows*) between the anterior tibial border (*TI*) and the anterior capsule (*AC*) (*M* medial malleolus, *T* talus). **b, c** The band is resected with a shaver (*S*)

Therapeutic Management

If conservative measures (external taping, immobilization, nonsteroidal anti-inflammatory medications) do not significantly improve symptoms, arthroscopic resection is indicated in patients with a history and clinical manifestations of a lateral ankle sprain.

As early as 1950, Wolin described the treatment of "talofibular internal derangement" by the operative removal of fibrotic tissue. The current treatment of choice is arthroscopic removal of the impinging structures.

Operative Technique

Clearing the Impingement
(Figs. 4.2-2 and 4.2-3)

1. **Inspection.** The anterolateral arthroscope portal and anteromedial instrument portal are established. The portals are switched to visualize the adhesion in the lateral part of the joint. In most cases the scar tissue is initially obscured by synovial villi.

2. **Probing.** An attempt is made to reach the anterior side of the fibula with the probe. Often this cannot be done because of adhesions.

3. **Partial synovectomy.** A partial synovectomy is performed with a shaver system (synovial resector from the small joint set) to demonstrate the soft-tissue structures.

4. **Function testing.** Dorsiflexion and plantar flexion will often demonstrate soft-tissue impingement on the lateral margin of the talus. This site is examined for cartilage damage and erosions (Fig. 4.2-2 a).

5. **Removing the scar tissue.** The offending scar tissue is debrided with a small synovial resector or with a small meniscus cutter if the tissue is very firm. Alternatively, a cautery probe (small hook or needle electrode) can be used to section the adhesive bands close to the talus.
   ▶ **Caution:** The anterior fibulotalar ligament must be preserved!
   A useful rule of thumb is to expose the fibula through about a 2-mm wide gap.

6. **Impingement testing.** The ankle is moved through dorsiflexion and plantar flexion to exclude further impingement.

Postoperative Care

An elastic compression bandage is applied postoperatively. Partial weightbearing on the operative limb at 50 % body weight is recommended for 2–4 days, followed by progression to full weightbearing according to pain tolerance and swelling.

Success rates from 60 % to 85 % have been reported in the literature following the arthroscopic resection of impingement tissue. Our own retrospective study of 135 patients showed that 69 % of the patients were completely free of complaints, 14 % had significant improvement, and 17 % had no improvement. Nine of the latter patients also had deep chondral damage, however.

4.2.2 Syndesmotic Impingement

According to Ferkel (1996), syndesmotic tearing occurs in 10 % of all ankle injuries. Tears may also occur in the anterior inferior tibiofibular ligament, posterior inferior tibiofibular ligament, transverse ligament, and/or the interosseous membrane.

Cause

A lateral ankle sprain may affect not only the lateral ligaments but also the ligaments that comprise the syndesmosis. These syndesmotic injuries are very difficult to diagnose clinically, and therefore many such injuries are not adequately treated. The primary mechanism is an external rotation injury with a dorsiflexion component.

Symptoms

Patients complain of anterior ankle pain that may radiate up the lower leg.

Clinical Diagnosis

Anterolateral joint tenderness is found over the anterior fibulotalar ligament and especially over the anterior portion of the syndesmosis. The squeeze test is positive in acute injuries. This test is performed by pressing the tibia and fibula together at the mid-tibia level. A positive test elicits pain in the distal lower leg, in the area of the ruptured interosseous membrane, and in the injured syndesmosis.

With a more chronic injury, the external rotation stress test is performed by forcibly externally rotating the foot with the knee flexed 90° and the fibula held in neutral rotation. Pain over the anterior and posterior inferior tibiofibular joint and interosseous membrane signifies injury to these structures.

Arthroscopic Findings

It is not always possible to differentiate syndesmotic impingement from lateral impingement syndrome, as both conditions may coexist. Synovitis and fibrous bands involve the anterior inferior tibiofibular ligament and the distal tibiofibular joint, which can be arthroscopically visualized with distraction. This joint may also contain chondral fragments occurring as intraarticular loose bodies.

Impingement testing should always be performed at arthroscopy by externally rotating the ankle and moving it through plantar/dorsiflexion. This will demonstrate the impingement of soft-tissue structures on the talus. Cartilage lesions and erosions are found on the talus, with occasional sites of exposed subchondral bone.

Therapeutic Management

Treatment is the same as for lateral impingement. Arthroscopic resection is necessary for removal of the impinging tissue.

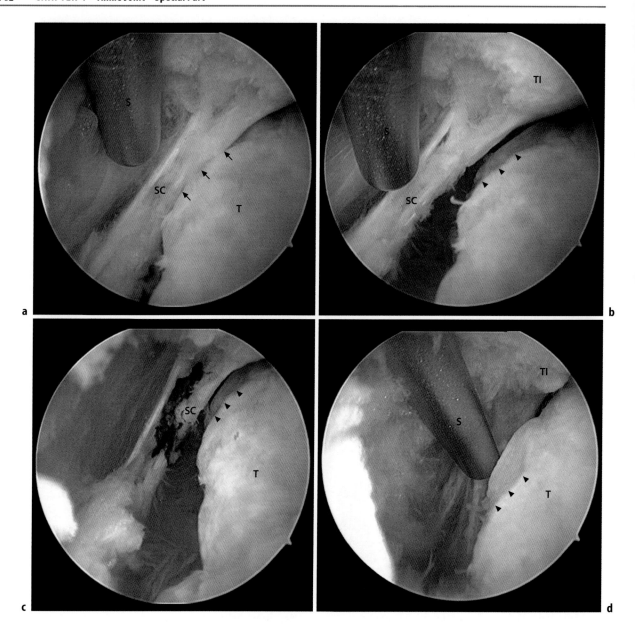

Fig. 4.2-4a–d. Syndesmotic impingement. **a** A stout anterolateral fibrous band (*SC*) impinges on the lateral margin of the talus (*arrows*) in dorsiflexion (*T* talus). Exposure of this scartissue band required preliminary anterolateral synovectomy with a shaver (*S*). **b** On plantar flexion, the fibrous band separates from the lateral talar dome, which is indented (*arrowheads*) from the chronic pressure. **c** The scar tissue is well vascularized. **d** After the band is removed with a shaver, the depression in the talus (*arrowheads*) is seen more clearly

Operative Technique

The resection technique is essentially the same as for lateral impingement syndrome, except that the scar-tissue bands are located distal and anterior to the distal tibiofibular joint (Fig. 4.2-4).

4.2.3 Posterior Impingement Syndrome

Posterior soft-tissue impingement is less common than the other two syndromes.

Cause

Posterior impingement syndrome is caused by injuries to the posterior fibulotalar ligament and posterior syndesmotic ligament (posterior tibiofibular ligament). These structures are commonly injured in lateral ankle sprains (partial rupture).

Symptoms

The symptoms are like those in lateral impingement but occur at a more posterolateral site.

Clinical Diagnosis

The physical findings are like those in lateral syndesmotic impingement (see above). Additionally, local tenderness is found over the posterior tibiofibular ligament in the posterolateral compartment behind the fibula.

Arthroscopic Findings

Often the posterior scar tissue is not visible on inspection from the anterior joint space. If posterior impingement is suspected, the posterior joint space should be inspected through a posterolateral portal.

Therapeutic Management

See Lateral Impingement Syndrome (Sect. 4.2.1).

Operative Technique

Resection of Scar Tissue from the Posterior Joint Space
The technique is essentially the same as in a posterior synovectomy (see Sect. 4.1).

4.3 Loose Bodies

Cause

Loose bodies in the ankle joint originate from basically the same types of lesion as in the knee (see Sect. 2.9). Detached osteophytes and osteochondral fragments are more common in the ankle than in the knee.

Symptoms

The predominant symptoms are pain and catching. Some patients have intermittent swelling accompanied by capsular irritation. Asymptomatic intervals are not uncommon, as the loose bodies often become fixed to the synovium. Certain movements may tear the fragments from their attachment, creating free loose bodies with associated symptoms.

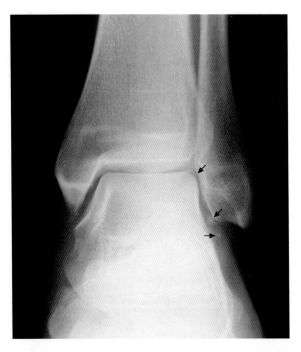

Fig. 4.3-1. Free intraarticular loose bodies (*arrows*) in the lateral recess of the ankle joint

Clinical Diagnosis

Besides causing tenderness and limited motion, loose bodies may be palpable in a few cases. The differential diagnosis includes extraarticular causes of pain and catching (peroneal tendon subluxation, tarsal tunnel syndrome, stress fractures, tendinopathies).

Radiographs

Most loose bodies are not visible on radiographs, so attention must be given to contour irregularities in the joint surfaces (detached osteochondral fragments) and degenerative changes. If an osteochondral loose body is found, its true intraarticular size is usually larger than its apparent radiographic size (Fig. 4.3-1).

▶ **Note:** Calcifications in the lateral and medial capsule and ligaments are easily mistaken for intraarticular loose bodies, but most are intraligamentous or intracapsular.

MRI

MRI is helpful for excluding osteochondral lesions as the cause of loose bodies.

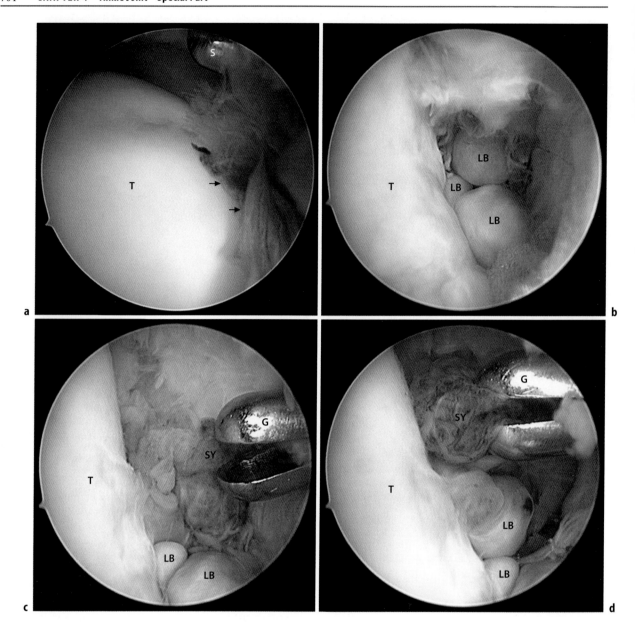

Fig. 4.3-2 a–d. Free loose bodies and chronic synovitis. **a** Vision is obscured by brownish synovial villi (*arrows*) overlying the talus (*T*). Anterolateral synovectomy is performed with a shaver (*S*). **b** This exposes several loose bodies (*LB*) on the floor of the anterolateral recess. **c, d** First synovial tissue (*SY*) is removed with a grasping forceps (*G*), followed by extraction of the loose bodies

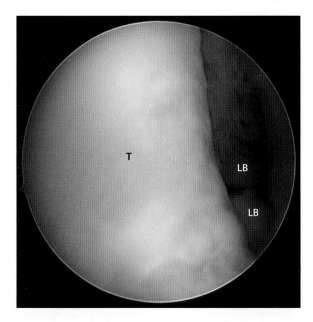

Fig. 4.3-3. Free loose bodies (*LB*) on the floor of the anteromedial recess. Loose bodies such as these are easily missed at arthroscopy (*T* talus)

Arthroscopic Findings

Loose bodies are not always immediately detectable at arthroscopy, as they may be partly or completely obscured by local synovitis. Thus, a preliminary partial synovectomy should be performed so that the loose bodies can be accurately located and evaluated (Fig. 4.3-2).

Loose bodies may be found in the anterior compartment, posterior compartment, or both, although posterior loose bodies are rare. Anterior loose bodies may occur in the anterior joint space or in the inferior portions of the anterolateral and/or anteromedial compartment (Fig. 4.3-3). Loose bodies in these areas may be fixed by connecting strands to the synovium or joint capsule.

Multiple loose bodies are common, and therefore the search should not end when an initial loose body is found. The rest of the joint cavity should be carefully scrutinized.

It is also important to determine the origin of the loose bodies. Arthroscopically detectable causes are detached osteophytes, osteochondral lesions (see Sect. 4.7), chondral flake fractures, bony ligament avulsions, and in rare cases synovial chondromatosis.

Therapeutic Management

A free loose body detected radiographically should be removed. A second goal is to determine and treat the cause in the same sitting. The principal causes are displaced osteochondral fractures of the talus, chondral lesions due to intermittent catching, and degenerative osteophytes on the anterior tibial border.

Operative Technique

Removal of Free or Fixed Loose Bodies
(Figs. 4.3-4 to 4.3-6)

1. **Inspection.** It is not always easy to find a loose body, which is often covered by synovium (Fig. 4.3-4). If the body is floating freely within the joint, the surgeon should always look for additional loose bodies.

2. **Fixation of the loose body.** A free loose body that has slipped into the anteromedial or anterolateral compartment can be fixed in that area with a needle if necessary. This technique is particularly recommended in a loose or chronically unstable ankle, for otherwise the body may slip into the posterior part of the joint, where it would be very difficult to retrieve.

3. **Partial synovectomy.** After the anteromedial instrument portal has been established, a partial synovectomy is performed. Often this is necessary to fully expose a loose body that has become fixed to the synovium or capsule (see Figs. 4.3-2 b–d and 4.3-4).

4. **Extraction.** The technique for loose body removal is the same as described in the knee (see Sect. 2.9).
   If multiple free loose bodies are present, the smaller bodies are removed before the larger. The bodies should be carefully extracted under arthroscopic vision to avoid losing them in the subcutaneous tissue, which may already be distended by extravasated irrigating fluid. Finding the loose bodies in the subcutaneous tissue is a tedious process. The blind grasping of a loose body can cause injury to subcutaneous nerves and veins.
   It is not uncommon for small loose bodies to collect in the dependent portions of the anteromedial and anterolateral compartments (see Fig. 4.3-3). If the loose bodies cannot be reached through the standard instrument and arthroscope portals, an accessory low anteromedial or anterolateral portal should be established.
   If multiple loose bodies are found, the posterior joint space should also be inspected. This requires the creation of a posterolateral portal (see Sect. 3.13-8 for technique).

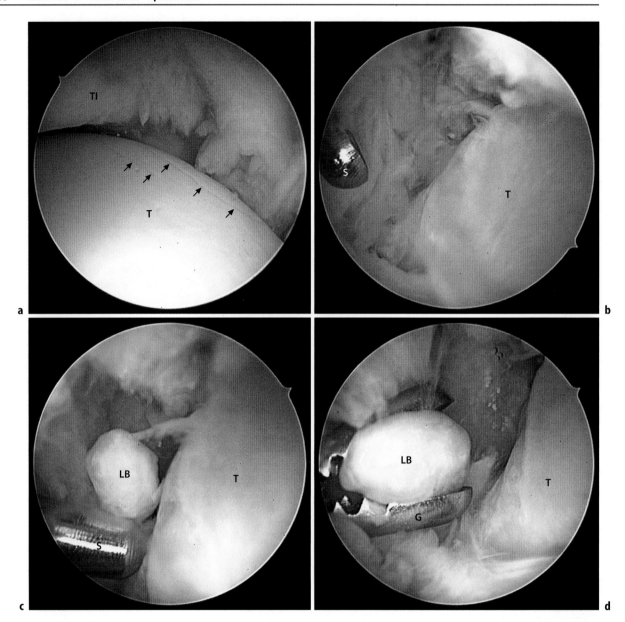

Fixed loose bodies must be freed from the synovium, capsule, or scar tissue prior to extraction (see Figs. 4.3-5 and 4.3-6). The cautery knife is useful for this purpose but must be handled with caution (see Fig. 4.3-5).

5. **Identifying and treating associated lesions.** It is always important to identify and treat the cause of the loose bodies (see Fig. 4.3-4). Unstable cartilage areas on the talus caused by intermittent catching of the loose body, often appearing as longitudinal cartilage grooves, are removed. The cartilage can be debrided with a small curette or small ronguer. A synovial resector often removes more cartilage tissue than intended.

Fig. 4.3-4a–d. Removal of a free loose body. **a** Longitudinal bony fissures (*arrows*) in the talus (*T*) may be caused by the intermittent entrapment of loose bodies (*T* talus, *TI* tibia). **b, c** Partial synovectomy with a shaver (*S*) exposes a free loose body (*LB*) in the lateral part of the joint. **d** The loose body is grasped and removed with a grasping forceps (*G*)

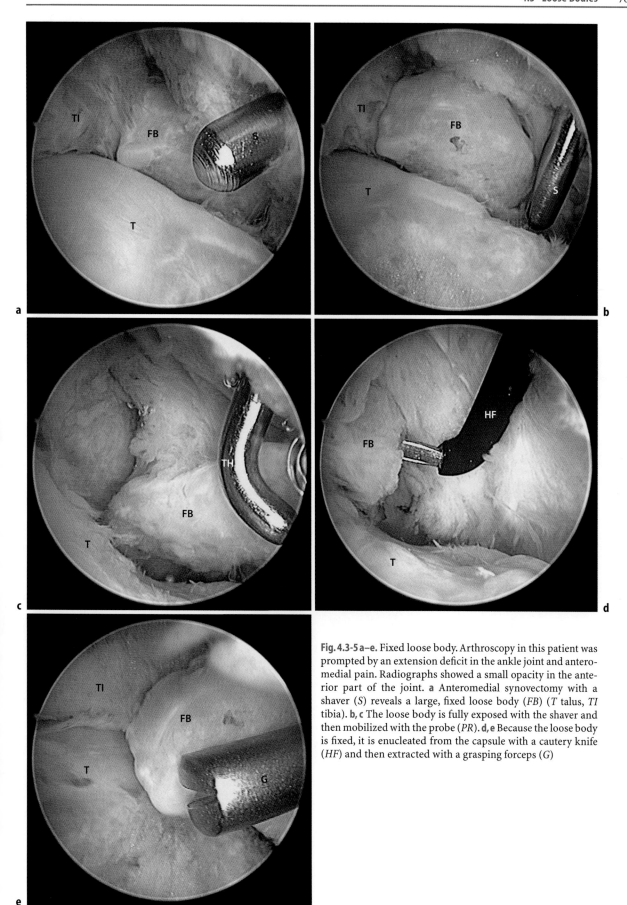

Fig. 4.3-5 a–e. Fixed loose body. Arthroscopy in this patient was prompted by an extension deficit in the ankle joint and antero-medial pain. Radiographs showed a small opacity in the anterior part of the joint. **a** Anteromedial synovectomy with a shaver (*S*) reveals a large, fixed loose body (*FB*) (*T* talus, *TI* tibia). **b, c** The loose body is fully exposed with the shaver and then mobilized with the probe (*PR*). **d, e** Because the loose body is fixed, it is enucleated from the capsule with a cautery knife (*HF*) and then extracted with a grasping forceps (*G*)

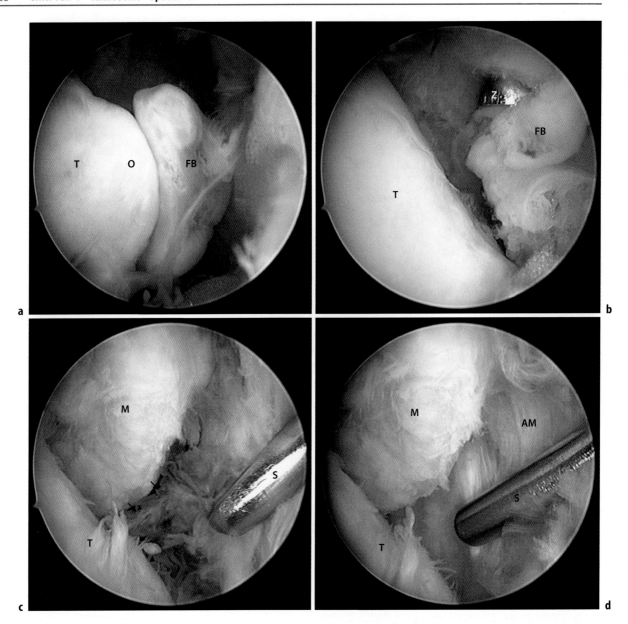

Fig. 4.3-6a–f. Fixed body in the anteromedial compartment. **a** The fixed body (*FB*) abuts anteromedially on a talar osteophyte (*O*) (*T* talus). **b** The loose body is extracted with a grasping forceps (*G*). **c** Posterior to the removal site is a brownish area of synovitis (*arrows*), which is resected with a shaver (*S*). Accompanying small, free loose bodies (*arrowheads*) should not be overlooked (*M* medial malleolus). **d** After the synovectomy is completed, the anterior circumference of the medial malleolus (*M*) and the anteromedial capsule (*AM*) can be seen

The joint is taken through a maximum range of dorsiflexion and plantar flexion to allow complete inspection of the talar dome. If no defects are found, the loose body may have originated from a defect at a far posteromedial site (check the radiographs closely!). This lesion is excluded by creating a posterolateral portal to inspect the posterior talus.

Postoperative Care

If free loose bodies were found and removed in the absence of other significant intraarticular pathology, progressive weightbearing may be started two days after surgery. Weightbearing at 50 % body weight is permitted for the first two days.

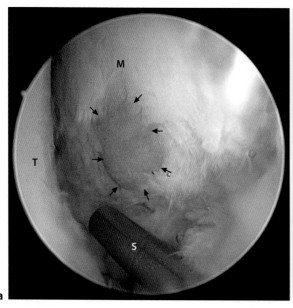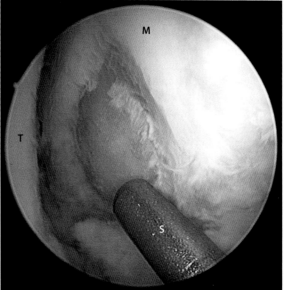

a   b

4.4 Cartilage Lesions

Cause

The causes of chondral lesions in the ankle joint are basically the same as in other joints (see Sect. 2.2). Osteochondral lesions are considerably more common (see Sect. 4.7).

Symptoms

Symptoms are nonspecific and consist of pain and swelling. There are no known symptoms that are specific for a traumatic or degenerative cartilage lesion.

Clinical Diagnosis

Besides checking for tenderness and excluding intraarticular effusion, the examiner should look for palpable osteophytes or decreased range of motion that would signify degenerative changes. No specific tests for diagnosing chondral lesions are known, and therefore many of these lesions are not detected prior to surgery.

Radiographs

Joints with advanced osteoarthritis will show degenerative changes such as joint space narrowing, subchondral sclerosis, and osteophytes. Most traumatic cartilage lesions are not visible on radiographs.

Fig. 4.4.1a, b. Cartilage defect on the medial malleolus. **a** A denuded area (*arrows*) is found on the anterior aspect of the medial malleolus (*M*) (*T* medial talar surface). **b** Treatment consists of stabilizing the edges of the defect with a shaver (*S*)

MRI

MRI provides valuable additional information on displaced chondral fragments. Not infrequently, the arthroscopic findings will differ significantly from the MR images.

Arthroscopic Findings

The full spectrum of traumatic and degenerative cartilage changes may be observed at arthroscopy (see Sect. 2.2). Bony involvement should always be considered when evaluating chondral lesions on the talus or tibial border. Osteochondral lesions are much more common in the ankle joint than in the knee.

Chondral lesions are located most often on the talar dome and anterior tibial border. Inspection of the anterolateral and anteromedial compartments may reveal deep cartilage lesions with craterlike areas of denuded bone (Fig. 4.4-1).

Therapeutic Management

Cartilage treatment follows the same principles as in the knee joint (see Sect. 2.2). As in the knee, it is always necessary to correlate the morphologic condition of the cartilage with the patient's symptoms.

If large areas of exposed subchondral bone are present, careful debridement of the unstable cartilage areas is recommended. Subchondral abrasion is unlikely to be of value in defects of the talus that measure 8–10 mm in their greatest diameter. This technique is appropriate only for smaller, traumatic chondral defects of the type that often occur in athletes (soccer players).

Cartilage defects on the medial or lateral margins of the talus are suspicious for osteochondral lesions (see Sect. 4.7). These areas should be carefully palpated with the probe.

Operative Technique

The operative techniques are basically the same as in the knee joint (see Sect. 2.2, p. 201) and consist of cartilage debridement, techniques to promote fibrocartilage formation (subchondral abrasion, microfracture technique), and cartilage grafting.

Postoperative Care

The cartilage treatment determines the postoperative protocol. If simple cartilage debridement was performed, it is sufficient to maintain partial weightbearing for two days. After drilling or subchondral abrasion, several weeks of non-weightbearing or partial weightbearing is advised, depending on the size and location of the defect. Shoe inserts can also be used to help relieve stress on the affected joint area.

4.5 Osteophytes

The ankle joint is second only to the elbow joint in the frequency of occurrence of symptomatic osteophytes.

Cause

Osteophytes (spurs) are mostly degenerative lesions caused by repetitive direct or indirect trauma. Tibial spurs in soccer players are very often caused by direct trauma to the front of the ankle during plantar flexion. Athletes who are subject to forced hyperflexion or twisting injuries (javelin throwers, high jumpers, long jumpers) are also at risk.

Symptoms

The cardinal symptoms are anterior ankle pain and limitation of dorsiflexion. Osteophytes on the medial or lateral malleolus can cause pain localized to the medial or lateral side.

Clinical Diagnosis

Local tenderness is found in the joint capsule over the osteophytes as a result of local reactive synovitis. Large osteophytes are palpable. Forced dorsiflexion is often painful due to the catching of synovium or capsular tissue between a tibial osteophyte and the talus or between tibiotalar osteophytes. Pain is aggravated by palpation of the anterior capsule during dorsiflexion.

Radiographs

The size of osteophytes on the anterior tibia and talus can be estimated on lateral radiographs. Medial or lateral osteophytes are considerably more difficult to detect, and talar osteophytes frequently go undiagnosed.

Normally the lateral radiograph should show an anterior angle of more than 60° between the anterior border of the distal tibia and the talar neck (tibiotalar angle). An angle less than 60° indicates tibial or tibiotalar spurring (Fig. 4.5-1).

Scranton and McDermott (1992) developed the following classification system for tibiotalar osteophytes (Fig. 4.5-2):

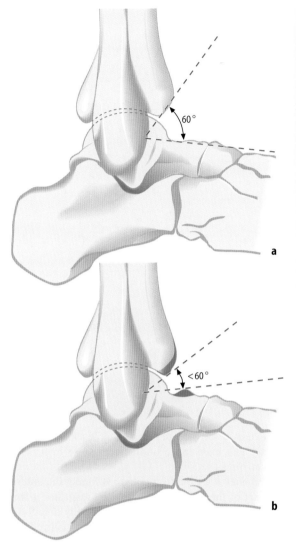

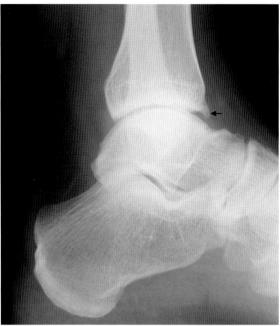

Fig. 4.5-1a–c. Tibiotalar angle. **a** The normal tibiotalar angle is greater than 60°. **b** The presence of tibiotalar spurring reduces this angle to less than 60°. **c** Lateral radiograph clearly demonstrates an anterior tibial spur (*arrow*)

Grade I. Synovial impingement: osseous reaction with up to 3-mm spur formation on the anterior tibia (Fig. 4.5-2a).

Grade II. Anterior tibial spur formation greater than 3 mm in size, with no talar spur (Fig. 4.5-2b).

Grade III. Large anterior tibial spur with or without fragmentation, accompanied by spur formation on the talar neck, often with fragmentation (Fig. 4.5-2c).

Grade IV. Osteoarthritic destruction of the anterior ankle joint. Radiographs also show medial, lateral, or posterior degenerative changes (Fig. 4.5-2d).

If the extent of spur formation is unclear, a lateral radiograph of the opposite limb should be obtained and compared with the involved limb to determine the tibiotalar angle.

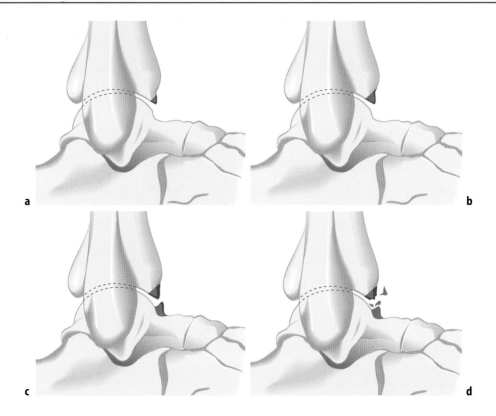

Fig. 4.5-2a–d. Scranton-McDermott classification of anterior tibiotalar degenerative changes (see text for explanation)

MRI

MRI is useful for determining the extent of small and moderate-grade osteophytes. Anterior spurs can be adequately evaluated on radiographs, however. MRI can also be used to confirm localized osteophytes in the anteromedial, anterolateral, and posterior compartments.

Arthroscopic Findings

Osteophytes appear considerably larger at arthroscopy than on radiographs. The following are sites of predilection for spur formation:

- **Anterior tibial border (most common site).** Lesions on the anterior border of the distal tibia range from small local spurs a few millimeters in diameter to large, extensive exostoses that prevent visualization of the tibiotalar joint. These osteophytes often incite a reactive synovitis on the anterior capsule. Capsular fibrosis may also be present. Usually a partial synovectomy must be performed to determine the true

extent of the osteophytes. Unstable osteophytes may act like fixed loose bodies and cause intermittent catching.

Whenever a tibial osteophyte is found, the anterior part of the ankle joint should be inspected arthroscopically while the ankle is maximally dorsiflexed. Even small spurs can impinge on the talus, producing cartilage fissures or deep chondral lesions on the opposing dorsal surface of the talus. Secondary talar spurs are found in advanced cases.

- **Talar osteophytes.** These lesions most commonly occur on the medial and lateral aspects of the talus and usually coexist with anterior tibial spurring. They range in size from a few millimeters to extensive exostoses that create a mechanical block to dorsiflexion. Usually a partial synovectomy must be performed to appreciate the full extent of these osteophytes.

- **Medial malleolus.** Less common than anterior spurs, osteophytes on the medial malleolus can hamper or prevent arthroscopic visualization of the anteromedial compartment. Determining their extent usually requires a partial synovectomy.

- **Lateral malleolus.** Spur formation rarely involves the lateral malleolus. Scarring is far more common in this area (see Sect. 4.2, Impingement Syndromes).

- **Posterior tibial border.** Osteophytic bone at this location usually coexists with anterior spurs. Posterior spurs generally are not diagnosed, because the posterior tibia is rarely evaluated arthroscopically.

With advanced degenerative disease, spur formation is accompanied by deep cartilage lesions and a generalized reactive synovitis (see Sect. 4.8, Osteoarthritis).

Therapeutic Management

The treatment of choice for isolated, symptomatic osteophytes is arthroscopic removal. The indications for osteophyte removal should be carefully considered in patients with clinical and radiographic evidence of advanced degenerative disease. Often the osteophytes will recur within a few months, depending on the patient's level of physical activity.

Osteophyte removal is sometimes done as a secondary measure while treating an osteochondral defect in the talus, for example.

The goals of treatment are discussed with the patient prior to surgery. In patients with severe pain, the primary goal of treatment is to relieve or reduce the pain. The goal in patients with decreased motion is to improve range of motion. The patient should always be informed of the potential for osteophyte recurrence, however.

Osteophytes on the posterior tibia rarely cause limitation of motion; hence they should be removed only if definite clinical symptoms are present. Posterior tibial spur resection is also a technically demanding procedure.

Operative Technique

Removal of an Anterior Tibial Osteophyte
(Figs. 4.5-3 and 4.5-4)

1. **Arthroscope portal.** Very large anterior tibial osteophytes can make it difficult to pass the sheath through the arthroscope portal, and the scope must be advanced at a lower angle to avoid contact with the osteophyte. Large osteophytes can seriously interfere with the rest of the procedure.

2. **Inspection.** The osteophyte is visualized. Usually a partial synovectomy must be performed before the full extent of the osteophyte can be appreciated.

3. **Partial synovectomy.** Partial synovectomy is performed with a shaver (small synovial resector). The anterior capsule is very often involved, and the synovial resector should be used very carefully in that area.
   ▶ **Caution:** Injury to the anterior tibial artery.

4. **Probing.** The extent of the osteophyte is assessed by probing. Unstable fragments, which may be present as fixed loose bodies, are excluded. If an unstable fragment is found, it should be removed first to avoid creating a free loose body during the osteophyte resection. The technique for removing the fixed portion is like that for a fixed loose body (see Sect. 4.3).

5. **Impingement testing.** While the ankle joint is moved from maximum plantar flexion to maximum dorsiflexion, the surgeon watches for sites of osteophyte impingement. During dorsiflexion, the osteophyte often impinges on the talus and produces a corresponding chondral lesion. A secondary talar spur may also be present. If possible, the impingement mechanics are documented with video prints.

6. **Complete visualization of the osteophyte.** The full extent of the osteophyte is visualized. Anterior tibial osteophytes usually extend farther proximally than assumed. Also, a relatively firm attachment may exist between the proximal part of the osteophyte and the anterior joint capsule. Therefore the anterior capsule should be carefully separated from the osteophyte, either by sweeping it proximally or dissecting it from its attachment to the osteophytic bone.

7. **Removing the osteophyte** (Fig. 4.5-3). Various techniques are available for osteophyte removal. A spherical bur (shaver) can be used, but the tight joint space often requires using a small bur of limited capacity. There is also a risk of the bur slipping from the tibial border and damaging the talar cartilage. This risk increases with proximity to the talus. As a result, power shavers are of limited use for osteophyte removal. Another technique is to detach the osteophyte with an arthroscopic chisel (see Fig. 1.6-17). The chisel has rounded edges so that it can "glide" over the talus without scratching the articular cartilage. Removal starts by detaching the medial portion of the osteophyte. Usually this part can be mobilized with the chisel and broken off with a prying motion of the chisel blade. The detached piece is grasped with a forceps and extracted under arthroscopic control. With a very large osteophyte, care should be taken not to detach the entire osteophyte with a single "chisel blow," as this would create a large fragment that is difficult to remove. Large osteophytes should be removed piecemeal.
   When the medial portion of the osteophyte has been removed, the arthroscope and instrument portals are switched, and the chisel is passed through the anterolateral portal. After resecting most of the osteophyte, the surgeon should check for proximal remnants that are attached to the anterior capsule. Any remnants in this area can be removed with a chisel or shaver (see

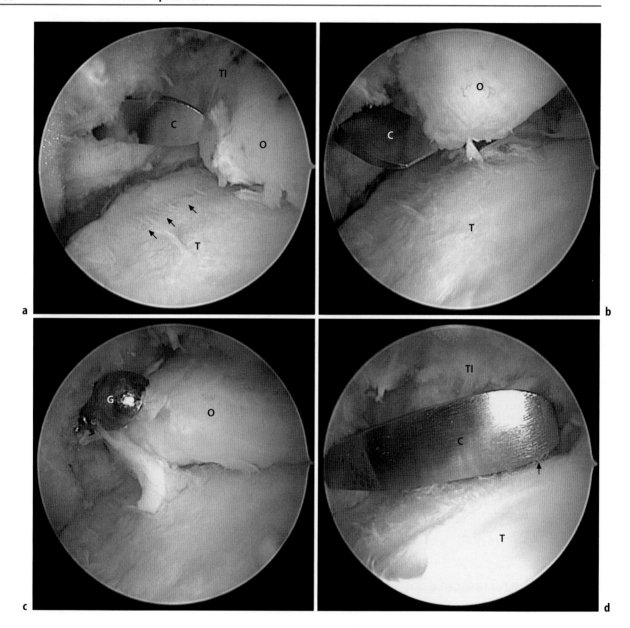

Fig. 4.5-4). Contour irregularities are smoothed first with the shaver and then with an arthroscopic file. (These files are designed to avoid scuffing the adjacent talar cartilage.) The entire resection site should be filed smooth.

8. **Hemostasis.** The final step is to cauterize the resection site with a ball-tipped electrode. Another option is the laser, which delays osteophyte recurrence by producing a deeper level of osteocyte necrosis. Our own initial findings in 37 patients confirm this advantage of laser cauterization, although long-term results are still lacking.

Fig. 4.5-3a–d. Removal of an anterior tibial osteophyte. **a** Following partial synovectomy, the osteophyte (*O*) can be seen on the anterior tibial border (*TI*). Numerous cartilage lesions (*arrows*) are visible on the talus (*T*). The osteophyte is partially detached from the tibia with a chisel (*C*). **b, c** The partially detached osteophyte is mobilized with the chisel and extracted with a grasping forceps (*G*). **d** A rounded chisel blade (*arrow*) avoids damage to the talar cartilage

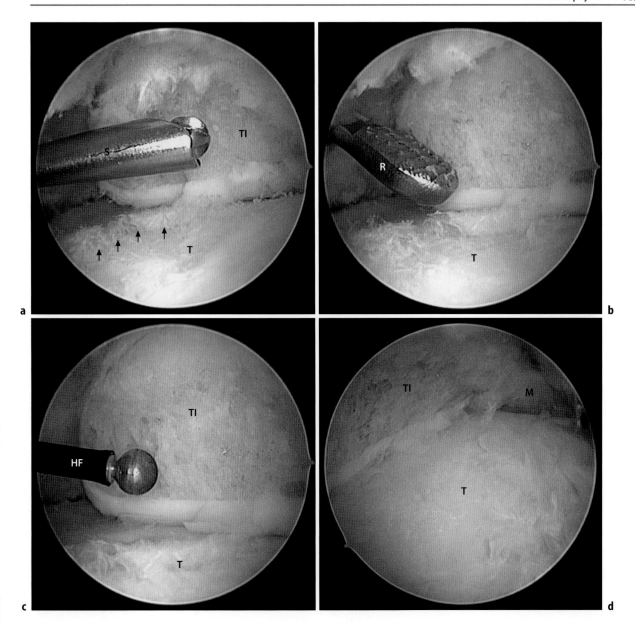

Fig. 4.5-4 a–d. Removal of an anterior tibial osteophyte (continued from Fig. 4.5-3). **a** The resection site is smoothed with a shaver (spherical bur) (*S*). Note the residual cartilage lesions (*arrows*) on the talus (*T*). **b** The resection site is smoothed with a rasp (*R*). **c** Exposed cancellous bone spaces are cauterized with a ball-tipped electrode (*HF*). **d** The spur resection has significantly expanded the anterior joint space (*M* medial malleolus)

9. **Impingement testing.** After the osteophyte has been removed, the joint is again moved through maximum dorsal and plantar flexion. The endpoints of the movement should be soft rather than firm.

10. **Treatment of associated lesions.** Often it is necessary to treat associated chondral lesions (see Sect. 4.4).

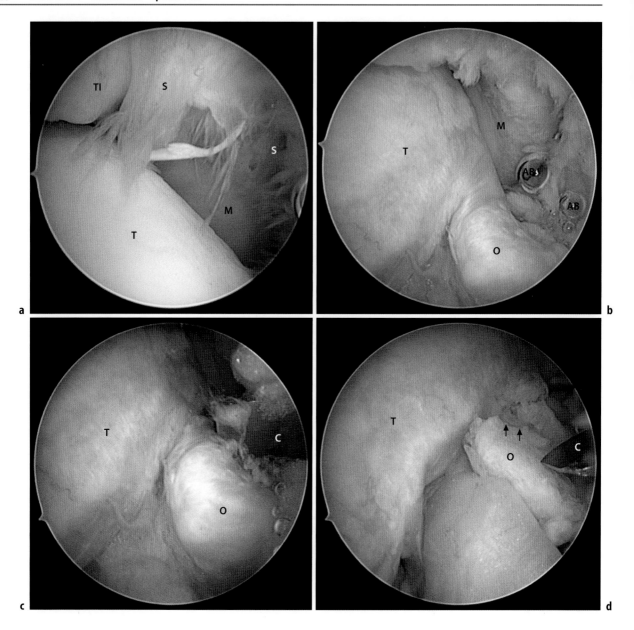

a

b

c

d

Removal of an Talar Osteophyte
(Figs. 4.5-5 and 4.5-6).

If a talar spur is also present, it is removed using the same technique, and the resection site is smoothed and cauterized. It is technically more difficult to reach and visualize osteophytes on the talus than on the tibia. The joint must be held in a position of "optimum dorsiflexion" during the surgery. This does not mean maximum dorsiflexion but the degree of dorsiflexion that is best for visualizing the spur.

Treatment of associated lesions. Often it is necessary to treat associated chondral lesions (see Sect. 4.4).

Fig. 4.5-5 a–d. Anteromedial talar osteophyte. **a** Synovitis (*S*) obscures the medial malleolus (*M*) (*T* talus, *TI* tibia). **b** Partial synovectomy exposes the medial malleolus and an anteromedial talar osteophyte (*O*) (*AB* air bubbles). **c, d** A chisel (*C*) is introduced, and the osteophyte is partially resected (*arrows*)

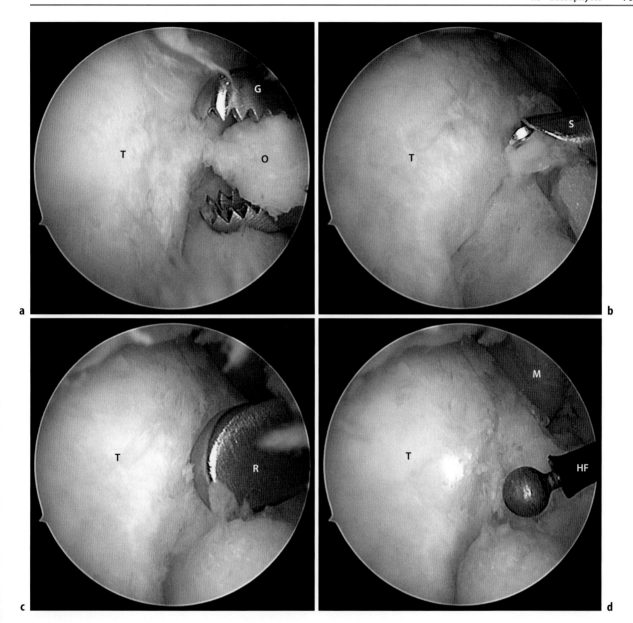

Fig. 4.5-6 a–d. Resection of a talar osteophyte (continued from Fig. 4.5-5). **a** The detached osteophyte (*O*) is extracted with a grasping forceps (*G*), and **b** the resection site is smoothed with a shaver (spherical bur) (*S*). **c** The site is fine-smoothed with a rasp (*R*). **d** Finally the site is cauterized with a ball-tipped electrode (*HF*) for definitive hemostasis (*M* medial malleolus)

Postoperative Care

Partial weightbearing at 50 % body weight is maintained for 2–4 days, followed by progression to full weightbearing according to pain tolerance. Graded physiotherapeutic stretching of the posterior joint capsule is advised to improve range of motion.

4.6 Arthrofibrosis, Scarring

Cause

Scarring and arthrofibrosis can result from surgery, trauma (often with prolonged immobilization), or joint infection. Adhesive bands of variable extent can also develop as a sequel to lateral ankle sprains.

Extensive intraarticular adhesions and anterior capsular fibrosis commonly develop following open operations on the ankle joint (e. g., for the open reduction and internal fixation of a tibial pilon fracture, talar fracture, or lateral malleolar fracture).

Symptoms

The principal complaints are pain and painful limitation of motion, depending on the location and extent of the scarring. Many patients describe a "tight belt" sensation in the anterior part of the ankle joint.

Clinical Diagnosis

Physical examination consists of range of motion testing and palpation for tenderness. Beyond this, there are no clinical tests that can accurately determine the location and extent of scarring.

If intraarticular adhesions are presumed to be present, the intraarticular injection of a local anesthetic can help advance the diagnosis. If only a few milliliters of solution can be injected into the joint, extensive fibrosis must be present and will make it more difficult to create the arthroscope and instrument portals.

Radiographs

The sequelae of bony injuries or surgical procedures can be demonstrated. Radiographs cannot define the extent of adhesions, however.

MRI

The thickened, fibrotic anterior capsule can be appreciated on MR images. The very small anterior joint space can also be seen.

Arthroscopic Findings

Findings are highly variable and range from isolated scar-tissue bands traversing the joint space (see Fig. 4.6-1) to the almost complete obliteration of the joint space by scar tissue. It should be noted that the extent of the scarring does not necessarily correlate with the degree of motion loss. It is remarkable how extensive intraarticular adhesions can sometimes cause only mild limitation of motion.

Therapeutic Management

Refractory pain and decreased motion in a patient with relatively normal-appearing X-ray films may have causes other than an impingement syndrome (see Sect. 4.3) or cartilage damage (see Sect. 4.4). Many of these patients have extensive intraarticular scars that produce severe clinical symptoms by exerting tension on the anterior capsule. Anterior capsular fibrosis in the ankle joint appears to occur easily in response to trauma or surgery. This constricts the size of the anterior joint space, leading to synovial impingement in the tibiotalar joint (see Fig. 4.1-1). Additionally, adhesive scar-tissue bands can exert direct traction on the "sensitive" joint capsule.

The treatment of choice is arthroscopic removal of the scar tissue. An anterior capsular release should be performed in patients with significant capsular fibrosis.

Associated lesions such as deep cartilage damage or bony deformities adversely affect the prognosis. Nevertheless, it is remarkable how well some patients do following arthroscopic arthrolysis, even when severe chondral lesions are also present.

It should be kept in mind that extensive adhesions will make it more difficult to establish a satisfactory arthroscope portal.

Operative Technique
(Figs. 4.6-1 to 4.6-3)

1. **Arthroscope portal.** Difficult joint distention may provide the first clue to intraarticular scarring. If only a few milliliters of irrigating fluid can be injected and produces little or no joint distention, it may be assumed that significant intraarticular scarring is present, provided the needle has been positioned within the joint.

   Even with minimal distention, it is still necessary to establish an arthroscope portal. Our standard technique is to pass the arthroscope posteriorly at a somewhat steeper angle than usual in order to reach the anterior tibia or talus as quickly as possible. If the sheath were advanced more anteromedially, the fibrotic anterior capsule could deflect it away from the joint space. Turning on the inflow would then distend the subcutaneous tissue and make the rest of the procedure more difficult.

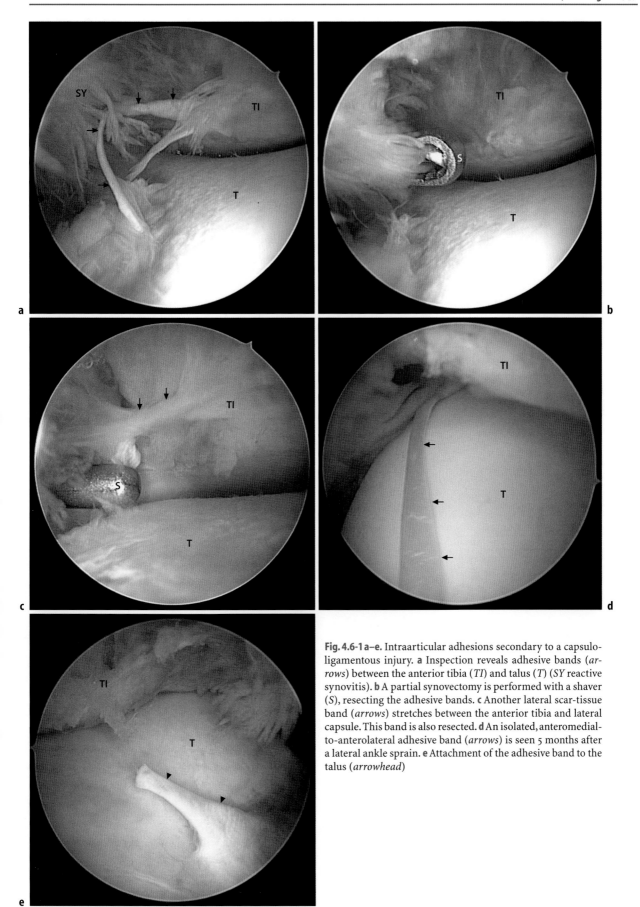

Fig. 4.6-1 a–e. Intraarticular adhesions secondary to a capsulo-ligamentous injury. **a** Inspection reveals adhesive bands (*arrows*) between the anterior tibia (*TI*) and talus (*T*) (*SY* reactive synovitis). **b** A partial synovectomy is performed with a shaver (*S*), resecting the adhesive bands. **c** Another lateral scar-tissue band (*arrows*) stretches between the anterior tibia and lateral capsule. This band is also resected. **d** An isolated, anteromedial-to-anterolateral adhesive band (*arrows*) is seen 5 months after a lateral ankle sprain. **e** Attachment of the adhesive band to the talus (*arrowhead*)

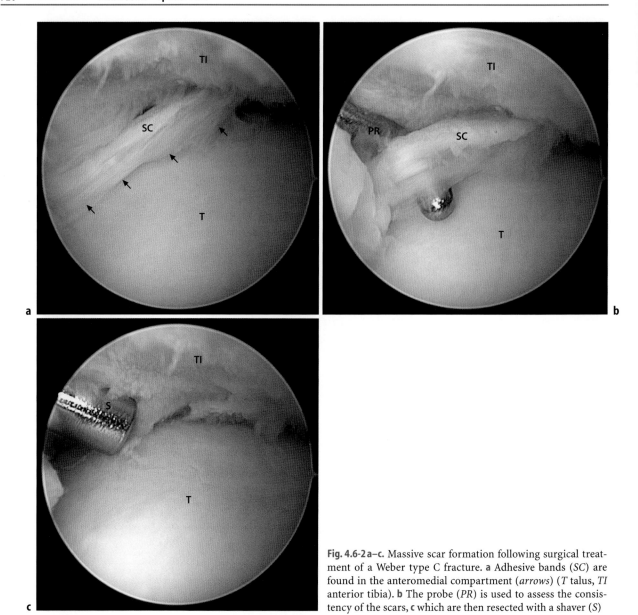

a

b

c

Fig. 4.6-2 a–c. Massive scar formation following surgical treatment of a Weber type C fracture. **a** Adhesive bands (*SC*) are found in the anteromedial compartment (*arrows*) (*T* talus, *TI* anterior tibia). **b** The probe (*PR*) is used to assess the consistency of the scars, **c** which are then resected with a shaver (*S*)

When the sheath has been positioned within the joint, the distention medium will dribble out through the opened spigot. When the arthroscope is in place, sometimes only a white-out or yellow-out image is seen on the monitor.

2. **Instrument portal.** Despite the difficult situation, an instrument portal must be created. The site is established by trying to place the needle tip directly in contact with the scope tip. Then the skin is incised, and the subcutaneous tissue and joint capsule are spread open until the clamp is in contact with the arthroscope. The clamp is moved back and forth in an effort to push the scar tissue aside and create a small joint space. Extensive scar tissue may extend directly between the anterior tibial border and the talus, and the scar must be pushed aside before the tibiotalar joint space and articular cartilage can be identified.

3. **Debridement.** The probe is used in an attempt to push the scar tissue aside. If the tissue is positively identified as scar, it is resected with a small synovial resector and the anterior joint space is carefully dissected free (see Fig. 4.6-2). The dissection proceeds anteromedially in small steps until the medial malleolus is visualized. The same technique is used on the lateral side after switching the arthroscope and instrument portals.

If vision is limited, isolated bands or plaques of scar tissue are most easily sectioned with a basket forceps.

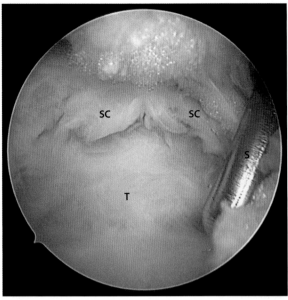
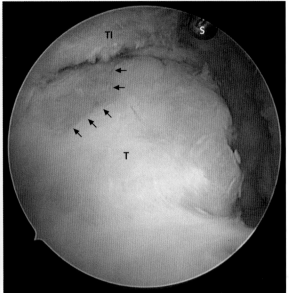

a   b

Fig. 4.6-3 a,b. Massive arthrofibrosis following a tibial pilon fracture. **a** Since the anterior joint space was completely filled with scar tissue (*SC*), it was difficult to pass a sheath into the joint. Scar tissue had to be resected with a shaver (*S*) to visualize the talus (*T*). **b** Extensive cartilage defects (*arrows*) are visible on the talar surface (*TI* anterior tibia)

Residual scar tissue and synovitis are removed with a synovial resector. After clearing the anterior joint space of scar tissue, the surgeon will usually find medial and lateral fibrous tissue responsible for causing lateral and/or medial soft-tissue impingement (see Sect. 4.2).

4. **Capsular release.** After removing the most prominent adhesions, the surgeon should determine how large the intraarticular space is. In most cases it is markedly reduced in size, and sometimes the joint capsule is adherent to the anterior talar surface. A probe or cautery knife can be used to free the capsule from the talus, using careful and meticulous technique.
   Not infrequently, the anterior tibial border cannot be identified because the joint capsule appears to arise directly from it. In this case the anterior tibial border is freed of capsular tissue. This is done with a small synovial resector, or a small meniscus cutter can be used if the capsule is fibrotic (see Fig. 4.6-3). Another option is the cautery probe (small hook electrode).

5. **Treatment of associated lesions.** Any chondral lesions and reactive synovitis are also treated (see Fig. 4.6-3 b).

Postoperative Care

Patients with localized scarring often describe a reduction in pain immediately after surgery and state they can move the joint more freely. Partial weightbearing at 50 % body weight is allowed for 2–4 days, followed by progression to full weightbearing. Intensive but gentle physical therapy is also recommended to stretch the joint capsule. Overvigorous therapeutic exercises are contraindicated, as they could incite a new fibrotic reaction in the anterior capsule. As in the postoperative management of arthrofibrosis in the knee joint, close cooperation between the physical therapist and surgeon is essential. We therefore recommend that inpatient therapy be provided in a special rehabilitation center. While the range of motion is still limited, strengthening and jumping exercises are prohibited for the first 4–6 weeks to avoid unnecessary capsular irritation.

4.7 Osteochondral Lesions

Osteochondral lesions are more common in the ankle than in any other joint. It is still common for authors to differentiate these lesions as osteochondritis dissecans, osteochondral fractures, transchondral fractures, and flake fractures. This is not useful from the standpoint of differential diagnosis and treatment, however, and it is better to characterize all of these conditions as "osteochondral lesions" (OCL).

Cause

In 1856, Munro became the first surgeon to observe and describe loose bodies in the ankle joint (Guhl 1993). He attributed the loose bodies to trauma. In 1888, König coined the term osteochondritis dissecans to describe a similar condition that he observed in the knee.

The precise cause of osteochondral lesions is controversial, especially since a variety of terms are used. The traumatic etiology of flake fractures and osteochondral elevations is undisputed. Osteochondritis dissecans on the medial edge of the talus have been variously ascribed to individual factors (growth, endocrine factors, vascular microemboli) and repetitive trauma. Single or repetitive trauma can lead to subchondral fracturing and perhaps to chondral surface fractures. An analysis of trauma mechanisms has shown that forced supination combined with dorsiflexion and internal tibial rotation can cause lateral osteochondral lesions of the talar dome. Lesions of the medial talar dome may be caused by forced supination of the plantar-flexed foot with external rotation of the tibia in relation to the talus.

Symptoms

Symptoms may occur acutely after an injury, but chronic cases are much more common. Patients complain of pain, swelling, and/or intermittent or persistent locking. Pain usually occurs in response to loading (prolonged standing, job-related activity, sports) and is relieved or reduced by rest (weekend). Intraarticular clicks and snaps may occur.

Clinical Diagnosis

Tender areas and motion-dependent pain are evaluated along with range of motion and joint swelling. Lateral or medial instability is excluded.

The various potential causes of pain (see Sect. 4.2) are included in the differential diagnosis.

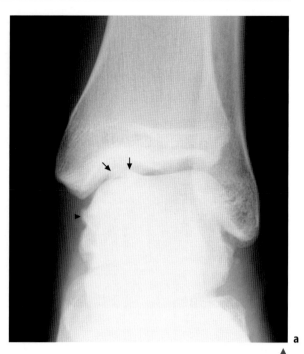

a

Fig. 4.7-1. a Osteochondral lesion of the medial talar dome (*arrows*) and spur formation on the talus (*arrowhead*). **b** Berndt and Harty staging system for transchondral lesions (Berndt and Harty 1959)

Radiographs

The lesions can be appreciated on AP radiographs (Fig. 4.7-1). CT can also be used to evaluate the various stages of transchondral lesions (Berndt and Harty staging system) (Fig. 4.7-1b).

MRI

MRI provides valuable information on lesion extent (Fig. 4.7-2). Anderson et al. (1989) devised the following MRI staging system for osteochondral fractures:

Stage I: subchondral compression, negative radiographs (in AP projection), positive bone scan, edema ("bone bruise").
Stage II A: subchondral cyst.
Stage II B: incomplete separation of the fragment.
Stage III: fragment detached and surrounded by synovial fluid but not yet displaced.
Stage IV: displaced fragment (intraarticular loose body).

MRI can define the location of the osteochondral lesions. Lesions of the medial talar dome tend to be more posterior and lateral lesions more anterior. This explains why many medial lesions cannot be adequately evalu-

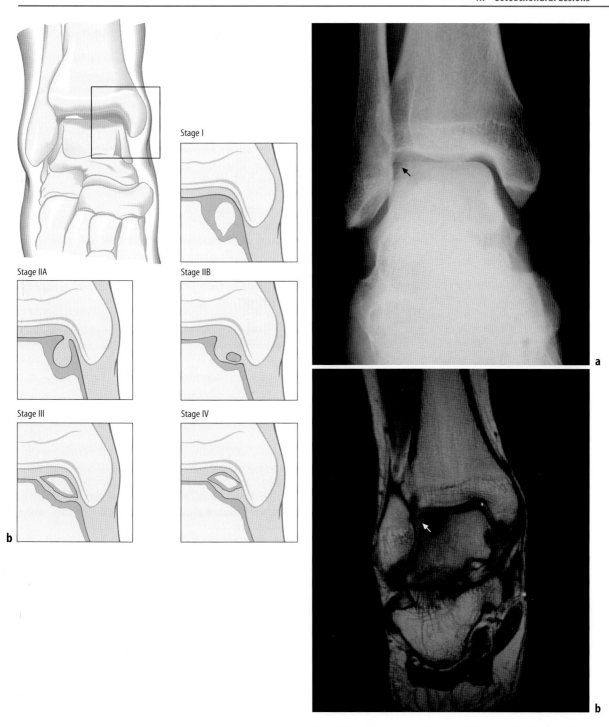

Fig. 4.7-2. a Osteochondral lesion of the lateral talar dome (*arrow*) (2 weeks old) in a 19-year-old male. **b** MRI more accurately defines the extent of the lesion (*arrow*)

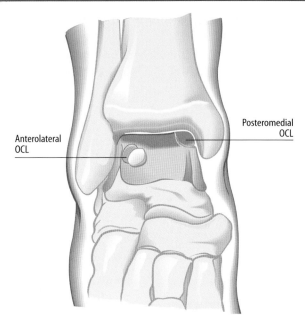

Fig. 4.7-3. Sites of occurrence of talar osteochondral lesions (anterior aspect)

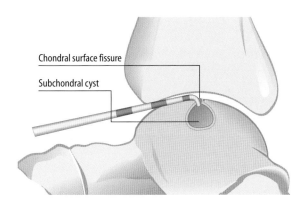

Fig. 4.7-4. Probing of a subchondral bone cyst

ated with arthroscopy from an anterior approach (Fig. 4.7-3).

Arthroscopic Findings

The condition of the cartilage over the lesion is variable and ranges from softening to a chondral defect with a displaced fragment. It is not uncommon to find chondral fractures with foci of cartilage separation. If a cystic area is found beneath the disrupted cartilage on probing, it may represent a subchondral bone cyst (Fig. 4.7-4).

Therapeutic Management

The approach to treatment depends on the cartilage changes found at arthroscopy, the subjective clinical symptoms, and the acute or chronic nature of the complaints.

With a recent osteochondral injury, it may be possible to reattach the fragment to its bed with screws or Ethipins, depending on the fragment size. Small, acutely displaced chondral fragments are removed if they do not involve the bone.

Local softening of cartilage (Fig. 4.7-5). If no cystic changes are found and the fragment is stable in the absence of clinical symptoms, a trial of conservative treatment is justified. The patient does not bear weight for several weeks and returns at 6 months for clinical and radiographic follow-up. If severe clinical symptoms are present, antegrade or retrograde drilling of the lesion is recommended. Often the underlying bone is very unstable, however, and drilling is unlikely to be of long-term benefit in these patients. Consequently, it may be necessary to remove softened cartilage areas in order to expose and debride the underlying focus.

Softened but intact cartilage layer with a slightly mobile fragment. Besides antegrade or retrograde drilling, an option for large fragments is reattachment with Ethipins or cannulated small-fragment screws if significant clinical symptoms are present. Retrograde cancellous bone grafting is recommended for a large unstable fragment located beneath an intact cartilage layer (Fig. 4.7-6). Another option for these cases is osteochondral autografting.

Partially detached fragment. Small chondral fragments with a very thin wafer of bone are removed and the base abraded (subchondral bone with microfracture technique). With larger fragments, it is worthwhile to attempt reattachment despite the limited prospect for an optimum result.

Displaced fragment. Small fragments are removed and the base treated by subchondral abrasion and microfracturing. Reattachment should be considered for larger fragments and may reduce the size of the talar defect. Both the fragment and its bed should be thoroughly freshened prior to reattachment. Another option in young patients with large defects is osteochondral autograft transfer. The osteochondral plug can be harvested from a non-weightbearing area in the ipsilateral knee joint.

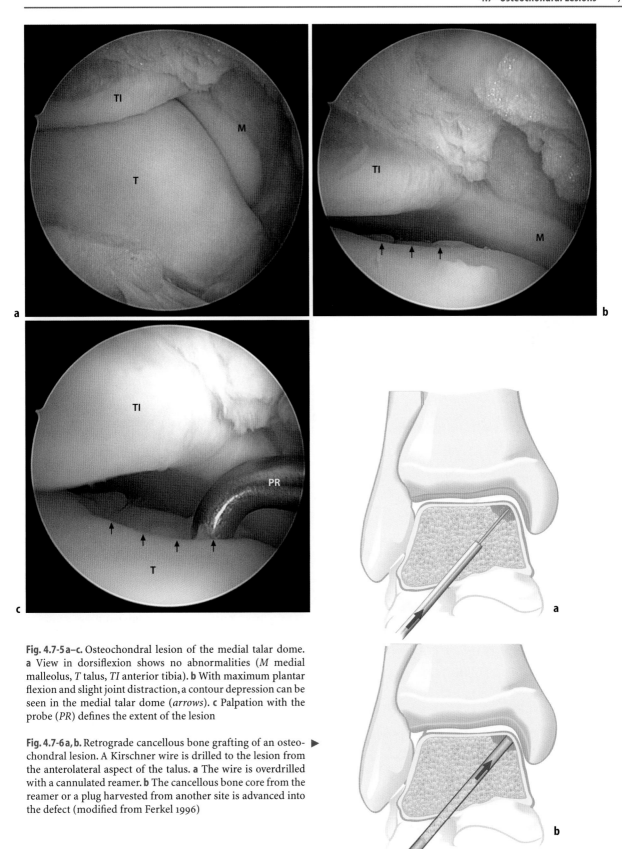

Fig. 4.7-5 a–c. Osteochondral lesion of the medial talar dome. **a** View in dorsiflexion shows no abnormalities (*M* medial malleolus, *T* talus, *TI* anterior tibia). **b** With maximum plantar flexion and slight joint distraction, a contour depression can be seen in the medial talar dome (*arrows*). **c** Palpation with the probe (*PR*) defines the extent of the lesion

Fig. 4.7-6 a, b. Retrograde cancellous bone grafting of an osteochondral lesion. A Kirschner wire is drilled to the lesion from the anterolateral aspect of the talus. **a** The wire is overdrilled with a cannulated reamer. **b** The cancellous bone core from the reamer or a plug harvested from another site is advanced into the defect (modified from Ferkel 1996)

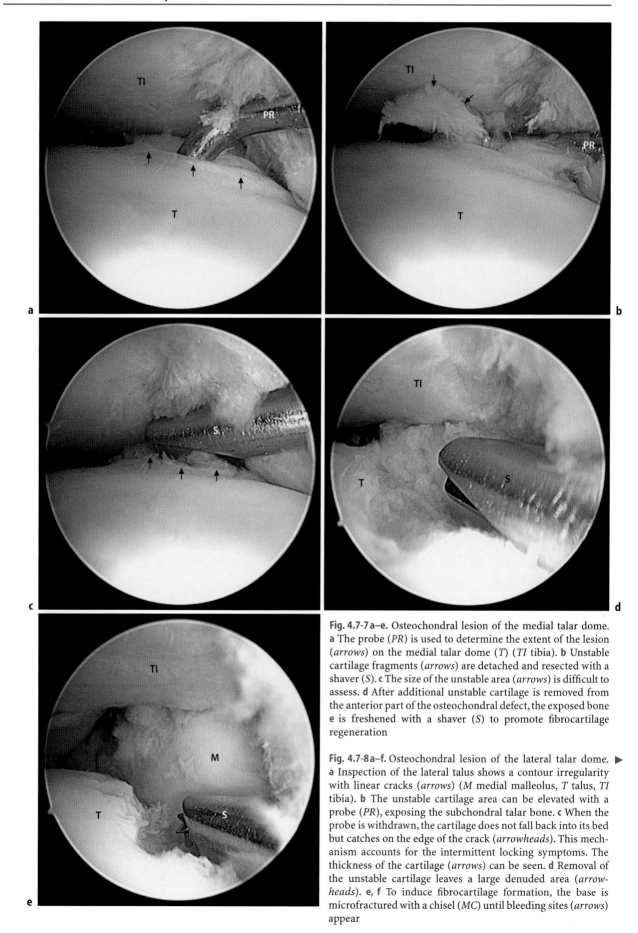

Fig. 4.7-7 a–e. Osteochondral lesion of the medial talar dome. **a** The probe (*PR*) is used to determine the extent of the lesion (*arrows*) on the medial talar dome (*T*) (*TI* tibia). **b** Unstable cartilage fragments (*arrows*) are detached and resected with a shaver (*S*). **c** The size of the unstable area (*arrows*) is difficult to assess. **d** After additional unstable cartilage is removed from the anterior part of the osteochondral defect, the exposed bone **e** is freshened with a shaver (*S*) to promote fibrocartilage regeneration

Fig. 4.7-8 a–f. Osteochondral lesion of the lateral talar dome. ▶ **a** Inspection of the lateral talus shows a contour irregularity with linear cracks (*arrows*) (*M* medial malleolus, *T* talus, *TI* tibia). **b** The unstable cartilage area can be elevated with a probe (*PR*), exposing the subchondral talar bone. **c** When the probe is withdrawn, the cartilage does not fall back into its bed but catches on the edge of the crack (*arrowheads*). This mechanism accounts for the intermittent locking symptoms. The thickness of the cartilage (*arrows*) can be seen. **d** Removal of the unstable cartilage leaves a large denuded area (*arrowheads*). **e, f** To induce fibrocartilage formation, the base is microfractured with a chisel (*MC*) until bleeding sites (*arrows*) appear

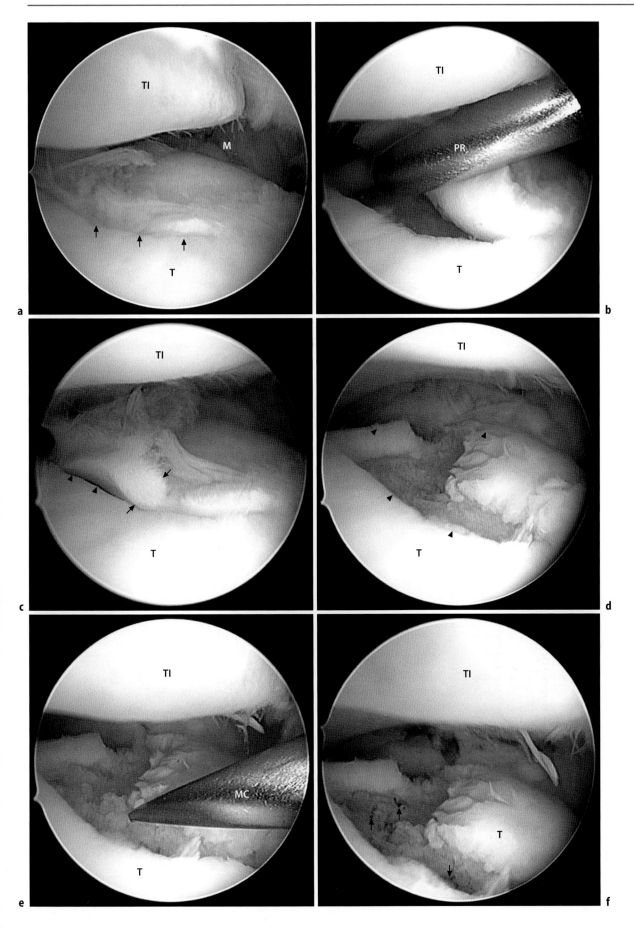

Operative Technique

Removal of Osteochondral Fragments
(Figs. 4.7-7 and 4.7-8)

The removal of loose chondral fragments or osteochondral fragments not suitable for reattachment follows the
same technique used for intraarticular loose bodies (see
Sect. 4.3).

Drilling

1. **Inspection and probing.** The softened cartilage area is
   arthroscopically visualized and probed to determine
   its extent.

2. **Drilling.** Antegrade drilling is performed with a
   Kirschner wire (1.2 or 1.5 mm) through the "standard"
   instrument portal, provided plantar flexion will move
   the chondral lesion far enough anterior to the tibia
   that it can be reached through that portal. Otherwise
   a medial or lateral transmalleolar portal should be
   created (see Sect. 3.13-4 for technique).
   Medial osteochondral lesions are often located on the
   posterior part of the talar dome, and therefore a posterolateral portal is sometimes necessary for drilling
   or debriding the lesion (Fig. 4.7-9). Drilling is performed to a depth of approximately 10–15 mm. The
   Kirschner wire is withdrawn, the flexion angle is
   changed, and the wire is drilled back into the softened cartilage area at a slightly different angle. Various areas of the talus can be drilled through a transmalleolar portal.

Postoperative Care

The patient does not bear weight for 4–8 weeks, depending on the size of the defect.

Reattachment

1. **Inspection and probing.** The probe is used to define
   the extent of the osteochondral fragment and determine whether it is completely or partially detached
   from its bed. Unstable cartilage fragments are identified and removed (Fig. 4.7-10 a).

2. **Placing the instrument portal.** Osteochondral lesions
   of the anterior talus can be reached through a standard anterolateral or anteromedial portal, but if reattachment is proposed, it will be necessary to create an
   instrument portal that gives perpendicular access to
   the lesion site. Thus a high anterolateral or high
   anteromedial portal is established just anterior to the

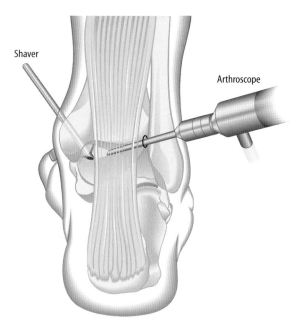

Fig. 4.7-9. Treatment of an osteochondral lesion of the posteromedial talus using a posterolateral arthroscope portal and a
medial transmalleolar portal. (Modified from Ferkel 1996)

anterior tibial border, using a percutaneous needle to
locate the optimum portal site (Fig. 4.7-10). If optimum access is not obtained even in maximum plantar flexion, it must be decided whether to establish a
transmalleolar portal or cut a small notch in the anterior tibial border with a bur. The latter technique
causes minimal trauma and is very useful if the high
anterolateral or anteromedial portal barely misses
the target site (Fig. 4.7-10 c).

3. **Freshening the lesion.** The bony component of the
   lesion and its talar bed are thoroughly freshened. Scar
   tissue can be removed with a small curette. Other
   freshening is performed with a small bur (shaver).

Fig. 4.7-10 a–e. Osteochondral lesion of the lateral talar dome, ▶
treated by reattaching the fragment. The patient sustained an
ankle sprain 14 days earlier while playing soccer (see Fig. 4.7-2).
a The extent and stability of the unstable osteochondral fragment (*F*) are evaluated (*PR* probe, *T* talus, *TI* tibia). **b** Unstable
anterior cartilage fragments are removed (*arrows*). A percutaneous needle (*N*) is used to determine if the center of the osteochondral fragment can be reached through a high lateral
instrument portal placed just anterior to the tibia. **c** When it is
confirmed that this cannot be done, a notch is cut into the
anterolateral tibial border with a shaver (*S*). **d** Now the needle
(*N*) can reach the center of the fragment. **e** The fragment and
its bed are freshened with the shaver

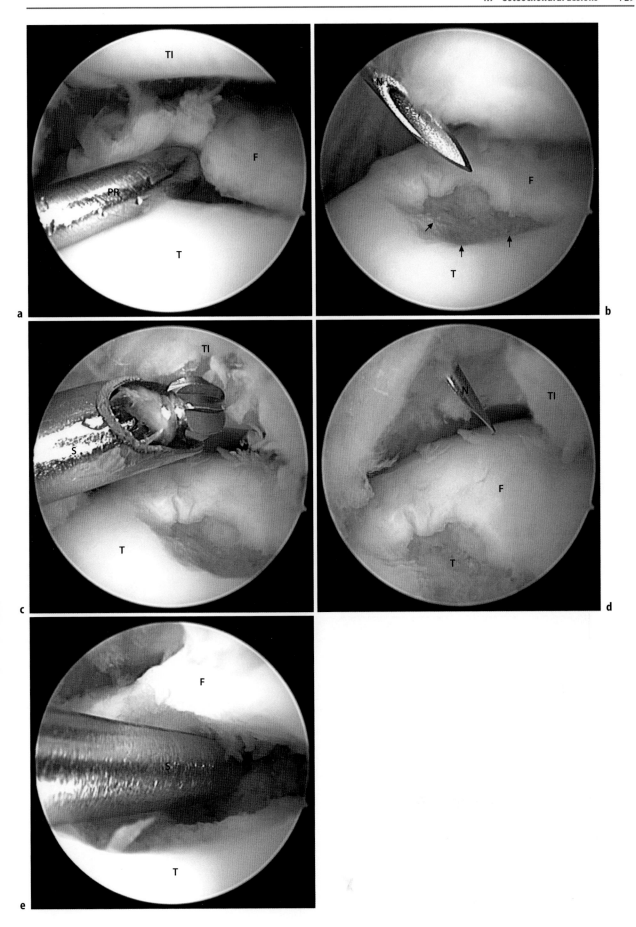

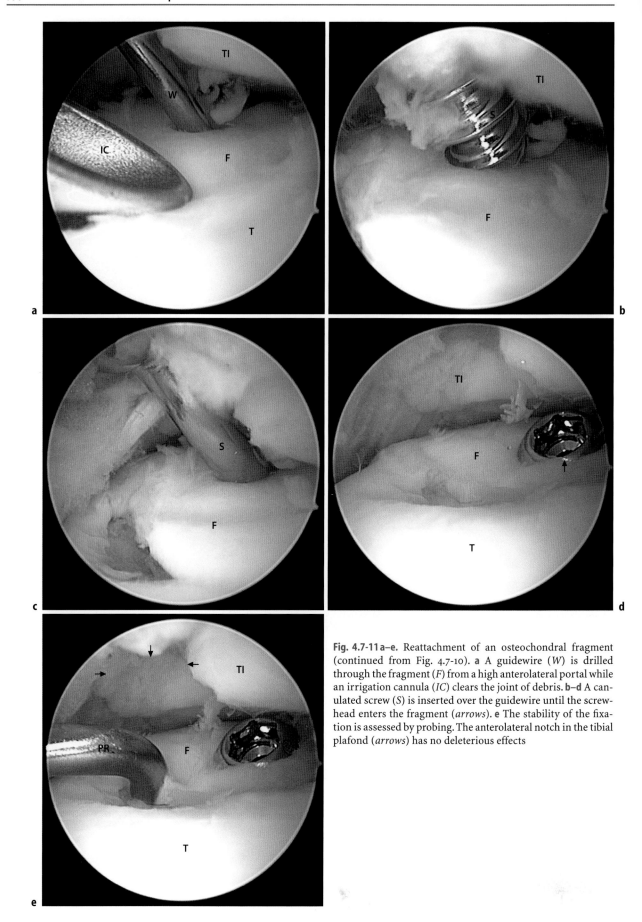

Fig. 4.7-11a–e. Reattachment of an osteochondral fragment (continued from Fig. 4.7-10). **a** A guidewire (*W*) is drilled through the fragment (*F*) from a high anterolateral portal while an irrigation cannula (*IC*) clears the joint of debris. **b–d** A canulated screw (*S*) is inserted over the guidewire until the screwhead enters the fragment (*arrows*). **e** The stability of the fixation is assessed by probing. The anterolateral notch in the tibial plafond (*arrows*) has no deleterious effects

4. **Reattaching the fragment** (Fig. 4.7-11). Various fixation materials can be used. Biodegradable screws are now being tested for graft fixation in ACL reconstructions but are not yet available for use on osteochondral fragments. A cannulated Herbert screw (Herbert-Whipple screw) could also be used. One problem with this screw is difficult removal; if portions of the fragment become detached, they may leave projecting screw parts that could damage the articular cartilage on the tibial plafond. Secure fixation with compression of the fragment can be achieved with a cannulated small-fragment screw. Usually a wire is inserted first and the reduction of the fragment is checked. Care is taken during wire insertion and manual predrilling that the fragment is not displaced or rotated in its bed. The fragment can be additionally stabilized with a Kirschner wire, but since the fragments are relatively small, they can easily be damaged by extra fixation hardware. After the hole has been drilled and tapped, the screw is carefully inserted until the screwhead is flush with the fragment surface (Fig. 4.7-11b–d). The ankle joint is flexed and extended to exclude screw impingement on the tibial plafond.

One small-fragment screw is sufficient for a small fragment (up to 1×1 cm in size). With a larger fragment, a biodegradable pin (e.g., Ethipin) may be added to prevent rotation or a second screw may be placed next to the first.

5. **Probing.** After the fragment has been reattached, it is checked for position and compression. Unstable, projecting cartilage fragments are removed.

Postoperative Care

The patient bears no weight on the operated ankle for 8–10 weeks. Before weightbearing is started, the screw is arthroscopically removed to avoid cartilage damage on the tibial plafond.

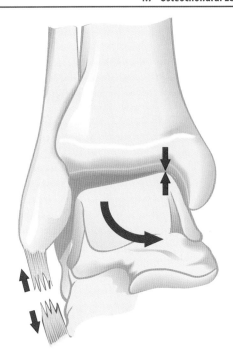

Fig. 4.7-12. Impaction of the medial talar dome in a supination-inversion ankle injury

4.7.1 Anteromedial Bony Impingement

Cause

Supination trauma leads to impaction of the talar dome against the anteromedial tibial border (Fig. 4.7-12).

Symptoms

Typical symptoms are anteromedial joint pain and tenderness over the anteromedial tibial border. Chronic or acute lateral capsuloligamentous instability is the dominant feature in some cases.

Clinical Diagnosis

The anteromedial joint line is tender to pressure. Sites of local firmness are sometimes palpable, requiring differentiation from fixed loose bodies and osteophytes. Many cases show clinical evidence of lateral instability.

Radiographs

Standard radiographic views are often unrevealing. Increased subchondral sclerosis in the medial portion of the anterior tibia may provide a radiographic clue.

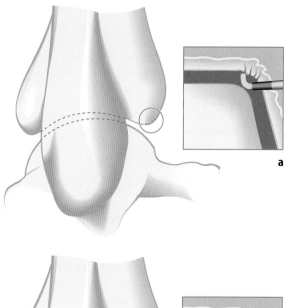

a

Arthroscopic Findings

Lundeen (1992) classified medial impingement lesions into three types (Fig. 4.7-13):

Type A: Superficial cartilage degeneration, often with erosion of the subchondral bone.

Type B: Deep degenerative cartilage changes with separation of the cartilage from the subchondral bone. This type of lesion may be covered by scar tissue or synovitis, and partial synovectomy or scar removal is necessary to evaluate lesion extent.

Type C: Complete separation of the cartilage and underlying subchondral bone, creating a defect that extends toward the tibiotalar joint. This type of lesion is often covered by scar tissue.

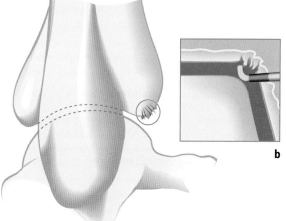

b

Therapeutic Management

Unstable cartilage fragments are removed. With a type C lesion, the separated subchondral bone is also removed. In most cases the initial stages of medial bony impingement are detected incidentally in a patient with chronic lateral instability. Unstable cartilage fragments and scar tissue are removed with a motorized shaver (small synovial resector) or small curette (Fig. 4.7-14).

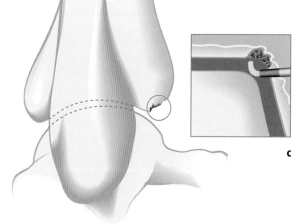

c

Fig. 4.7-14 a–c. Anteromedial bony impingement. **a** Anteromedial synovectomy is performed with a shaver (*S*) so that the anterior tibia (*TI*) can be more clearly evaluated (*SY* synovitis, *T* talus). **b** Inspection reveals an irregular anterior tibial contour with foci of chondral expansion (*arrows*). **c** The prominence and other cartilage changes are debrided with the shaver

Fig. 4.7-13 a–c. Medial bony impingement, Lundeen classification (1992) (see text for explanation)

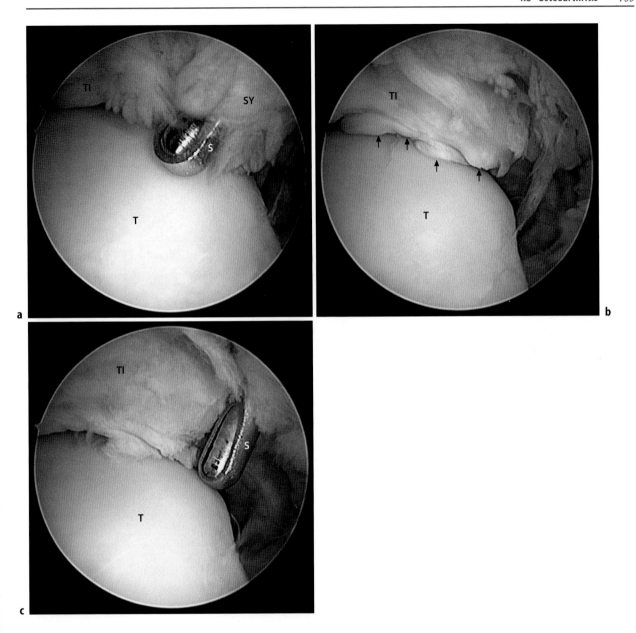

4.8 Osteoarthritis

Cause

Degenerative joint changes may be caused by trauma, chronic ligamentous instabilities, or individual wear and tear.

Symptoms

The cardinal symptoms are pain (cold pain, pain on exertion), crepitation, and limitation of motion.

Clinical Diagnosis

Clinical examination shows decreased range of motion and local tenderness. Osteophytes are palpable in some cases.

Radiographs

Bony deformity or even fractures may be found, depending on the etiology. In other respects, radiographs display the typical features of degenerative joint disease such as joint space narrowing, subchondral sclerosis, and marginal osteophytes (Fig. 4.8-1). The lateral view should be taken in maximum dorsal extension. It may be

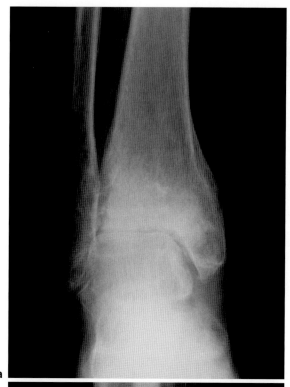

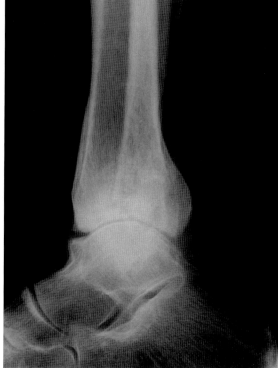

Fig. 4.8-1 a, b. Advanced osteoarthritis of the ankle joint

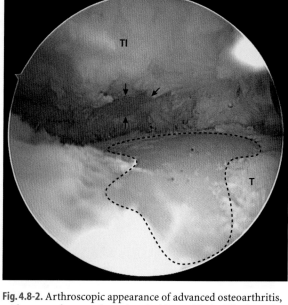

Fig. 4.8-2. Arthroscopic appearance of advanced osteoarthritis, with areas of exposed subchondral bone (*dashed line*) on the talar surface and tibial plafond (*TI, arrows*)

necessary to remove tibial osteophytes or a talar osteophyte intraoperatively to restore a neutral position of the tibiotalar joint and improve access before arthrodesis is performed.

Arthroscopic Findings

Arthroscopy reveals high grades of cartilage damage with denuded bone areas, osteophytes, chronic synovitis, and occasional loose bodies (see Sections 4.1–4.5) (Fig. 4.8-2).

Therapeutic Management

The lavage effect of fluid arthroscopy will improve acute pain symptoms in some patients. Often, however, lasting benefit is not achieved without cartilage treatment, osteophyte removal, and synovectomy, and the complains may recur within a few months. Thus, while strict criteria should be followed in selecting osteoarthritis patients for arthroscopy, this technique can still be helpful in assessing the need for arthrodesis.

If advanced osteoarthritis does not improve in response to conservative and operative treatment (arthroscopic debridement) and the patient is having significant pain, ankle arthrodesis must be considered. In an analysis of gait patterns following arthrodesis in the neutral position, Masur (1979) found that patients were able to walk at normal speed with no visible compensatory movements of the trunk and legs. Mild gait changes were seen during running, stair climbing, and uphill walking, however.

Ankle arthrodesis may be performed as an open or arthroscopic procedure. The latter is preferred for its lower morbidity and, according to initial results, its higher fusion rate. A study in 75 patients showed a fusion rate of 91%, with 84% of results rated good or excellent. Bony consolidation took an average of 9 weeks, or 4 weeks less than in an open ankle fusion (Blick 1996). The tissue-conserving arthroscopic technique is particularly recommended in cases that are at risk for wound healing problems (e.g., dermatologic diseases, prolonged cortisone therapy, rheumatoid disorders, peripheral vascular disease).

Adequate distraction is necessary to permit the complete removal of articular cartilage and sclerotic bone from the tibiofibular joint surfaces (see Sect. 3.5).

Operative Technique

Debridement and Lavage

The procedure consists of synovial treatment, osteophyte removal, cartilage treatment, and if necessary the removal of free loose bodies (see above).

Arthrodesis (Figs. 4.8-3 to 4.8-5)

1. **Inspection and probing.** While adequate distraction is applied to the joint, the arthroscope and instrument portals are established and the articular surfaces examined.

2. **Removing the articular cartilage and sclerotic subchondral bone.** Adequate joint distraction is necessary for expeditious removal of the remaining articular cartilage and sclerotic bone. A tight joint capsule is particularly common in patients with significant arthrofibrosis or advanced, long-standing degenerative changes.
The articular surfaces of the talus, tibia, and medial and lateral malleoli are systematically denuded of their hyaline articular cartilage (Fig. 4.8-3). Care is taken to include the lateral and medial aspects of the talus. The cartilage can be removed with a motorized bur or with a curette, which is a swift and precise instrument for exposing the subchondral bone (Fig. 4.8-3). Though difficult to reach, the posterior aspect of the talus should also be completely denuded of articular cartilage. A mirror can be used to confirm complete removal of the posterior cartilage. Next the subchondral bone is abraded with a spherical bur to bleeding bone (Fig. 4.8-4). Care is taken to preserve the bony contours for better coaptation of the tibial and talar surfaces.

▶ **Caution:** Make certain to expose the talar cancellous bone and vascular bed.
In removing the subchondral bone, no attempt is made to create a flat surface on the talus or tibia. This would require considerably more bone removal than preserving a "normal" convex-concave architecture of the tibiotalar surfaces.
The bur is passed through a posterolateral portal to debride the posterior articular surfaces. When adequate distraction is maintained, the posterior part of the joint can be viewed arthroscopically from an anterior portal.

3. **Arthrodesis.** The distraction is released, and the coaptation of the articular surfaces is checked with fluoroscopy. In the early days of arthroscopic arthrodesis, the fused position of the ankle was maintained by external skeletal fixation. When radiographs confirmed union, the external fixation was removed.
Today, cannulated cancellous bone screws are increasingly used for the internal fixation of arthroscopic ankle fusions (Fig. 4.8-5).
First the medial and then the lateral guidewire (over which the cannulated screws will be placed) are inserted into the residual tibiotalar joint space under fluoroscopic control. They are not yet drilled into the talus. The foot is then placed in the definitive position of fusion, again using fluoroscopic control. The optimum ankle position is the neutral position between pronation and supination, with a slight degree of plantar flexion (5°). While the foot is held in the desired position, the guidewires are drilled into the talus under fluoroscopic control. The placement of the wires is checked under fluoroscopy to confirm that the wires are actually in the talus. After the ankle has been rechecked with fluoroscopy to exclude positioning errors, the guide holes are threaded with a cannulated tap, the cannulated cancellous bone screws (6.5 mm) are placed over the guidewires, and the wires are removed. The position of the joint and screws is rechecked with fluoroscopy in the AP and lateral projections.

Postoperative Care

A below-knee plaster splint or rigid cast brace is worn for one week, bearing no weight on the operated limb. When joint swelling has subsided, a short leg cast is applied, or the cast brace may continue to be worn in cooperative patients. Progressive weightbearing is allowed starting in the 4th to 6th postoperative week. Bony consolidation is checked radiographically.

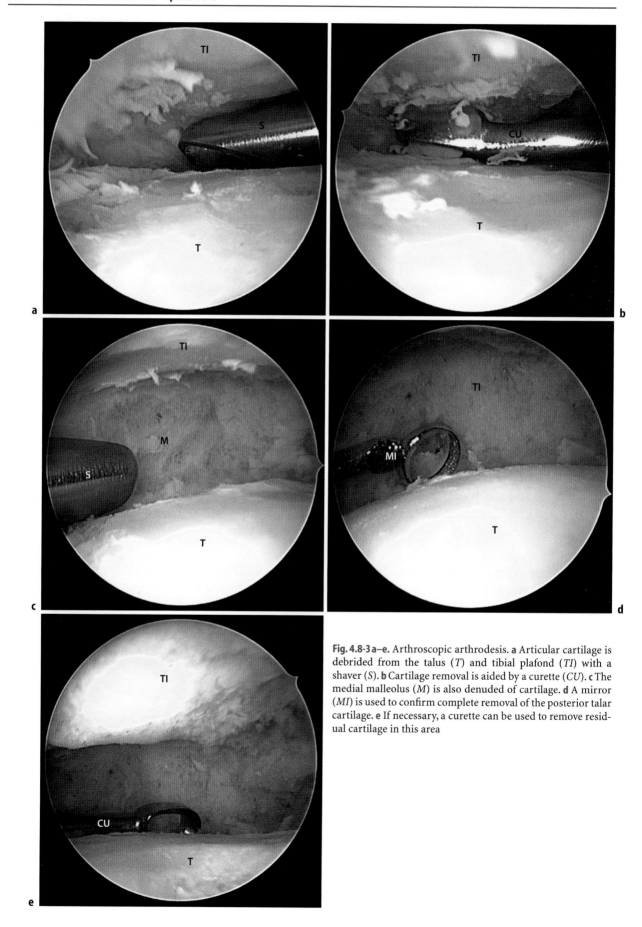

Fig. 4.8-3 a–e. Arthroscopic arthrodesis. **a** Articular cartilage is debrided from the talus (*T*) and tibial plafond (*TI*) with a shaver (*S*). **b** Cartilage removal is aided by a curette (*CU*). **c** The medial malleolus (*M*) is also denuded of cartilage. **d** A mirror (*MI*) is used to confirm complete removal of the posterior talar cartilage. **e** If necessary, a curette can be used to remove residual cartilage in this area

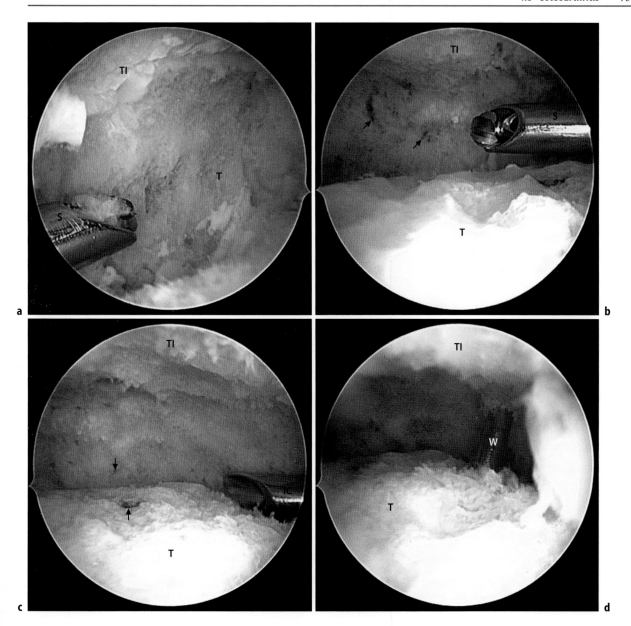

Fig. 4.8-4a–d. Arthroscopic arthrodesis (continued from Fig. 4.8-3). **a** Sclerotic subchondral bone is removed with a shaver (spherical bur, *S*) **b** until bleeding points (*arrows*) appear. **c** The field is cleared of debris with an irrigation cannula (*IC*). **d** A Kirschner wire (*W*) is inserted for preliminary fixation and to define the position for arthrodesis

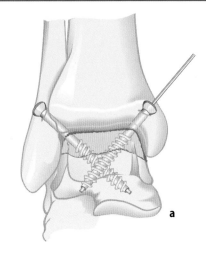

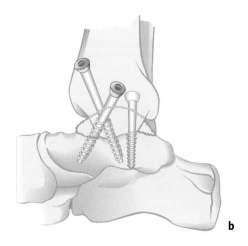

Fig. 4.8-5 a, b. Fixation of arthroscopic ankle fusion with cannulated screws

4.9 Chronic Lateral Instability

Cause

Lateral ankle sprains are the most common ligamentous injury in general, and the majority will heal with conservative treatment. Recurrent lateral ankle sprains may result in chronic instability.

Symptoms

The cardinal symptoms are subjective instability, repeated inversion episodes, and predominantly lateral ankle pain. Giving-way symptoms are also described.

Clinical Diagnosis

Instability is assessed by anterior drawer testing of the distal tibia (to test the integrity of the anterior tibiofibular ligament) and varus stress (tilt) testing. It is very common to find anterolateral tenderness suggestive of lateral impingement.

Radiographs

Standard radiographic views may show calcifications (including rounded ossicles distal to the lateral malleolus) consistent with an old lateral ankle sprain. Concomitant osteochondral lesions may be seen on the lateral or medial border of the talus.

The degree of pathologic mobility in chronic instability can be documented with comparative stress radiographs.

Arthroscopic Findings

Marked opening of the lateral joint space is observed when manual distraction is applied (Figs. 4.9-1). Sometimes the joint space can be inspected as far back as the posterior capsule. This is always suggestive of lateral ankle instability or congenital ligament laxity. Associated chondral and osteochondral lesions are found. It is common to find local synovitis and adhesive bands anterior to the fibula (lateral impingement) and in the area of the syndesmosis (syndesmotic impingement) (see Sect. 4.2).

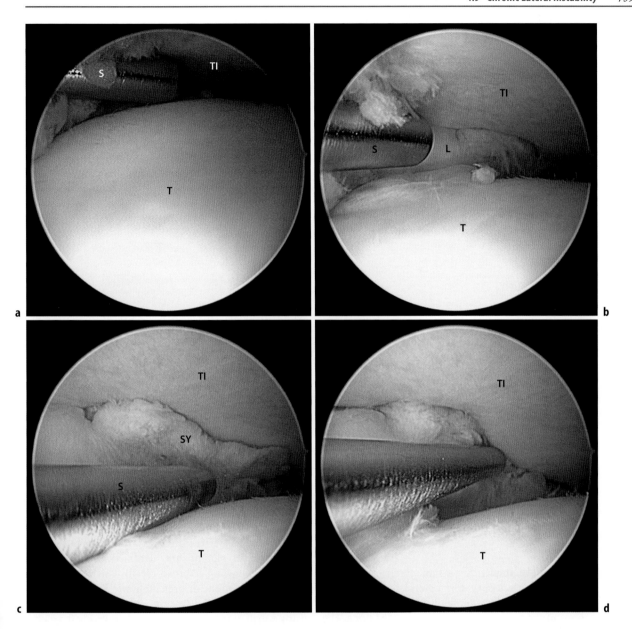

Fig. 4.9-1 a–d. Lateral ankle instability. **a** Anterolateral synovectomy is performed to improve visualization in the lateral part of the joint (*S* shaver, *T* talus, *TI* tibial plafond). **b, c** Distraction with a slight varus stress exposes the lateral malleolus (*L*) and, farther posteriorly, synovial tissue (*SY*) interposed between the tibial and talar articular surfaces. If these surfaces are sufficiently distracted, the posterior synovial tissue can be resected with a shaver. **d** Distraction and varus opening of this magnitude are characteristic of lateral ankle instability

Therapeutic Management

In patients with recurrent inversion trauma and increased lateral opening, lateral ankle stabilization is recommended to prevent further joint wear due to repetitive subluxation. Both open and arthroscopic techniques are available. Open treatments include reconstruction of the lateral ligaments with a pedicled peroneal tendon (peroneus brevis transfer). Another option is arthroscopic ankle stabilization. This technique was first described by Hawkins (1987), who recommends practicing the arthroscopic technique in cadaveric joints and models.

Operative Technique

Lateral Stabilization
(Figs. 4.9-2)

1. **Inspection.** The anterolateral portion of the joint is inspected, and the ligament instability is documented while the joint is distracted and a varus stress applied. It is not uncommon to find chondral and osteochondral lesions of the talus.

2. **Debridement.** The anterolateral joint space is cleared of local synovitis and scar tissue (impingement).

3. **Abrasion.** About 1 cm anterior to the tip of the fibula, an area of talus 6–8 mm in diameter is abraded to bleeding cancellous bone. Later a staple will be placed in this area to fix the anterolateral ligaments. Obstructing soft tissues are debrided with a synovial resector.

4. **Inserting the staple.** A 5.5-mm staple is inserted through an accessory low anterolateral portal to secure the anterior tibiofibular ligament and portions of the lateral capsule to the abraded bone. The foot should be in a neutral position to ensure adequate tightening of the lateral ligaments.

5. **Checking staple placement.** The position of the staple is checked arthroscopically and fluoroscopically. Suture anchor techniques (Mitek anchors) can also be used as an alternative to stapling.

▶ **Note:** Due to published reports on staple breakage and loosening, we do not use staples at our institution. Another problem is the considerable difficulty and surgical trauma associated with staple removal. When Hawkins removed his staples at 3 months, he often found that they were very firmly embedded in the bone and could not be removed without causing additional trauma to the lateral capsule. The results from larger clinical series are still pending.

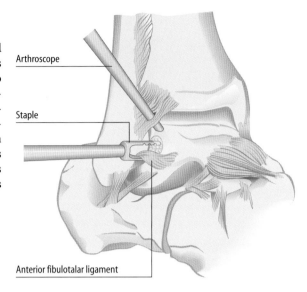

Arthroscope

Staple

Anterior fibulotalar ligament

Fig. 4.9-2. Chronic lateral instability treated by stapling the anterior fibulotalar ligament to the talus. (Modified from Ferkel 1996)

4.10 Fractures

Arthroscopically assisted reduction and internal fixation is an option for ankle fractures that show mild to moderate displacement. Ferkel et al. (1996) reported on the arthroscopic stabilization of fractures of the medial malleolus and the anterior and posterior Volkmann triangle (Fig. 4.10-1).

The fracture site is inspected arthroscopically after joint has been cleared of debris. Cartilage lesions on the talus or tibial plafond are identified and treated as required. Following arthroscopically assisted reduction of the fragment, one or preferably two Kirschner wires are placed across the fracture site under fluoroscopy using a drill guide. The fracture is definitively fixed and compressed by inserting cannulated lag screws over the guidewires under fluoroscopic control. The reduction and fixation are assessed arthroscopically and radiographically.

There is no doubt that the arthroscopically assisted treatment of ankle fractures will become more widely practiced in the next few years. For the present, surgeons are acquiring initial experience with this modality and are defining the range of its indications.

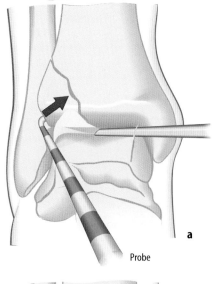

Probe

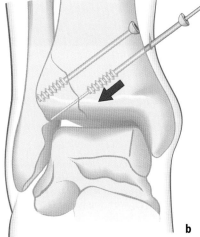

Fig. 4.10-1 a, b. Arthroscopically assisted internal fixation of an ankle fracture. **a** The displaced fragment is reduced with the probe (*PR*) and secured with two Kirschner wires. **b** Cannulated lag screws are placed over the wires. (Modified from Ferkel 1996)

4.11 Infection

The causes, symptoms, and clinical diagnosis are the same as in other joints (see Sect. 2.18).

Arthroscopic Findings

The synovial and cartilage changes are like those encountered in other joints (see Sect. 2.18).

Therapeutic Management

Whenever an intraarticular infection is suspected, regardless of the cause, it constitutes an emergency indication for surgical treatment. The treatment principles are the same as those described for other joints (see Sect. 2.18).

If the infection is secondary to a percutaneous aspiration, injection, arthroscopic procedure, or hematogenous spread, arthroscopy is preferred over an arthrotomy. As in the knee, both the anterior and posterior portions of the ankle joint must be irrigated and debrided.

Limitation of ankle motion is common after infections, and the arthroscopic lysis of adhesions should therefore be considered. Unstable osteochondral fragments are sometimes found as late sequelae of chronic joint infection (Fig. 4.11-1). When these fragments are removed, they leave more or less pronounced defects for which arthrodesis may be the only remaining option.

4.12 Tumors

Cause

Unknown.

Symptoms

Ankle tumors present with local pain and swelling, which may be detected incidentally.

Clinical Diagnosis

The only clinical findings are nonspecific tenderness and possible local swelling. Some patients have no clinical manifestations.

Radiographs

Contour irregularities, lytic areas, and local calcifications may suggest the diagnosis. Tumors are also detected incidentally in many cases.

MRI

MRI is usually necessary to define the location and extent of a tumor involving the talus or tibiotalar joint (Fig. 4.12-1).

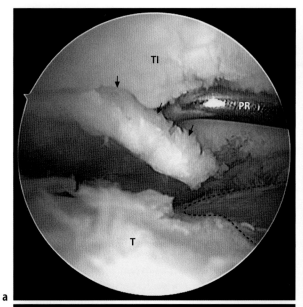

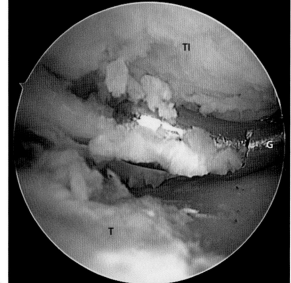

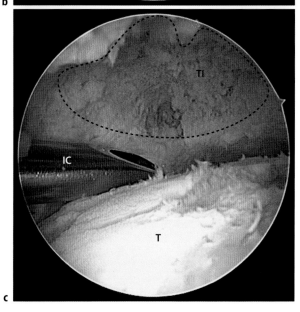

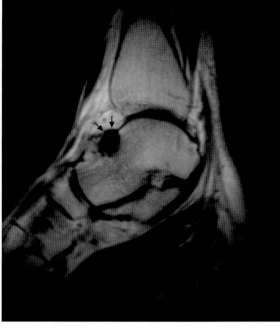

▲
Fig. 4.12-1. Tumor of the talar neck in a 39-year-old patient with severe anterior ankle pain on dorsiflexion. Radiographs showed a slight irregularity in the contour of the talar neck. MRI demonstrates the tumor as a large, rounded area of low signal intensity (*arrows*)

◄
Fig. 4.11-1 a–c. Posttraumatic osteochondral necrosis following a tibial pilon fracture and osteitis in a 36-year-old woman. **a** Osteochondral fragments (*arrows*) are easily separated from the tibial plafond (*TI*) with the probe (*PR*). A large denuded area (*dashed line*) is visible on the talus (*T*). **b** Loose osteochondral fragments are removed with a grasping forceps (*G*). **c** The resulting defect extends into the cancellous bone of the tibia (*dashed line*). Loose chondral fragments and small bony particles are removed with an irrigation cannula (*IC*)

Therapeutic Management

Most tumors cannot be treated arthroscopically. Only circumscribed tumor masses that extend into the ankle joint are suitable for arthroscopic treatment, but these are uncommon (Fig. 4.12-2).

Fig. 4.12-2 a–f. Arthroscopic tumor removal. **a** The tumor site ▶ (*T*) is overgrown by synovial tissue (*T* talus, *TI* tibia). **b** Synovium and tumor tissue (*TU*) are removed with a grasping forceps (*G*). Destructive tumor growth is evidenced by the color variations and variable pore size of the cancellous tissue. **c** Finely porous areas of involved cancellous bone (*arrows*) are resected with a shaver (*S*). **d** A mirror (*MI*) shows residual involved cancellous bone (*arrows*) in the anterior talar neck. **e** The involved areas are extracted with the grasping forceps (*G*). **f** Final inspection shows a denuded area (tumor bed) with a normal-appearing cancellous bone structure in the talar neck (*dashed line*)

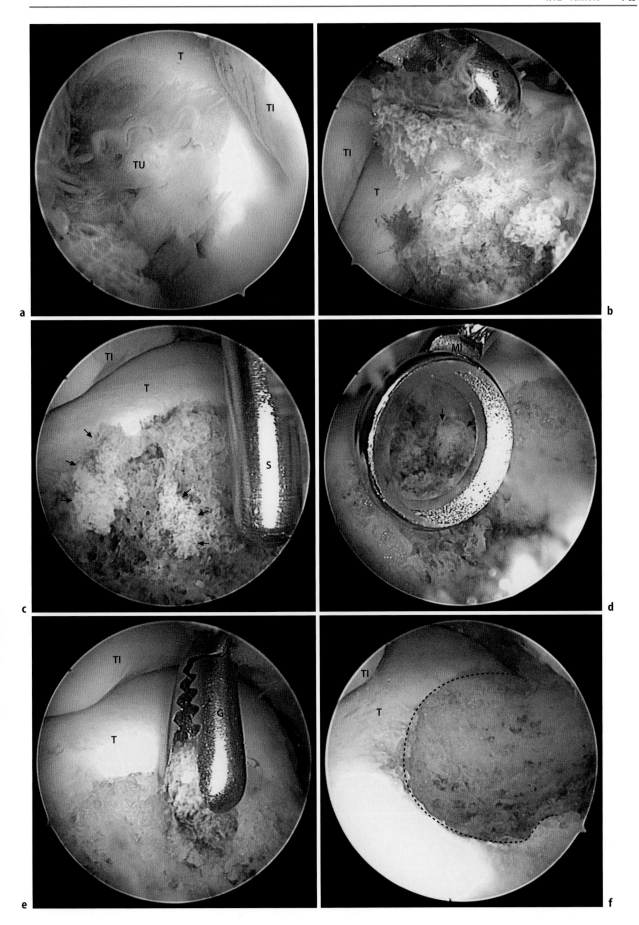

PART III

Wrist

Wrist – General Part

5.1 Historical Development

In 1931, Michael Burmann, considered the pioneer of arthroscopy in the United States, developed an arthroscope that incorporated some of the basic features found in modern instruments. Using a sheath 4 mm in diameter, Burmann distended cadaveric joints with Ringer lactate solution and inspected them with a 3-mm 0° scope. He examined 20 hips, 25 shoulders, 100 knees, 15 elbows, 4 wrists, and 3 ankles. Wrist arthroscopy was difficult at that time due to the relative large size of the instruments. While Burmann realized that the eventual development of narrower scopes would make it possible to examine small joints (Burmann 1931), he felt that only knee arthroscopy had a realistic chance of practical clinical use in the foreseeable future.

Smaller arthroscopes, then, were the key to the evolution of arthroscopy. Watanabe worked for years on the development of smaller scopes. A rigid fiberscope (No. 23 arthroscope) with an outer diameter of 2 mm was introduced in 1967, and an improved successor was introduced the following year. However, structures closer than 3 mm to the scope tip could not be viewed clearly with these fiberscopes. A new rod lens system with the trade name Selfoc was developed in 1968 (Watanabe 1985). In 1970, Watanabe worked intensively with the Selfoc system to develop a practical arthroscope for small joints. In the same year, manufacturers succeeded in producing an arthroscope with an outer diameter of only 1.7 mm. This resulted in a total diameter of just 2 mm for the arthroscope/sheath system and provided an instrument (No. 24 arthroscope) that could be used to examine small joints. Manufacturers also developed biopsy forceps small enough to pass through the sheath (operating arthroscope).

As early as 1971, Watanabe reported on a series of 19 clinical arthroscopic examinations performed in small joints (Jackson 1987).

In the years that followed, oblique arthroscopes were developed to expand the field of view. By 1972, while these scopes were being developed, small-joint arthroscopic examinations were performed in 188 patients. These examinations included 21 wrists, 3 distal radioulnar joints, 1 carpometacarpal joint, 21 metacarpopha-langeal joints, and 4 interphalangeal joints (Watanabe 1985).

Thus, smaller scopes have been the key to making arthroscopy of the wrist and other small joints a reality. The most modern scopes currently available are 1 mm in diameter (see Chap. 12, Fig. 12.2-1), and recent advances suggest that the indications for arthroscopy will be extended to even smaller joints.

5.2 Instrumentation (Arthroscopy System)

5.2.1 Arthroscope

The significance of the development of small arthro-scopes has been alluded to. Wrist arthroscopy requires an arthroscope diameter in the range of 1.9 to 2.5 mm. The outer diameter of the sheath/arthroscope system should not exceed 3.5 mm (Fig. 5.2-1).

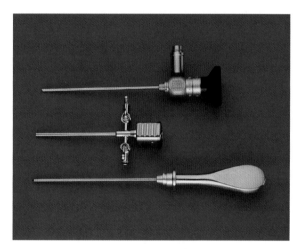

Fig. 5.2-1. Scope for wrist arthroscopy (diameter 2.4 mm) and matching sheath (Karl Storz, Germany)

An arthroscope for small-joint use should satisfy the fol-lowing requirements:

- **Short barrel.** The barrel length should not exceed 60 mm, as this would place the surgeon too far from the joint and make it difficult to brace the hand or fore-arm against the patient, resulting in less precise manipulations and greater fatigue. It should also be considered that the video camera and light cable will be connected to the scope.

- **Image brightness.** Even thin scopes should provide adequate image brightness.

- **Image size.** Despite the small diameter and short bar-rel length, adequate image size is an important con-sideration. Modern scopes 2.4 mm in diameter have an image size comparable to that of a standard 4-mm arthroscope.

The recommended instrument for wrist arthroscopy is a 30° oblique scope with an outer diameter of 2.4 mm (see Fig. 5.2-1).

The same rules apply to the handling of small scopes as standard scopes (see Sect. 1.2.1).

5.2.2 Sheath

The sheath is matched to the arthroscope. The inflow and outflow ports for the irrigating fluid should be located very close to the tip of the arthroscope. If they are several millimeters from the scope tip, there is a risk of distending the subcutaneous tissue when the scope is retracted, causing restriction of intraarticular vision. Since the frequent portal changes in the wrist necessi-tate frequent cleaning of the scope tip, a fast and easy connect/disconnect mechanism is required. Also, the coupling system should permit the scope to be inserted into the sheath and secured in any desired position (see Sect. 1.2.2 and Fig. 5.2-1). The same types of light source and light cable are used as in other joints (see Sections 1.2.3 and 1.2.4).

5.3 Video System

The video camera for wrist arthroscopy should be small, lightweight, and of high optical quality. It is very helpful to have a zoom feature and manual sharpness adjust-ment. Optimum image sharpness is of prime impor-tance in the wrist.

Electronic contrast enhancement is useful for bring-ing out fine tissue differences (see Sect. 1.3.3). The latest generation of arthroscopic cameras come equipped with a digital image processor to enhance contrast (see Sect. 1.3.3, Fig. 1.3-5).

5.4 Probe

Wrist arthroscopy employs a special, small probing hook that has a maximum working length of 60 mm. Standard probes used in large-joint arthroscopy are poorly suited for wrist arthroscopy. A 60° tip angulation, rather than the standard 90°, is useful for very tight joints.

5.5 Mirrors

Mirrors have various applications in the wrist such as evaluating the ulnar head after osteotomy (wafer procedure) or inspecting the lunate bone from the distal aspect. This can eliminate the need to switch portals (see Fig. 5.6-3).

5.6 Operating Instruments

5.6.1 Mechanical Instruments

Arthroscopic wrist surgery requires small-size operating instruments whose working length (shaft length) does not exceed 70 mm. Consistent with the general requirements for mechanical instruments (see Sect. 1.6.1), small grasping forceps and small basket forceps must be used (Fig. 5.6-1). The basic instrument set for wrist arthroscopy includes the following:

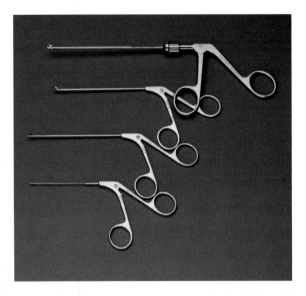

Fig. 5.6-1. Mechanical instruments with reduced jaw size and shaft length, compared with standard-size instruments (*top*)

- Straight basket forceps
- Up-angled basket forceps
- Straight grasping forceps
- Up-angled grasping forceps
- Small, straight grasping forceps
  (1.5 mm outer diameter)

The instruments should have an outer diameter less than 3 mm. A straight grasping forceps is recommended for grasping very fine tissue fragments or small, free intraarticular loose bodies. A very small grasping forceps is necessary for the arthroscopic repair of lesions of the triangular fibrocartilage complex (TFCC lesions).

Arthroscopic scissors and knives are not used in the wrist.

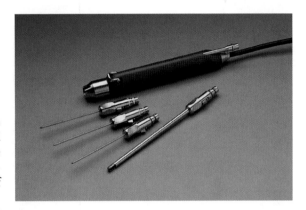

Fig. 5.6-2. Small-joint shaver (Karl Storz, Germany)

5.6.2 Motorized Instruments (Shaver)

A shaver system (see Sect. 1.6.2) is necessary in many procedures and should meet certain criteria:

- **Small handpiece.** A small handpiece is easier to handle and less fatiguing to the surgeon.

- **Short, thin blades.** The shaver blades should have a maximum working length of 70 mm and an outer diameter less than 3 mm.

- **Good cutting action.** An efficient cutting action is particularly important with small blades, since the repeated positioning of a tiny instrument in the confines of the wrist can be problematic. Frequent instrument changes should be avoided.

The following blades should be available:
- Synovial resector (small synovial resector)
- Lateral cutter (meniscus cutter)
- Spherical bur (abrader)

All these blades are consistently required in arthroscopic wrist surgery (Fig. 5.6-2). The small synovial resector is used for partial synovectomy and removing cartilage flaps (Fig. 5.6-3). Synovectomy is very often necessary to improve intraarticular vision. The small cutter is used to resect unstable portions of the articular disk. The spherical bur is used for removing osteophytes, shortening the ulnar head (wafer procedure), and for subchondral abrasion.

The small blades from the small joint set have also proven useful in other joints such as the ankle, elbow, posterior knee joint, subtalar joint, and smaller joints

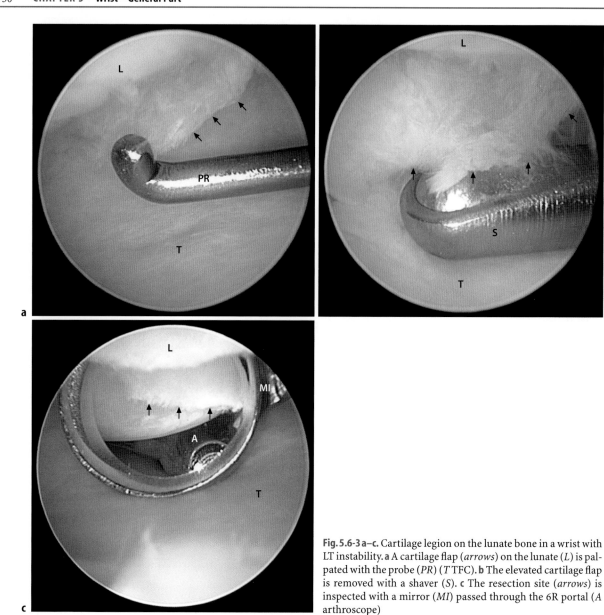

Fig. 5.6-3 a–c. Cartilage legion on the lunate bone in a wrist with LT instability. **a** A cartilage flap (*arrows*) on the lunate (*L*) is palpated with the probe (*PR*) (*T* TFC). **b** The elevated cartilage flap is removed with a shaver (*S*). **c** The resection site (*arrows*) is inspected with a mirror (*MI*) passed through the 6R portal (*A* arthroscope)

such as the toes and the metacarpophalangeal joints of the hand. Even in larger joints like the elbow and ankle, one should not hesitate to use these fine attachments, particularly since they can be introduced through an incision only 2–3 mm long. Standard attachments require a considerably larger incision.

5.6.3 Electrosurgical Instruments

Electrosurgical instruments can be used in wrist arthroscopy to divide scar tissue, remove unstable TFC fragments, and effect hemostasis (Fig. 5.6-4). They might also be used for the debridement of frayed degenerative cartilage.

The following electrodes are required:
- Ball-tipped electrode (2 mm ball diameter)
- Hook electrode (2 mm hook length)

As with mechanical instruments, the working length of the electrode should not exceed 70 mm.

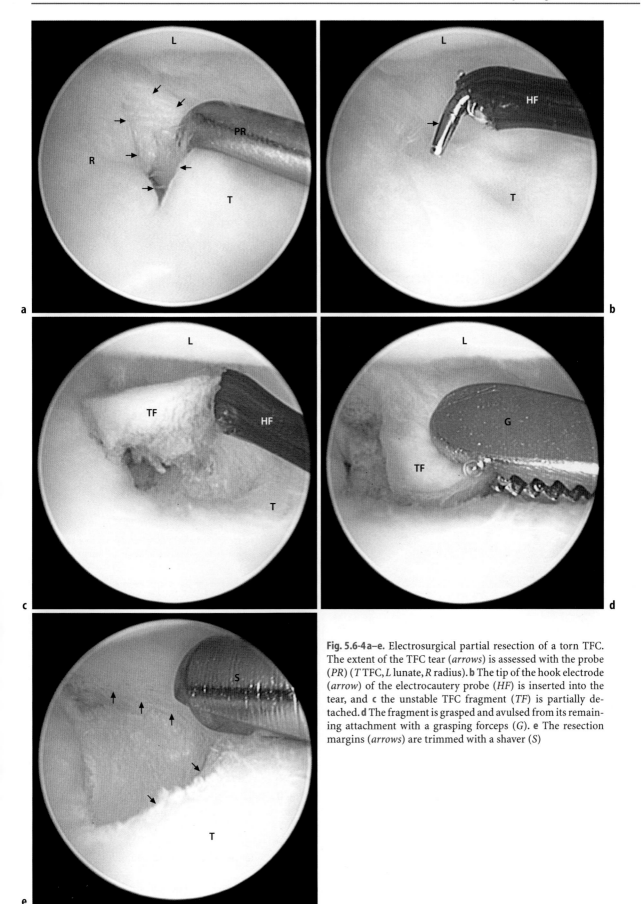

Fig. 5.6-4a–e. Electrosurgical partial resection of a torn TFC. The extent of the TFC tear (*arrows*) is assessed with the probe (*PR*) (*T* TFC, *L* lunate, *R* radius). **b** The tip of the hook electrode (*arrow*) of the electrocautery probe (*HF*) is inserted into the tear, and **c** the unstable TFC fragment (*TF*) is partially detached. **d** The fragment is grasped and avulsed from its remaining attachment with a grasping forceps (*G*). **e** The resection margins (*arrows*) are trimmed with a shaver (*S*)

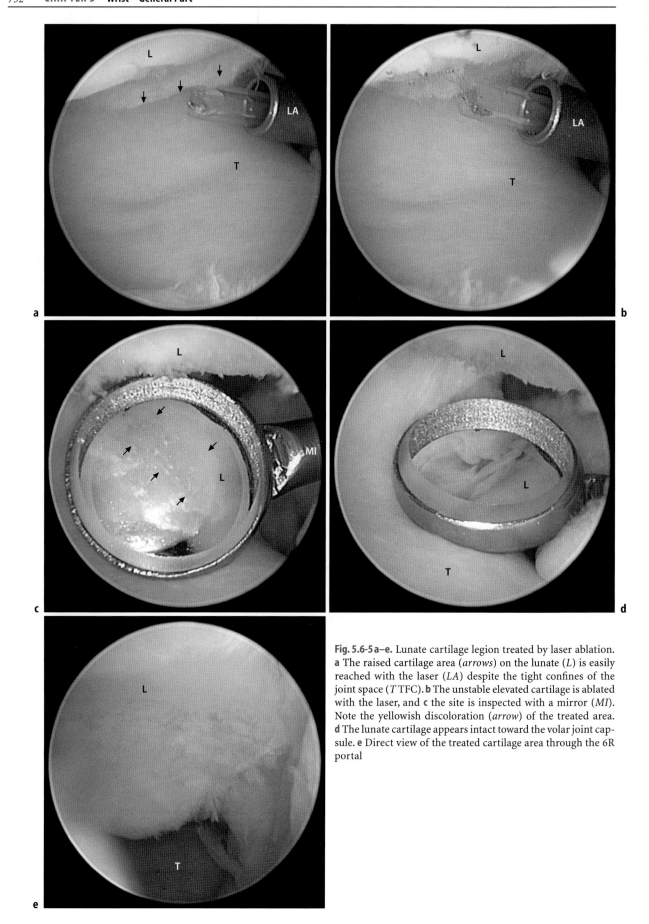

Fig. 5.6-5 a–e. Lunate cartilage legion treated by laser ablation. **a** The raised cartilage area (*arrows*) on the lunate (*L*) is easily reached with the laser (*LA*) despite the tight confines of the joint space (*T* TFC). **b** The unstable elevated cartilage is ablated with the laser, and **c** the site is inspected with a mirror (*MI*). Note the yellowish discoloration (*arrow*) of the treated area. **d** The lunate cartilage appears intact toward the volar joint capsule. **e** Direct view of the treated cartilage area through the 6R portal

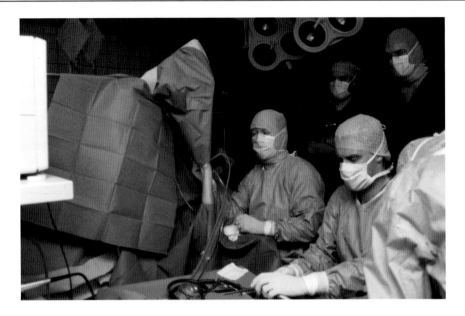

5.6.4 Lasers

The small diameter of laser fibers makes the laser a useful ablation instrument for small joints (Fig. 5.6-5). It should be considered, however, that laser use in a confined space will cloud the field of view, requiring frequent irrigation. Also, the close proximity of the laser probe may permanently damage the scope tip. "Laser hits" appear as small hazy spots on the video image.

5.7 Anesthesia

As in other joints, arthroscopy in the wrist can be performed under general anesthesia or various forms of regional anesthesia (i.v. regional anesthesia, plexus block). Since complete muscular relaxation facilitates joint distraction, general anesthesia is preferred.

5.8 Positioning

The patient is positioned supine, and the arm is positioned on a radiolucent hand table. Various techniques are available for wrist distraction.

5.8.1 Distraction by Countertraction

The fingers are secured to a frame with finger traps. The necessary traction is produced by hanging a weight on the upper arm with the elbow flexed 90°.

Fig. 5.8-1. The wrist is distracted by suspending the hand from finger traps and placing weights on the upper arm. This setup requires a complex draping arrangement

The advantages of this simple positioning technique are its easy setup and low-cost equipment (Fig. 5.8-1). There are also several disadvantages:

- **Complex draping.**
- **Unstable positioning.** Wrist manipulations cause a swinging of the elbow and upper arm that can be very troublesome in complex operations.
- **Lack of fine position control.** The wrist cannot be placed in a defined position of ulnar/radial deviation or dorsiflexion/volar flexion. An assistant or scrub nurse must hold the arm in the desired position.
- **Difficult adjustment of distraction force.** If it is necessary to increase or reduce distraction, an operating room attendant must "crawl" beneath the draped area to add or remove weights. This can make it difficult to maintain asepsis.

5.8.2 Traction Tower

The traction tower is an apparatus, developed by Terry Whipple, for distraction of the radiocarpal and midcarpal joints. It is mounted on the hand table at the side of the operating table. Sterile finger traps are placed on the fingers and connected to the traction tower. A spring scale indicates the distraction force. Since the entire apparatus can be sterilized, the examiner can use a ball joint to secure the wrist in any desired position of flexion or rotation during the operation. Traction adjust-

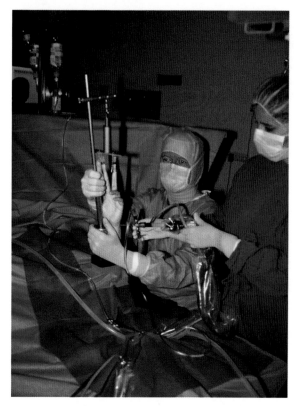

Fig. 5.8-2. Wrist distraction with a traction tower. This setup permits easy intraoperative adjustments of the wrist position

ments can be made by moving the finger traps or by increasing or reducing the distraction (Fig. 5.8-2).

Another advantage is a relatively simple and effective draping arrangement that eliminates sterility problems.

▶ **Note:** Because the traction tower is made entirely of steel, it requires at least a 90-minute cool-down period after sterilization. This must be considered in consecutive wrist arthroscopies to avoid burning the next patient.

We use plastic finger traps, because the wire-mesh type can damage the soft tissues when pulled tight. Special care must be taken in patients on chronic cortisone medication because of their "paper-thin" skin. Attention should also be given to projecting osteophytes in degenerative joints to avoid compressive nerve damage due to forcible or prolonged distraction. One solution in these cases is to apply the traction through a different finger that is free of osteoarthritic deformity.

As a rule, it is sufficient to place two finger traps on the index and middle fingers.

▶ **Tip:** In patients with skin problems (cortisone therapy, see above), use four finger traps to distribute the traction force over several fingers.

5.9 Tourniquet

Surgery is facilitated by using a tourniquet or exsanguination. Bleeding of sudden onset can cause significant clouding and vision obstruction. The lavage effect of fluid arthroscopy is much less efficient in the wrist than in larger joints because of the smaller flow-through volume and lower distention pressure. We therefore recommend exsanguination (250 mm Hg).

5.10 Draping

Because wrist arthroscopy is performed in a fluid medium, waterproof drapes are required. A pneumatic tourniquet is placed on the upper arm, and the hand and forearm are aseptically prepared to the elbow. Then the hand table is sterilely draped, a slit drape is secured to the upper arm, and the hand is sterilely positioned on the hand table. Next the traction tower is assembled (see Sect. 5.8). The upper arm should be secured to the hand table with sterile velcro tape, since the distraction force will be applied against the fixed upper arm.

An extremity drape of the kind used in knee arthroscopy is placed over the positioned and suspended hand. This setup provides for complete, simple, and effective sterile draping.

5.11 Distention Medium

Electrosurgical instruments are used in the wrist as in other joints. A nonelectrolytic solution (e.g., Purisole SM, Fresenius) is recommended, therefore.

5.12 Setup and Preparations for Arthroscopy

Since the hand is positioned on a traction tower, the back of the hand points toward the patient's head. The surgeon and assistant sit at the head of the operating table next to the hand table. The surgical nurse stands next to the instrument table at the narrow end of the hand table. The arthroscopy cart is placed opposite the surgeon, i.e., on the volar side of the positioned hand.

5.13 Portal Placement

The portals for accessing the radiocarpal, intercarpal, and distal radioulnar joints are placed on the dorsal side. Volar portal sites have been described but carry a significant risk of tendon and nerve injuries.

5.13.1 Anatomy

A knowledge of wrist anatomy is essential for correct portal placement.

Bones

The wrist is composed of 15 separate bones that allow motion in 6 degrees of freedom. The radiocarpal joint, midcarpal joint, and distal radioulnar joint are accessible to wrist arthroscopy.

Radiocarpal joint. The radiocarpal joint is formed by the proximal row of carpal bones (scaphoid, lunate, and triquetral), the distal articular surface of the radius, and the ulnar portion of the TFCC.

Midcarpal joint. The midcarpal joint (intercarpal joint) is located between the proximal and distal rows of carpal bones. The distal row consists of the trapezium, trapezoid, capitate, and hamate. These bones are interconnected by strong ligaments that permit little if any relative motion.

Distal radioulnar joint. This joint is formed by the undersurface of the articular disk (= TFC, part of the TFCC), the ulnar head, and the ulnar part of the radius. Between the ulna and radius is the sacciform recess.

Tendons

Because the portal locations are defined with respect to the extensor tendon compartments (ETC), these compartments must be positively identified. A total of six extensor tendon compartments are present:

First ETC:	Extensor pollicis brevis, abductor pollicis longus
Second ETC:	Extensor carpi radialis brevis and longus
Third ETC:	Extensor pollicus longus
Fourth ETC:	Extensor digitorum, extensor indicis
Fifth ETC:	Extensor digiti minimi
Sixth ETC:	Extensor carpi ulnaris

The third and fourth extensor compartments must always be clearly identified, because the primary portal for the arthroscope is placed between them (see below).

Ligamentous Structures

Since the articular surfaces of the bones comprising the wrist are either flat or only slightly concave or convex, the wrist cannot be adequately stabilized by its bony anatomy. It is stabilized chiefly by a complex ligamentous system consisting of both extrinsic and intrinsic ligaments. The extrinsic ligaments connect the radius and ulna to each other and connect the carpal bones to the metacarpals. These ligaments consist of both a dorsal and a volar group. The intrinsic ligaments connect adjacent carpal bones. These ligaments are of great clinical importance, and injuries to these structures have major clinical relevance.

Because some ligaments can be visualized arthroscopically, they will be described in connection with the arthroscopic examination sequence and the TFCC (see Sect. 5.14).

Anatomic Landmarks

Before arthroscopy is begun, the following landmarks must be palpated and positively identified. It is recommended that inexperienced examiners mark these structures on the skin.

- **Radial styloid process.** The radial styloid process is always palpable, even in obese patients.

- **Lister's tubercle.** Lister's tubercle (dorsal tubercle of the radius) is located about 1 cm proximal to the radiocarpal joint space. It is an extremely important landmark for placing the arthroscope portal.

- **Radiocarpal joint space.** The radiocarpal joint space is located about 1 cm distal to Lister's tubercle and is palpable in most patients. Palpation of the joint line is facilitated by alternately flexing and extending the wrist. The dorsal radial margin can usually be identified, even in obese patients.

- **Soft spot at the level of the midcarpal joint.** If a line is drawn connecting Lister's tubercle to the ulnar border of the third ray, a soft spot will be felt on that line approximately 2 cm distal to Lister's tubercle. It marks the level of the midcarpal joint. The soft spot is bounded on the ulnar side by the capitate, proximally by the scaphoid, and distally and radially by the trapezoid.

- **Ulnar styloid process.**

- **Extensor carpi radialis tendon.** This tendon should always be identified, as it is the essential landmark for the ulnar approaches to the radiocarpal joint and TFCC.

- **Distal radioulnar joint** (sacciform recess). The distal radioulnar joint is located on an imaginary line midway between the styloid process and Lister's tubercle. It can be difficult to palpate in obese patients.

- **Extensor tendon compartments.** The extensor compartments, especially the area between the third and fourth ETC, are identified.

5.13.2 Radiocarpal Portals

Five portals are available for accessing the radiocarpal joint (Fig. 5.13-1). They are positioned and designated on the basis of their relation to the dorsal tendon compartments. Thus, the 1–2 portal is located between the first and second ETC.

1–2 Portal

The 1–2 portal, located between the first and second ETC, is used only occasionally because of its proximity to the superficial branch of the radial nerve and the deep branch of the radial artery. Placement of this portal requires positive identification of the distal portion of the radial styloid process and the first and second ETC. The portal is created in the palpable "soft spot" of the capitate sulcus.

The 1–2 portal can be used as a viewing portal for inspecting the dorsal capsule. It can also be used for inflow and instrumentation (radial styloidectomy, osteophyte removal).

3–4 Portal

The 3–4 portal is located between the third and fourth ETC just distal to Lister's tubercle. It serves as the primary portal for the arthroscope.

For the arthroscopic treatment of a dorsal wrist ganglion in this area, a more ulnar portal site (e. g., 4–5 or 6 R portal) should be created first.

The 3–4 portal is just a few millimeters distal to the scapholunate (SL) ligament and is very close to the ridge on the radial articular surface that separates the lunate and scaphoid facets of the distal radius.

4–5 Portal

The 4–5 portal can be used for viewing or instrumentation. Radially and more ulnarly situated lesions can be inspected and treated through this portal.

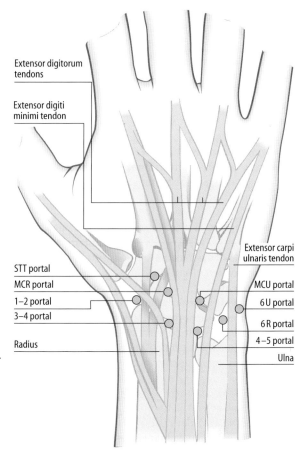

Fig. 5.13-1. Portal sites for accessing the radiocarpal, intercarpal, and distal radioulnar joints

6 R Portal

The 6 R portal is placed just radial to the extensor carpi ulnaris tendon (radial to the sixth extensor compartment). It is used chiefly as an instrument portal and is positioned under arthroscopic control.

This portal is located just distal to the TFC and is closely adjacent to the lunotriquetral (LT) ligament.

6 U Portal

The 6 U portal is placed under arthroscopic vision just ulnar to the extensor carpi ulnaris tendon (ulnar to the sixth extensor compartment). Since the creation of this portal risks injury to the superficial branches of the ulnar nerve, the 6 R portal is better suited for accessing the ulnar portion of the radiocarpal joint. The 6 U portal is established only in exceptional cases.

5.13.3 Midcarpal Portals

Three midcarpal portals are known (see Fig. 5.13-1).

Midcarpal Radial (MCR) Portal

This portal is located approximately 8–10 mm distal to the 3–4 portal at the palpable soft spot. It is level with the distal pole of the scaphoid. The capitate is ulnar to the MCR portal, the trapezium distal and radial to it.

Midcarpal Ulnar (MCU) Portal

This portal is located between the triquetral and hamate approximately 1 cm distal to the 4–5 portal. It is used as an instrument portal for the midcarpal joint and is slightly more proximal than the MCR portal. It enters the midcarpal joint at the "intersection" of the capitate (distal-radial), hamate (distal-ulnar), triquetral (proximal-ulnar), and lunate (proximal-radial).

Scaphotrapezial-Trapezoid (STT) Portal

This portal is located just ulnar to the extensor pollicus longus tendon at the level of the distal pole of the scaphoid and in line with the radial border of the second metacarpal. It is used primarily for instrumentation of the STT joint. Within the joint it is bounded proximally by the distal part of the scaphoid, distally and radially by the trapezium, and distally and ulnarly by the trapezoid.

5.13.4 Distal Radioulnar Portal

A small depression can be felt about 10 mm proximal to the 4–5 radiocarpal portal. The distal radioulnar (DRU) portal is placed at this site, which directly overlies the distal radioulnar joint (see Fig. 5.13-1).

5.13.5 Creating the Radiocarpal Arthroscope Portal: Technique

The smaller the joint and the more complex the surrounding anatomic structures, the more important it is to follow a precise technique for creating the arthroscopic portals. A standardized technique is particularly important in the wrist in order to establish effective, atraumatic access.

To date, we have not found it necessary to inject radiographic contrast medium into the joint space and create the portals under fluoroscopic control, as described by Hempfling (1995).

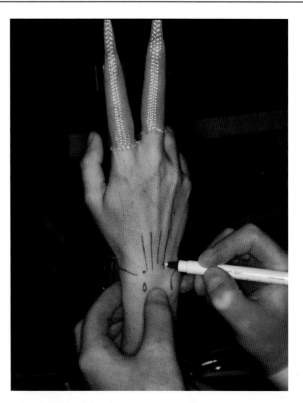

Fig. 5.13-2. Skin markings on the wrist indicate key anatomic landmarks

1. **Palpating and marking the anatomic landmarks.** Lister's tubercle, the radial and dorsal borders of the radius, and the styloid process with the extensor carpi ulnaris tendon are marked on the surface of the skin. On the dorsal side, the extensor tendon compartments are identified and marked while traction is applied. The traction displaces the skin several millimeters in relation to underlying ligaments and bony structures.
   The joint space is palpated about 1 cm distal to Lister's tubercle and marked between the third and fourth extensor compartments (3-4 portal) (Fig. 5.13-2).
   ▶ **Tip:** For arthroscopic treatment of a dorsal wrist ganglion in this area, first establish an arthroscope portal at a more ulnar site.

2. **Needle test.** An ordinary hypodermic needle is inserted into the marked joint space. On entering the radiocarpal joint, it should be considered that the radial articular surface has an approximately 15° volar slope relative to the horizontal plane. The needle is inserted freehand, without an attached syringe, to give the examiner a more accurate feel for the needle position. It is then moved very carefully in the radial and ulnar directions. In this way the examiner can easily determine whether the needle has entered the joint or is still in the soft tissues.

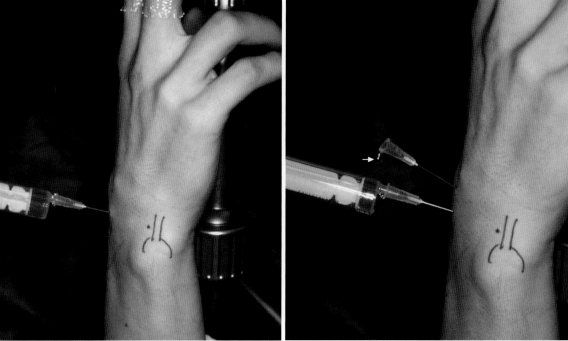

a   b

Fig. 5.13-3 a, b. Fluid distention of the radiocarpal joint. **a** When full distention is achieved, a bulge appears not only in the radiocarpal joint but also farther distally over the midcarpal joint. **b** If a needle is placed in the midcarpal joint, fluid drainage from the hub (*arrow*) confirms a communication between the midcarpal and radiocarpal joints. This usually results from an SL or LT lesion

▶ **Note:** Intraarticular adhesions or pronounced synovitis can reduce the mobility of the needle.

3. **Joint distention.** After intraarticular needle placement has been confirmed, the joint is slowly distended with irrigating fluid while the dorsal wrist contours are observed (Fig. 5.13-3). The contour changes can provide useful diagnostic information:

- **Intact ligaments.** The fluid enters and distends the radiocarpal joint, producing a curved, distally concave bulge in the joint capsule.

- **Torn interosseous ligament.** A tear in the SL or LT ligament creates a communication between the radiocarpal and midcarpal joints. This allows distention fluid to enter the midcarpal joint, producing a distinct bulge distal to the radiocarpal joint (see Fig. 5.13-3 b). This confirms the presence of a radiocarpal-midcarpal connection before arthroscopy is begun.

- **TFCC lesion.** Disruption of the TFCC creates a communication between the radiocarpal and distal

radioulnar joints. This leads to distention of the distal radioulnar joint, manifested by a contour change over and proximal to the ulnar head.

▶ **Tip:** If doubt exists, use the needle test to determine whether fluid has really entered the midcarpal or distal radioulnar joint. While distending the wrist through the 3-4 portal, insert a second needle into the midcarpal joint (MCR portal) or distal radioulnar joint (DRU portal). Fluid discharge from the second needle confirms a pathologic communication between the two joints.

Distend only the joint space, not the subcutaneous tissue. This is particularly important in the wrist, where pressure from the swollen subcutaneous tissue will push the capsule toward the joint space and hamper the rest of the procedure. As in all joints, adequate distention is confirmed by a spurt of fluid from the needle hub when the syringe is removed. To keep the joint distended, leave the syringe in place and maintain pressure on the plunger while withdrawing the needle. Creation of the arthroscope portal requires a well-distended joint.

4. **Skin incision.** A 2–3-mm skin incision is made with a pointed scalpel. The blade should cut only the skin, as a deeper incision could damage fine cutaneous nerves or extensor tendons.

5. **Spreading the subcutaneous tissue.** The subcutaneous tissue is spread to the joint capsule using a fine hemostat or blunt mosquito clamp. This pushes aside fine

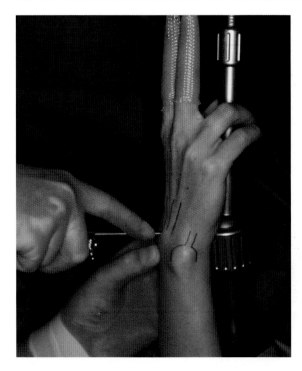

Fig. 5.13-4. Sheath insertion into the radiocarpal joint

cutaneous nerves and any accessory tendon fibers that may be present. The capsule is not yet perforated, however, as this would cause fluid extravasation and loss of distention. Creation of the arthroscope portal would then be more difficult and more traumatizing.

6. **Inserting the sheath and blunt obturator.** The sheath with blunt obturator is inserted into the joint with a gentle twisting motion (Fig. 5.13-4). In directing the sheath into the radiocarpal joint, one must take into account the volar slope of the distal radial articular surface. Also, the wrist capsule can be surprisingly tough even in young patients. Often a considerable capsular resistance must be overcome to enter the joint. Some surgeons may prefer to use a sharp obturator initially. However, this can cause deep, irreversible cartilage damage on the scaphoid or radial articular surface, and so it is better to use a semisharp or conical-tip obturator that can penetrate the tough joint capsule with less risk of cartilage injury.

Since the sheath is inserted with an open spigot, fluid discharge from the spigot will confirm joint entry. This has proven to be a very atraumatic technique. It avoids alternately withdrawing and reinserting the obturator to check for joint entry, which in turn avoids capsular injury and multiple perforations.

After insertion of the scope, the arthroscopic examination sequence is begun.

5.13.6 Midcarpal and Distal Radioulnar Portals

The technique is the same as for the radiocarpal portal. Because the radiocarpal joint is always entered first, portal placement in the midcarpal and distal radioulnar joints can be more difficult if fluid extravasation has occurred.

5.13.7 Creating the Instrument Portal: Technique

Radiocarpal Joint

The 6R instrumentation portal is created first, using the following technique:

1. **Palpating the extensor carpi ulnaris tendon.** Palpation of the extensor carpi ulnaris tendon is essential for portal localization, as the portal is positioned in relation to it. Care is taken not to injure the tendon during portal placement.

2. **Transillumination.** The dorsoulnar capsule is visualized, and the light spot from the scope is used to transilluminate the portal site.

3. **Trial needle.** A percutaneous needle is inserted distal to the articular disk, and its tip is visualized within the radiocarpal joint (Fig. 5.13-5). If the needle perforates the disk, it is withdrawn and repositioned. Piercing the disk is less serious than placing the instrument portal too far proximally, which could cause significant disk injury.
An attempt is made to reach the disk surface and, if possible, the radius with the needle. This can be difficult in very tight joints.
   ▶ **Tip:** Joint distraction should be checked several times during the operation, as a decrease in distraction leads to joint space narrowing.

4. **Skin incision.** A 3-mm longitudinal skin incision is made at the needle insertion site. A deep incision is avoided.

5. **Spreading the subcutaneous tissue and joint capsule.** The subcutaneous tissue is spread in the radial and ulnar directions with a blunt mosquito clamp. The clamp, with jaws closed, is then advanced to and through the joint capsule. The entry of the closed clamp is monitored arthroscopically. The clamp is then spread to create an adequate capsular opening (Figs. 5.13-5 and 5.13-6).

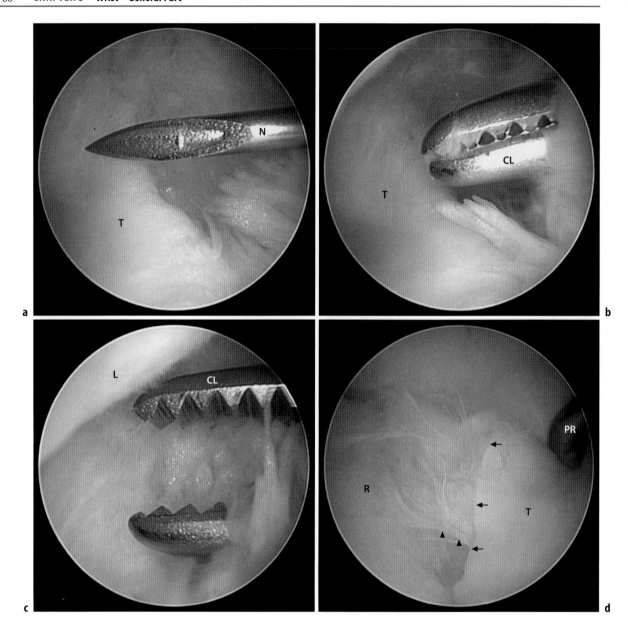

Fig. 5.13-5 a–d. Creating the instrument portal (6R portal). **a** The trial needle (*N*) is introduced distal to the TFC (*T*). **b** A stab incision is made in the skin, the subcutaneous tissue is spread open, and a closed clamp (*CL*) is passed into the joint. **c** The clamp is opened within the joint space. The probe (*PR*) is then inserted (e.g., for probing the TFC, *L* lunate). **d** Radial-side disk tear (*arrows*) (*R* radius). Sites of degenerative disk fibrillation (*arrowheads*) are visible in the depths of the tear

▶ **Tip:** Poor visualization due to pronounced synovitis or intraarticular adhesions can make it considerably more difficult to create the instrument portal. Proceed very carefully in this situation to avoid injuring the TFC. Obstructing air bubbles can be pierced and aspirated with the needle (Fig. 5.13-7).

Midcarpal Joint

The midcarpal instrument portal (MCU portal) is created using the same technique as in the radiocarpal joint. First the midcarpal joint is distended with irrigating fluid. After the skin incision and spreading of the subcutaneous tissue, a sheath with blunt obturator is inserted. The sheath should be directed more toward the index finger than toward the palm so that it will enter the dorsal portion of the midcarpal joint.

Fig. 5.13-6. The capsule is spread open with a blunt clamp during creation of the 6R portal (*L* lunate, *CL* clamp, *T* TFC)

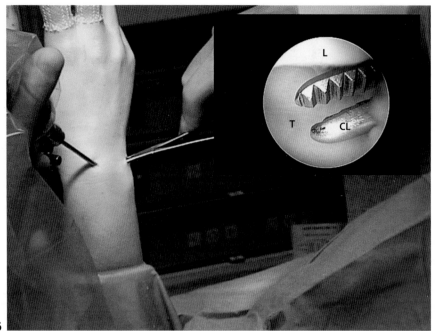

5.13-6

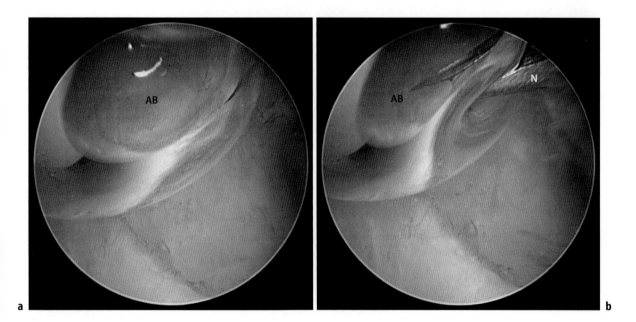

a   b

Fig. 5.13-7 a, b. Vision is obscured by reflections from an air bubble (*AB*), which is pierced and aspirated with a percutaneous needle (*N*)

5.13.8 Switching Portals

As in other joints, visual and instrument access to all areas of the wrist makes it necessary to switch portals. A switching rod is used, following the technique described for other joints (see Sect. 1.13.6).

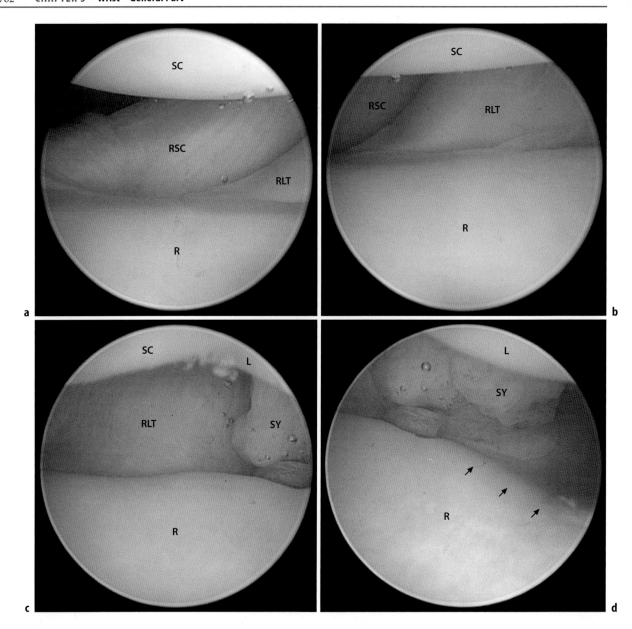

5.14 Anatomy and Examination Sequence

Understanding the intraarticular anatomy of the wrist is critical to making an accurate arthroscopic evaluation and diagnosis.

5.14.1 Extrinsic Ligaments

The extrinsic ligaments connect the carpal bones, radius, and ulna and also interconnect the metacarpals. This system is distinguished from the intrinsic ligaments that connect adjacent carpal bones.

The extrinsic system is composed of volar and dorsal structures.

Fig. 5.14-1 a–d. Extrinsic radiocarpal ligaments. **a** The radial-most structure in the field is the radioscaphocapitate ligament (*RSC*) (*RLT* radiolunotriquetral ligament, *R* radius, *SC* scaphoid). **b** Sweeping the scope medially demonstrates the radiolunotriquetral ligament (*RLT*) and **c** its intimate contact with a "cauliflower-like" synovial protrusion (*SY*), which covers the short radioscapholunate ligament (of Testut). **d** An elevation on the radial articular surface (*arrows*) marks the separation between the lunate and scaphoid facets of the distal radius

Dorsal Extrinsic System

This system consists of seven ligaments, three of which interconnect the distal row of carpal bones (trapezoid ligament, trapezocapitate ligament, capitohamate ligament).

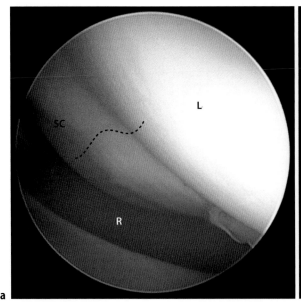
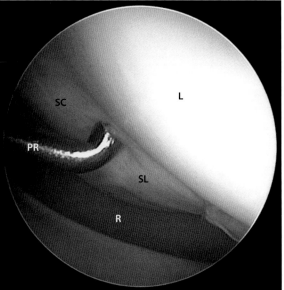

a   b

Fig. 5.14-2a,b. Probing of the SL ligament. a A homogeneous-appearing junction (*dashed line*) is found between the lunate (*L*) and scaphoid (*SC*) (*R* radius). Palpation with the probe (*PR*) confirms the integrity of the SL ligament (*SL*)

Located proximal to these structures are the dorsal intercarpal ligament, the radiotriquetral ligament, and radiolunate ligament, and the radioscaphoid ligament. The strongest ligament of this group is the dorsal radiotriquetral, which combines with the dorsal intercarpal ligament (between the scaphoid and triquetral bones) to form a V-shaped ligament system that is based on the triquetral bone and opens in a proximal-radial direction. The dorsal extrinsic ligaments may be injured by hyperextension trauma.

Extrinsic Volar Ligaments

The volar ligament group has a considerably more complex arrangement. It includes the very strong volar radiocarpal ligament, which is composed of a thin superficial and thicker deep capsular layer. The deep capsular component is visible arthroscopically and divides on the radial aspect into three separate structures (Fig. 5.14-1):

- **Radioscaphocapitate (RSC) ligament**
- **Radiolunotriquetral (RLT) ligament**
- **Radioscapholunate (RSL) ligament** (of Testut)

The radially situated RSC ligament is of clinical importance in scapholunate lesions, because it transmits tensile forces during pronation and supination to the proximal scaphoid. Arthroscopy can demonstrate the stout RLT ligament, which is usually separated by a small sulcus.

The RSL ligament (of Testut) is located under synovial tissue that sometimes appears "cauliflower-like" on the volar capsule. Anterior to this ligament is a ridge on the radial articular surface that separates the radioscaphoid and radiolunate articular surfaces. Distal to this "synovial cauliflower" is the scapholunate (SL) ligament, which is part of the intrinsic system (see below).

Farther ulnarward is the ulnolunate (UL) ligament, which is identified by its oblique course toward the lunate bone. Farther radially is the ulnotriquetral (UT) ligament.

5.14.2 Intrinsic Ligaments

The principal intrinsic ligaments are the scapholunate (SL) ligament and the lunotriquetral (LT) ligament (Figs. 5.14-2 and 5.14-3).

SL Ligament

The strong SL ligament connects the scaphoid and lunate bones (see Fig. 5.14-2).

This ligament is frequently injured by falls onto the dorsiflexed hand. The treatment of SL injuries is very complex (see Sect. 6.5).

SL lesions are among the most common hand injuries, but many are overlooked and therefore undiagnosed. Only the "initiated" can appreciate the often

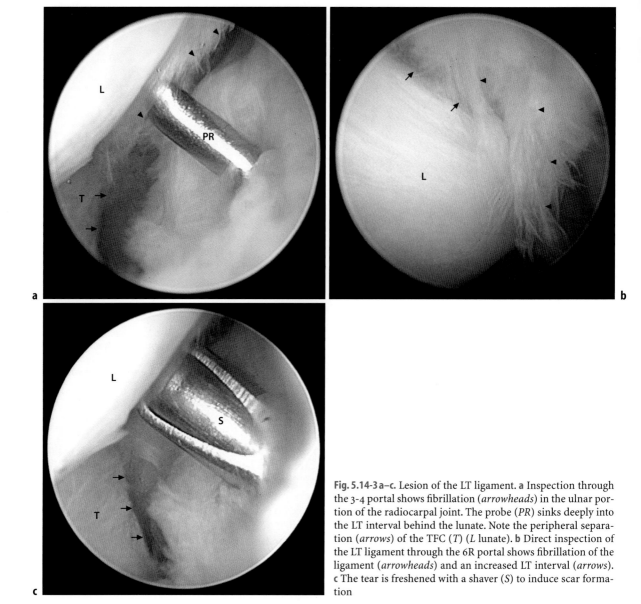

Fig. 5.14-3 a–c. Lesion of the LT ligament. **a** Inspection through the 3-4 portal shows fibrillation (*arrowheads*) in the ulnar portion of the radiocarpal joint. The probe (*PR*) sinks deeply into the LT interval behind the lunate. Note the peripheral separation (*arrows*) of the TFC (*T*) (*L* lunate). **b** Direct inspection of the LT ligament through the 6R portal shows fibrillation of the ligament (*arrowheads*) and an increased LT interval (*arrows*). **c** The tear is freshened with a shaver (*S*) to induce scar formation

subtle radiographic changes, and patients with normal-appearing X-rays are often classified as malingerers when they complain of persistent pain despite conservative treatment.

▶ **Note:** A scapholunate tear is the most frequently missed severe ligamentous injury in the wrist.

LT Ligament

The LT ligament connects the lunate and triquetral bones. Like the SL ligament, it is attached to the proximal poles of the bones that it connects. It therefore separates the radiocarpal and midcarpal joints. It may be

torn by a fall onto the hand or by a distal radial fracture (see Fig. 5.14-3).

5.14.3 TFCC

The articular disk (TFC) is part of the triangular fibrocartilage complex (TFCC), which also includes fibers of the extensor carpi ulnaris tendon sheath and the ulnar collateral ligament. Between the ulnar collateral ligament and the TFC is the variable triangular prestyloid recess.

The TFC arises from the dorsoulnar border of the radius and runs horizontally to the base of the fifth metacarpal. Thus, the TFC as a whole separates the ulnar head and distal radioulnar joint from the radiocarpal joint.

When the wrist is in the neutral position, the TFC is apposed to the lunate bone. With ulnar deviation, the disk comes into contact with the triquetral. The TFC presents a triangular shape in longitudinal section. Its center is very thin and is perforated in up to 25% of patients, creating a communication between the distal radioulnar joint and radiocarpal joint.

The average length of the TFC is approximately 15 mm. Its cross section is biconcave, with the thinnest area located centrally and radially. The TFC thickens to 5–6 mm at the volar and dorsal capsular attachments.

The TFC functions as a coupler for transmitting axial loads from the wrist to the forearm. When the TFC is intact, it distributes 60% of pressure loads to the radius and 40% to the ulna. When the disk is absent, 95% of the total pressure load is transmitted to the radius and only 5% to the ulna (Palmer 1990; Feldmeier 1988). This underscores the importance of the TFCC for wrist function.

5.14.4 Examination of the Radioulnar Joint

The following structures are systematically inspected from the 3-4 portal (arthroscope portal):

1. Radial articular surface
2. Radial capsule and scaphoid
3. Radial part of volar capsule, scaphoid, and scaphoid-lunate junction (SL ligament)
4. Junction of radial surface with articular disk
5. TFC
6. Ulnar part of volar capsule
7. Ulnar capsule and triquetral
8. Dorsoulnar capsule
9. Dorsal radial capsule after switching portals (arthroscope in 6R portal)

5.14.5 Examination of the Midcarpal Joint

The midcarpal joint is inspected from the MCR portal at the intersection of the capitate, scaphoid, and trapezoid. Looking radially demonstrates the distal part of the scaphoid and the proximal articular surfaces of the trapezoid, and looking ulnarly demonstrates the articular surface of the capitate. Looking proximally toward the radiocarpal joint brings the distal articular surface of the scaphoid and the proximal articular surface of the capitate into view. The scapholunate interval can be seen in the deepest part of the field. This gap is markedly widened in the presence of an SL lesion. With complete disruption of the SL ligament, a probe passed through the 3-4 radiocarpal portal is visible through the lesion,

and the ulnar midcarpal portal (MCU) can be placed under vision using the needle technique.

5.15 Complications

Wrist arthroscopy rarely leads to complications, despite the smallness of the structures. To date we have not had a serious complication in any of our wrist arthroscopy patients.

Besides general surgery-related complications, some specific complications may arise.

5.15.1 General Complications

Infection, postoperative bleeding, or reflex sympathetic dystrophy may develop in the wrist as in any other joint. The symptoms, diagnosis, and treatment are the same as in other joints (see Sect. 1.15).

5.15.2 Specific Complications

The following complications are specific to wrist arthroscopy.

Positioning- and Distraction-Related Complications

Excessive finger traction can cause skin lesions on the fingers, compression nerve injury, or traction injury to the metacarpophalangeal joints. If the patient is frail or has skin problems, the traction should be applied through four long fingers rather than two.

Another potential complication is skin burns caused by a traction tower that is still hot from sterilization.

Local Complications

Portal placement can cause injury to subcutaneous nerves, arteries, veins, and extensor tendons. The best prevention is following a systematic placement technique after first marking the anatomic landmarks on the skin.

Intraarticular Lesions

Cartilage damage, TFC lesions, and bony injuries may occur. Careless insertion of the arthroscope can gouge or scuff the articular cartilage. Therefore, portals are created using careful atraumatic technique (blunt obturator) while adequate distraction is applied. Instruments should be handled carefully in hard-to-see joint regions, especially when a relatively large instrument is used.

The TFC may be injured by incising the capsule with the scalpel during creation of the instrument portal. The forcible insertion of operating instruments into the joint space can also injure the TFC. Bony injuries may occur during the arthroscopic stabilization of SL or LT lesions, and therefore this type of surgery should be performed under fluoroscopic control.

Arthroscopy-Specific Complications

Besides instrument breakage, the subcutaneous extravasation of irrigating fluid during the arthroscopic treatment of acute fractures can lead to a compartment syndrome.

5.16 Documentation

Documentation requirements are the same as in the arthroscopy of other joints (see Sect. 1.16).

5.17 Outpatient Arthroscopy

Most arthroscopic procedures on the wrist can be performed on an ambulatory basis. Patients should be hospitalized, however, for the surgical stabilization of fractures (image intensification fluoroscopy is unavailable in most outpatient settings) and for the treatment of intraarticular infections. An image intensifier should also be available for treating an interosseous ligament injury by percutaneous pinning.

5.18 Indications

As wrist arthroscopy has become more widely practiced, its range of indications has expanded. Arthroscopic experience has made it possible to elucidate the pathomechanics of numerous disorders that affect the wrist.

As in other joints, it is counterproductive to draw a distinction between diagnostic and therapeutic arthroscopy in the wrist.

▶ **Note:** A surgeon who performs wrist arthroscopy must be able to carry out any and all therapeutic measures that are found to be necessary.

The indications for arthroscopy are not symptom-oriented but should be based on objective findings. In most cases, an accurate presumptive diagnosis can be made on the basis of clinical examination techniques.

5.18.1 Chronic Pain

The most common symptom that leads patients to seek medical attention is pain. It is common for patients with chronic pain to be referred for arthroscopy even though a detailed wrist examination has not been performed. But accurate history taking (a fall onto the wrist), the correlation of point tenderness with specific anatomic structures, and function tests supported by radiographic findings will usually furnish a presumptive diagnosis. Arthroscopy is indicated only if the examiner, having exhausted the entire palette of clinical diagnostic studies, still cannot formulate an acceptable working diagnosis.

Numerous potential causes of wrist pain should be included in the differential diagnosis:

Radial-Sided Pain
- Tenosynovitis
- Tenosynovitis stenosans
- Osteoarthritis between the radius and scaphoid
- Radial styloiditis
- Scaphotrapezial-trapezoid osteoarthritis (STT osteoarthritis)
- Scaphoid fracture

Dorsoradial Pain
- Ganglion (intra- or extraarticular)
- Partial or complete rupture of the extensor carpi radialis longus or brevis tendon
- Scaphoid cartilage damage
- SL lesion
- SL dissociation
- Radial styloid fracture
- Scaphoid fracture

Dorsal Pain
- Extensor tenosynovitis
- Lunate cartilage damage
- Capitate cartilage damage
- Osteoarthritis between the lunate and capitate
- Osteoarthritis between the scaphoid and lunate
- Synovitis
- Kienböck disease
- SL lesion
- Distal radial fracture
- Lunate fracture
- Capitate fracture

Dorsoulnar Pain
- TFCC lesion
- LT tear
- Midcarpal instability
- Cartilage lesion on the proximal hamate
- Distal radioulnar osteoarthritis

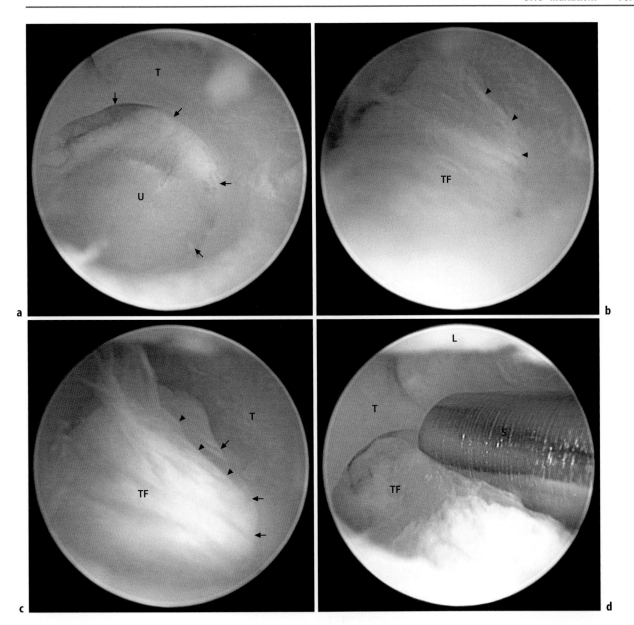

- Free loose body in the distal radioulnar joint or ulnar part of the radiocarpal joint
- Dissociation of the distal radioulnar joint (e.g., after a distal radial fracture)
- Extensor carpi ulnaris tenosynovitis
- Subluxation of the extensor carpi ulnaris tendon

Fig. 5.18-1 a–d. Central TFC lesion with a mobile flap. **a** The 36-year-old patient was evaluated for intermittent wrist locking with dorsoulnar pain. Arthroscopy reveals a central tear in the TFC (*T*) with smooth margins (*arrows*) (*U* ulnar head). **b, c** With alternating pronation and supination, a fibrillated flap of TFC tissue (*TF, arrowheads*) displaces into the distal radioulnar joint, obscuring the ulnar head. **d** The mobile flap is resected with a shaver (*S*) (*L* lunate)

5.18.2 Locking

Intermittent locking of the wrist may be caused by intraarticular loose bodies (very rare in the wrist), articular disk tears, mobile flaps in capsuloligamentous injuries, scar-tissue bands, or hyperlaxity of the capsule and ligaments (Fig. 5.18-1). Except for constitutional ligament laxity, all of these causes can be verified and treated arthroscopically.

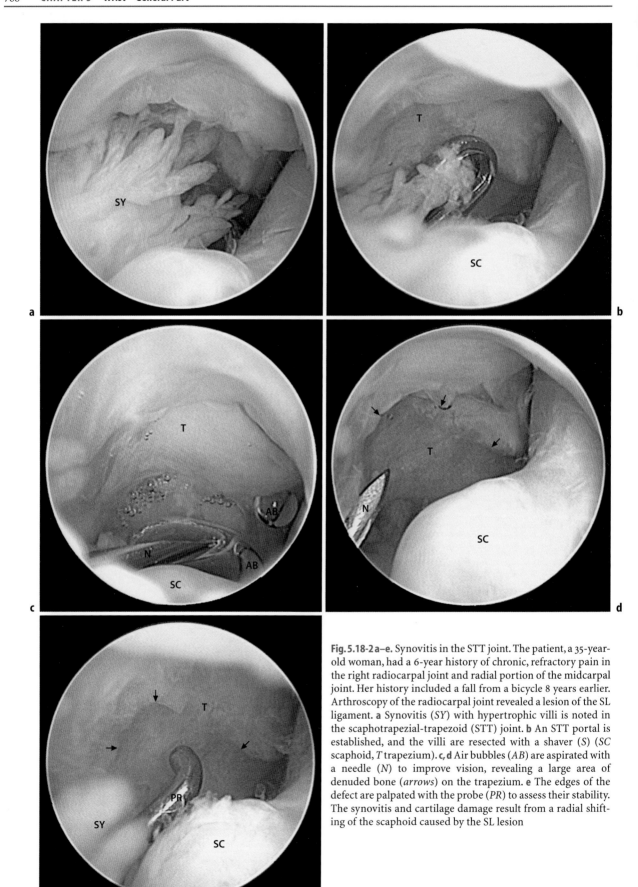

Fig. 5.18-2 a–e. Synovitis in the STT joint. The patient, a 35-year-old woman, had a 6-year history of chronic, refractory pain in the right radiocarpal joint and radial portion of the midcarpal joint. Her history included a fall from a bicycle 8 years earlier. Arthroscopy of the radiocarpal joint revealed a lesion of the SL ligament. **a** Synovitis (*SY*) with hypertrophic villi is noted in the scaphotrapezial-trapezoid (STT) joint. **b** An STT portal is established, and the villi are resected with a shaver (*S*) (*SC* scaphoid, *T* trapezium). **c, d** Air bubbles (*AB*) are aspirated with a needle (*N*) to improve vision, revealing a large area of denuded bone (*arrows*) on the trapezium. **e** The edges of the defect are palpated with the probe (*PR*) to assess their stability. The synovitis and cartilage damage result from a radial shifting of the scaphoid caused by the SL lesion

5.18.3 TFC Lesion

Pain, snapping, and/or swelling in the ulnar joint region may by symptomatic of a TFC lesion. Arthroscopic treatment options consist of resection or repair. An accompanying reactive synovitis, which often contributes to the pain, can also be treated arthroscopically by partial synovectomy.

5.18.4 Synovitis

The pain associated with synovitis may be localized to the capsule or generalized, and intermittent swelling may occur. Arthroscopic options are synovial biopsy, partial synovectomy, or complete synovectomy (if indicated). The radiocarpal joint, midcarpal joint, or STT joint may be involved (Fig. 5.18-2).

5.18.5 Chondral and Osteochondral Lesions

Osteochondral fractures and chondral flake fractures can occur in the wrist as in other joints. Clinical examination can furnish only a presumptive diagnosis; no specific clinical tests are known. Osteochondritis dissecans of the scaphoid has also been diagnosed and treated in the wrist.

5.18.6 Ligamentous Lesions

Arthroscopy is the most accurate technique for evaluating injuries of the interosseous ligaments (SL and LT ligaments).

5.18.7 Ganglia

Arthroscopy can be used to determine the cause of wrist ganglia (intraarticular lesions are often responsible for ganglion formation), and the ganglia can be treated arthroscopically. Arthroscopy is particularly useful in patients with recurrent ganglia to exclude or treat an intraarticular cause (e.g., osteoarthritis, ligament lesions, TFCC lesions).

5.18.8 Fractures

Scaphoid fractures, avulsion-fractures of the radial and ulnar styloid, and distal radial fractures with articular involvement can be reduced and fixed under arthroscopic control (arthroscopically assisted procedure). The extent of concomitant cartilage damage – usually more serious than presumed – can be assessed arthroscopically. Partial arthrodesis of the carpal bones (scaphoid-lunate, lunate-triquetral) can also be performed under arthroscopic control.

5.19 Contraindications

Besides the general contraindications to elective surgery, one should also give consideration to local infectious foci. The potential for transmission to the wrist is the same as in other joints (see Sect. 1.19).

Wrist – Special Part

6.1 Synovitis

Cause

The principal causes of synovitis are the same in the wrist as in other joints (see Sect. 2.3). Localized synovitis is commonly found in association with ligament instabilities, TFCC lesions, cartilage lesions, or scarring. Some cases result from chronic overuse. In other cases a history of rheumatoid disease or psoriasis may underlie a generalized synovitis.

Symptoms

The complaints may arise from the underlying disorder (e. g., a TFC lesion) or from the synovitis itself. The most common symptom is pain. Less common features are local warmth and recurrent swelling. Localized pain (e. g., at the dorsoulnar joint line) is frequently caused by local synovitis.

Clinical Diagnosis

The purpose of the clinical examination is to exclude associated injuries (TFC lesion, see Sect. 6.4), ligament injuries (see Sect. 6.5), and ulnocarpal impingement (see Sect. 6.7) and to evaluate the wrist for point tenderness, capsular tenderness, and capsular swelling.

Pain on terminal dorsiflexion and volar flexion and a painful "shake test" may indicate synovitis. In the shake test, the patient relaxes the arm while the examiner fixes the distal forearm and shakes the hand. Pain or apprehension signifies irritation. With synovitis of the distal radioulnar joint, pain is elicited by passive relative motion of the distal radius and distal ulna. Crepitation signifies degenerative change. Pain on compression of the wrist is more suggestive of a chondral or ligamentous lesion.

Local midcarpal tenderness and pain in response to passive relative movements of the carpal bones (e. g., the scaphoid relative to the lunate, the lunate to the triquetrum) indicate synovitis in the midcarpal joint.

Radiographs

In the absence of rheumatoid deformity or other bony abnormalities, synovitis is not associated with specific joint changes on radiographs. Lytic areas or cyst formation are occasionally seen at ligament origins as a sign of accompanying ligamentous lesions. Specific attention is given to conditions that can cause synovitis:

- Widening of the scapholunate interval (SL lesion)
- Positive ulnar variance (ulnocarpal impingement)
- Degenerative changes (e. g., following a distal radial fracture)
- Intraarticular calcifications

MRI

MRI may show further evidence of the underlying disorder. Localized or generalized changes in the synovial membrane can be seen. In many cases, however, the importance of MRI is overestimated in examinations of the wrist.

Arthroscopic Findings

The arthroscopic features of synovitis are basically the same as in other joints (see Sect. 2.3).

It is not uncommon to find localized synovitis in the dorsoulnar part of the wrist (Fig. 6.1-1). The affected

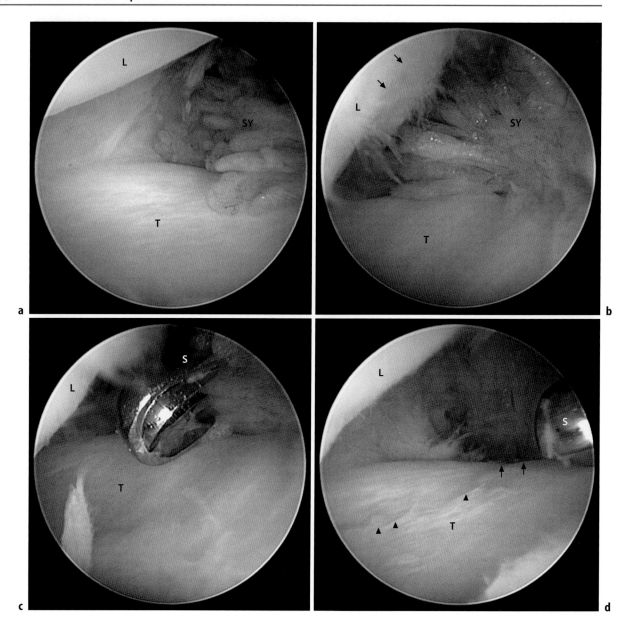

synovium may occupy part of the dorsoulnar or ulnar joint space and obscure visualization of the TFC.

Therapeutic Management

In many cases of local and generalized synovitis, a partial synovectomy is performed so that adjacent intraarticular structures can be adequately inspected. With localized synovitis of unknown cause, a synovial biopsy should be obtained.

Generalized synovitis in the wrist can be treated by partial or complete synovectomy. Pronounced synovitis can also occur in the midcarpal joint, but a synovectomy is more technically demanding at this level and cannot

Fig. 6.1-1 a–d. Synovitis. The patient, a 26-year-old woman, had an 8-month history of ulnar-sided wrist pain. Several conservative therapies were tried without success. **a** Arthroscopy reveals synovitis (*SY*) in the ulnar portion of the joint (*T* TFC, *L* lunate). **b** A cartilage lesion (*arrows*) is also visible on the lunate. **c** Affected synovial villi are removed with a shaver (*S*). **d** The synovectomy reveals a large prestyloid recess (*arrows*). A peripheral ulnar-sided TFC avulsion should be included in the differential diagnosis. Note the fine degenerative irregularities (*arrowheads*) on the disk

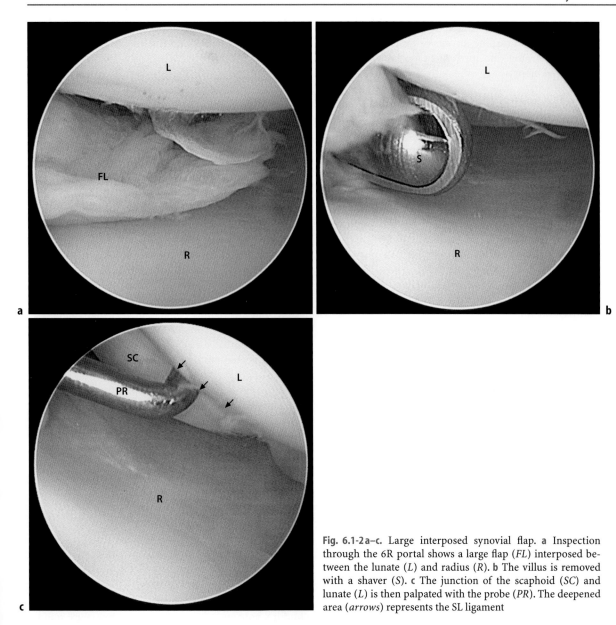

Fig. 6.1-2a–c. Large interposed synovial flap. **a** Inspection through the 6R portal shows a large flap (*FL*) interposed between the lunate (*L*) and radius (*R*). **b** The villus is removed with a shaver (*S*). **c** The junction of the scaphoid (*SC*) and lunate (*L*) is then palpated with the probe (*PR*). The deepened area (*arrows*) represents the SL ligament

be performed as completely as in the radiocarpal joint. The same applies to the distal radioulnar joint. If the synovitis is caused by a rheumatoid or other systemic disease, it should be noted that the tendons surrounding the wrist have synovial sheaths that are also affected by the changes. This should be considered in selecting patients for arthroscopic synovectomy and should be discussed with the patient so that realistic expectations are maintained.

Operative Technique

Partial Synovectomy
(Figs. 6.1-1 and 6.1-2)

The extent of the synovitis is assessed, and the synovial villi are removed with a small synovial resector, taking care not to injure the joint capsule. Very often the synovitis is present as an associated feature, and the rest of the procedure depends on the coexisting pathology.

Complete Synovectomy in the Radiocarpal Joint

1. **Inspection.** The extent of the synovitis is assessed and documented.

2. **Synovial biopsy.** Before a complete synovectomy is performed, a grasping forceps or ronguer should be passed through the instrument portal to obtain a synovial biopsy.

3. **Synovectomy.** The synovial villi are resected from the ulnar portion of the joint using a small synovial resector. The dorsal capsule is done first, followed by the ulnar capsule. The surgeon should proceed very carefully if synovium has encroached on the articular disk (triangular fibrocartilage disk). Next the synovectomy proceeds to the volar side and is carried as far radially as possible. The portals are switched, and the synovectomy is completed on the dorsal capsule before proceeding to the radiopalmar portion of the joint. This can be difficult through the 3-4 portal, and the 1-2 portal may have to be used.

   The wrist capsule is very delicate, and the surgeon should be particularly careful when completing the dorsal portion of the synovectomy.

4. **Wound closure.** After the intraarticular instillation of a local anesthetic (5 mL), the sheath is removed from the joint. During portal closure, care is taken to pass the sutures through the skin only. Deeper suture passes could fix or injure subcutaneous nerves, resulting in painful neuroma formation.

6.2 Cartilage Lesions

Cause

Cartilage lesions in the wrist may be caused by trauma (chondral flake fractures), distal radial fractures, ligamentous lesions (SL or LT lesions), or degenerative chondropathy.

Symptoms

Pain and limited motion in acute injuries are usually caused by the dominant injury (e.g., a distal radial fracture). Degenerative changes are often characterized by limited motion and pain. The pain in degenerative cases may occur during loading of the wrist, at rest, or during initial use of the wrist after prolonged rest. Intermittent swelling may occur. Cartilage lesions have been discovered in 54% of patients with chronic wrist pain.

Clinical Diagnosis

The wrist is palpated for point tenderness that may direct suspicion of a chondral lesion to specific structures. It is important to exclude the various potential causes of a cartilage lesion (ligament instabilities, TFC lesions, etc.).

Radiographs

Radiographs show posttraumatic changes such as fracture lines, postfracture deformities, signs of ligamentous injury (e.g., an increased SL interval), as well as degenerative changes such as joint space narrowing, subchondral sclerosis, and spurring of joint margins. Degenerative changes in the midcarpal joint are often caused by ligamentous instability (see Sect. 6.5).

MRI

MRI can sometimes demonstrate localized cartilage lesions, but this requires images of very high quality.

Arthroscopic Findings

Like other joints, the wrist may display the full spectrum of traumatic and degenerative cartilage lesions (see Sect. 2.2, Fig. 6.2-1). Chondral lesions are commonly found on the radius and lunate and occasionally on the triquetrum (Fig. 6.2-2). When ligamentous instabilities are present, cartilage lesions also may be found between the affected carpal bones.

Therapeutic Management

Treatment is based on the same principles that govern the management of traumatic and degenerative cartilage lesions in the knee (see Sect. 2.2, p. 201). Unstable cartilage fragments are removed. Sites of exposed subchondral bone usually have a degenerative cause, and so there is no rationale for inducing reparative fibrocartilage formation. Given the anatomic shape of the radiocarpal joint, current techniques of cartilage grafting would be of little value for the treatment of local defects. When cartilage fibrillations are present, the removal of unstable fragments is indicated simply to improve arthroscopic vision.

Operative Technique

Cartilage fibrillations and unstable chondral fragments in the wrist are treated using the same stabilization and resection techniques that are used in the knee joint (see Sect. 2.2, Fig. 6.2-2 and 6.2-3).

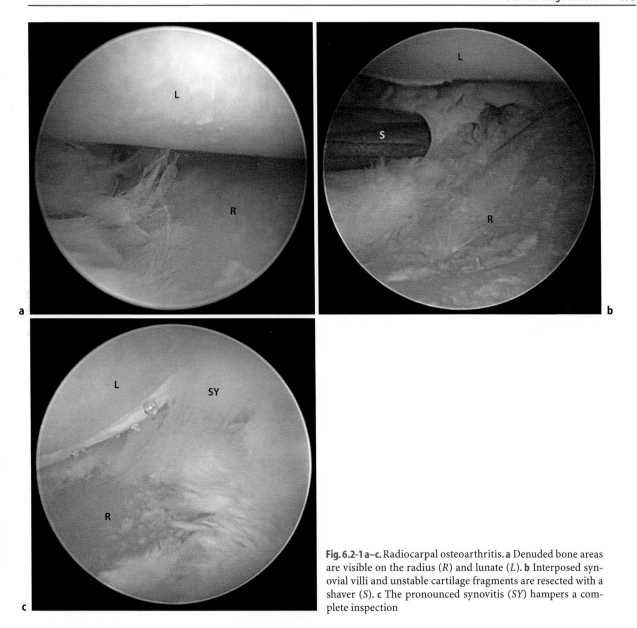

Fig. 6.2-1 a–c. Radiocarpal osteoarthritis. **a** Denuded bone areas are visible on the radius (*R*) and lunate (*L*). **b** Interposed synovial villi and unstable cartilage fragments are resected with a shaver (*S*). **c** The pronounced synovitis (*SY*) hampers a complete inspection

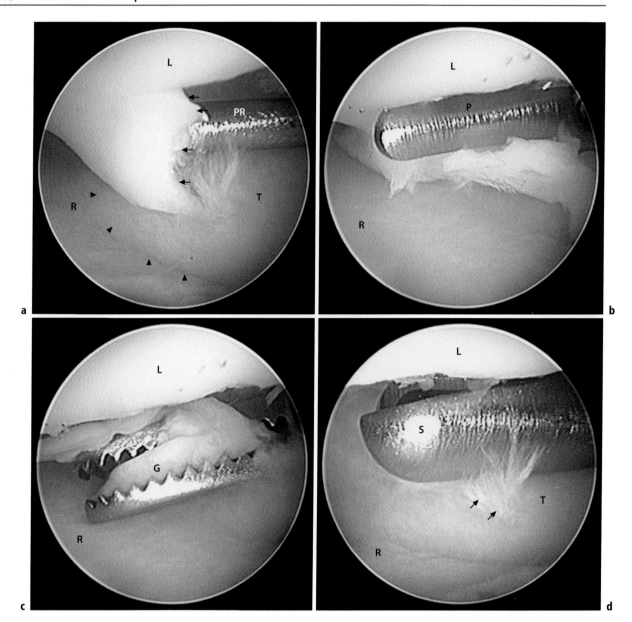

Fig. 6.2-2 a–d. Lunate cartilage lesions in UCIS. **a** A large cartilage tag (*arrows*) is elevated from the lunate (*L*) with the probe (*PR*). A depression (*arrowheads*) marks the junction between the radius (*R*) and TFC (*T*). **b, c** Unstable cartilage fragments are detached with a small punch (*P*) and extracted with a grasping forceps (*G*). **d** The edges are smoothed with a shaver (*S*). Note the central disk lesion with fibrillations (*arrows*)

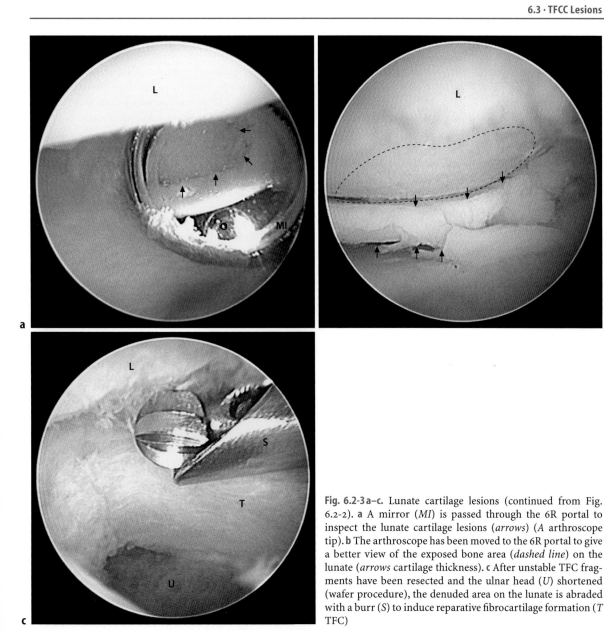

Fig. 6.2-3 a–c. Lunate cartilage lesions (continued from Fig. 6.2-2). **a** A mirror (*MI*) is passed through the 6R portal to inspect the lunate cartilage lesions (*arrows*) (*A* arthroscope tip). **b** The arthroscope has been moved to the 6R portal to give a better view of the exposed bone area (*dashed line*) on the lunate (*arrows* cartilage thickness). **c** After unstable TFC fragments have been resected and the ulnar head (*U*) shortened (wafer procedure), the denuded area on the lunate is abraded with a burr (*S*) to induce reparative fibrocartilage formation (*T* TFC)

6.3 TFC Lesions

Cause

TFC lesions can have various causes:

- **Avulsion of the ulnar styloid process.** An avulsion of the styloid process (e.g., in a distal radial fracture) deprives the TFC of its ulnar attachment.

- **Distal radial fracture.** The distal radial articular surface is often grotesquely displaced relative to the ulna, accounting for the very high incidence of articular disk injury.

The relative shortening of the radius that often results from this fracture causes a positive length discrepancy of the ulna relative to the radius (positive ulnar variance). This not only exerts a constant tension on the articular disk but also causes the ulnar head to press directly against the disk, especially with ulnar deviation of the hand.

- **Rheumatoid disease.** Chronic synovitis can lead to TFC lesions.

- **Degenerative changes.** Degenerative lesions of the TFC can result from repetitive microtrauma over time, combined with a declining diffusion capacity of the disk resulting in compromise of disk nutrition.

- **Direct pressure injury.** In a wrist with positive ulnar variance, regardless of the cause, the disk is chronically compressed between the ulnar head and lunate bone.

- **Congenital perforation.** Congenital perforations of the TFC have been observed.

- **Hyperflexion injury (rare).** A fall onto the flexed hand causes dorsal capsular injury with a dorsal TFC avulsion. The volar portions of the disk are compressed.

- **Hyperextension injury (common).** A natural impulse in falling is to use the hand to break or cushion the fall. At the time of impact, the hand is in a position of dorsiflexion and slight ulnar deviation. The TFC is subject to extreme axial compression, and forces are also transmitted to the SL ligament via the capitate.

Symptoms

Often the pain is localized to the ulnar side but may radiate throughout the joint. Sometimes a snap or click occurs intermittently or during certain movements. Loss of grip strength is also described.

Clinical Diagnosis

Local tenderness is noted in the dorsoulnar quadrant of the wrist. With an acute or fairly recent injury, ulnar deviation of the wrist produces ulnar-sided pain. This pain can also be elicited by the "hammer test," in which the patient is told to hold a reflex hammer in the hand while the hand is relaxed and ulnar-deviated. If this test is painful, a TFC lesion should be suspected. Letting the hand sag into maximal ulnar deviation intensifies the pain.

Another test is based on loading of the TFC by ulnar deviation and axial compression. The patient rests the flexed elbow on the examination table and relaxes the arm, and the forearm is fixed distally. The hand is ulnar-deviated at the wrist, and then the wrist is passively flexed and extended. Pain and a palpable or audible snap are suggestive of a TFC lesion. Sometimes the snap can be increased by pronation and supination.

▶ **Note:** An ulnar snap is very often detected in a wrist with hyperlax ligaments even though the TFC is free of demonstrable morphologic changes.

A degenerative TFC lesion should be suspected in a patient over age 30 who has ulnar-sided pain but no recollection of trauma to the wrist.

Radiographs

The TFC is visible radiographically only when it contains calcifications. Positive ulnar variance provides an indirect sign of TFC pathology, which is further demonstrated by AP function views in ulnar deviation.

MRI

MRI is not useful for the detection of small TFC lesions, but larger defects can be visualized. Thus, MRI is used only in highly selected cases for the investigation of a suspected disk lesion.

Arthroscopic Findings

The normal TFC has a smooth, yellowish-white surface that closely resembles the articular cartilage of the distal radius. Often a probe must be used to identify the radial attachment of the disk (Fig. 6.3-1). The TFC attachments to the volar and dorsal capsule are homogeneous. The small prestyloid recess on the ulnar side of the disk may be expanded as a result of complex dorsoulnar disk avulsions.

The disk is palpated with the probe to evaluate its consistency, resilience, and its dorsal and radial attachments.

Disk lesions range from local induration and superficial fibrillations to flaplike tears of varying size. When destructive changes are advanced and coexist with positive ulnar variance, arthroscopy reveals complex TFC lesions in which only the dorsal and volar condensations may still be intact.

Even if the disk appears grossly intact, it should always be probed to exclude hypermobility resulting from an old tear. Peripheral dorsoulnar tears are quickly covered over with synovial tissue, and function tests are necessary to detect the avulsion.

Various classifications of TFC lesions have been proposed.

Bittar (1988) distinguishes five types:

Type 1: Traumatic etiology, radioulnar lesion
Type 2: Central tear with ulnar involvement
Type 3: Complete absence of the TFC secondary to rheumatoid disease
Type 4: Radiodorsal tear
Type 5: Tear of the ulnar attachment

Palmer (1990) proposed a more comprehensive classification of TFC lesions that distinguishes between a traumatic (Class 1) or degenerative (Class 2) etiology.

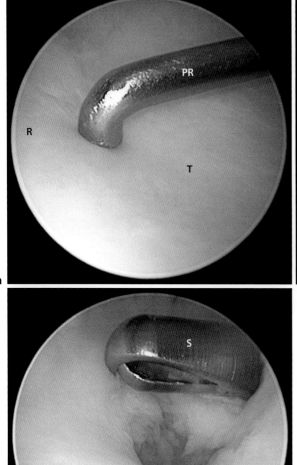

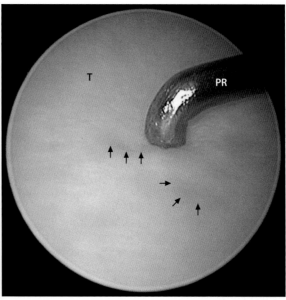

Fig. 6.3-1a–c. Probing the TFC. **a** The TFC (*T*) is carefully palpated with the probe (*PR*), giving particular attention to the disk attachment to the radius (*R*), which is frequently torn. **b** The residual depressions in the TFC (*arrows*) indicate loss of resilience due to incipient degenerative change. **c** After partial synovectomy with a shaver (*S*), the TFC attachment can be seen in the dorsoulnar portion of the joint (*arrows* prestyloid recess)

Class 1: Traumatic lesions

Stage A: Central perforation

Stage B: Ulnar TFC avulsion
- With a distal ulnar fracture (styloid process)
- Without a distal ulnar fracture

Stage C: Distal TFC avulsion from the lunate and triquetrum

Stage D: Radial TFC avulsion (with or without an associated radial fracture)

Class 2: Degenerative lesions

Stage A: TFC wear

Stage B: TFC wear plus lunate and/or ulnar chondromalacia

Stage C: TFC perforation plus lunate and/or ulnar chondromalacia

Stage D: TFC perforation plus lunate and/or ulnar chondromalacia plus tearing of the LT ligament

Stage E: TFC perforation plus lunate and/or ulnar chondromalacia plus tearing of the LT ligament plus ulnocarpal arthritis

While this classification covers a variety of TFC abnormalities, it is of limited practical clinical use. A more practical classification is that of Ostermann (1990), which distinguishes three types of TFC lesion:

Type 1: Traumatic radial tear
Type 2: Central degenerative perforation
Type 3: Traumatic peripheral tear

Ostermann examined 52 patients with isolated tears of the TFC and found a Type 1 lesion in 34 %, a Type 2 lesion in 46 %, and a Type 3 lesion in 20 %. This classification disregards structural changes in the TFC tissue, however.

Careful probing is necessary to verify a TFC lesion. Very often the tear is invisible on inspection because its margins reappose or overlap. This is particularly true with central degenerative lesions, which become symptomatic in response to a trivial injury or ordinary movement. Central perforations, by contrast, are easily diagnosed.

The following systematic probing technique has proven useful for confirming or excluding lesions in a normal-appearing TFC:

- Exclude a central tear.
- Exclude a peripheral (dorsoulnar, volar-ulnar) tear or laxity.
- Evaluate the TFC tissue (softening, induration, superficial fibrillations).
- Exclude impingement by the ulnar head.

▶ **Note:** The TFC is evaluated in an "unnatural condition," since the wrist is distracted during arthroscopy. It is necessary, therefore, to imagine the condition of the TFC in the absence of distraction. The pathomechanical sequelae of chronic impingement, due for example to positive ulnar variance, can then be easily determined.

Therapeutic Management

The TFC has an essential function in stabilizing the distal radioulnar joint and ulnocarpal joint. Complete resection of the TFC leads to disintegration of the distal radioulnar joint, like that resulting from a complete avulsion of the styloid process. Thus, surgical repair should be attempted for acute peripheral tears and for peripheral laxity due to an older tear. Central TFC tears and radial avulsions are not amenable to repair because of their relatively poor blood supply.

Five options are available for the management of a TFC lesion:

- Leaving the lesion alone
- Debriding TFC irregularities
- Resection of unstable flaps
- Repair
- Combined resection and repair

Most cases also require a partial synovectomy so that peripheral lesions can be evaluated. With a central lesion accompanied by positive ulnar variance (ulnocarpal impingement), an arthroscopic wafer procedure should be considered to shorten the ulnar head (see p. 801).

- **Leaving the lesion alone.** A central disk perforation with no unstable flaps or even a large disk defect without unstable flaps can be left alone. Fine superficial fibrillations or indurated areas, while not normal, are not necessarily an indication for debridement. A hypermobile disk that is asymptomatic and is detected incidentally should also be left alone. Positive ulnar variance should always be excluded, as it may be responsible for the disk pathology. Positive ulnar variance sometimes lead to bulging of an intact disk, in which case the ulnar head can be arthroscopically probed through the TFC. An arthroscopic wafer procedure is not indicated, as it would entail destruction of the central TFC. An open shortening osteotomy of the ulna is still an option, however.

- **Debriding TFC irregularities.** Superficial fraying of an otherwise intact disk is treated by carefully removing the fibrillations (e.g., with a small synovial resector) or by "melting down" the fibrillations with a cautery electrode (small ball-tipped electrode). Positive ulnar variance should be excluded, as it predisposes to disk pathology. If severe clinical symptoms are present, an ulnar shortening osteotomy is recommended.

- **Resection of unstable flaps.** Unstable flaps associated with a central TFC perforation or tear should be resected. The periphery of the TFC should be preserved owing to its functional importance.

- **Repair.** Even with an older tear or a hypermobile TFC, repair should be considered if clinical symptoms are present. The disk can be repaired using a modified outside-in suture technique. Radial TFC avulsions can also be repaired, but it must be decided whether repair is worthwhile given the sparse blood supply in that region.

- **Combined resection and repair.** A combined approach is recommended for concomitant central and peripheral TFC lesions. The periphery, which has a major role in stabilizing the distal radioulnar joint, is repaired while unstable central flaps are removed.

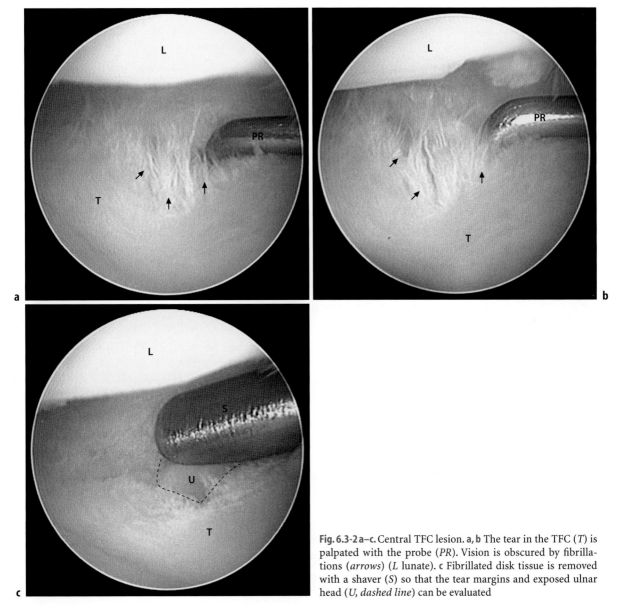

Fig. 6.3-2 a–c. Central TFC lesion. **a, b** The tear in the TFC (*T*) is palpated with the probe (*PR*). Vision is obscured by fibrillations (*arrows*) (*L* lunate). **c** Fibrillated disk tissue is removed with a shaver (*S*) so that the tear margins and exposed ulnar head (*U, dashed line*) can be evaluated

▶ **Note:** Because TFC lesions are often associated with partial or complete SL or LT ligament tears and with cartilage lesions, treatment of the TFC alone is unlikely to relieve all symptoms.

Operative Technique

Debriding Disk Irregularities
(Fig. 6.3-2)

1. **Inspection.** Inspection of the TFC is often hampered by accompanying dorsoulnar synovitis, making it necessary to perform a partial synovectomy.

2. **Probing.** The extent of degenerative changes, including fibrillations, is assessed by probing (Fig. 6.3-2 a,b).

3. **Debriding surface irregularities.** Superficial fibrillations are carefully removed with a synovial resector (from the small joint set). Another option is to "melt down" the fibrillations with a ball-tipped or hook-tipped electrocautery probe. Debridement of the fibrillations will sometimes reveal a TFC tear (Fig. 6.3-2 c).

Partial Resection
(Figs. 6.3-3 through 6.3-5)

1. **Inspection** (see above).

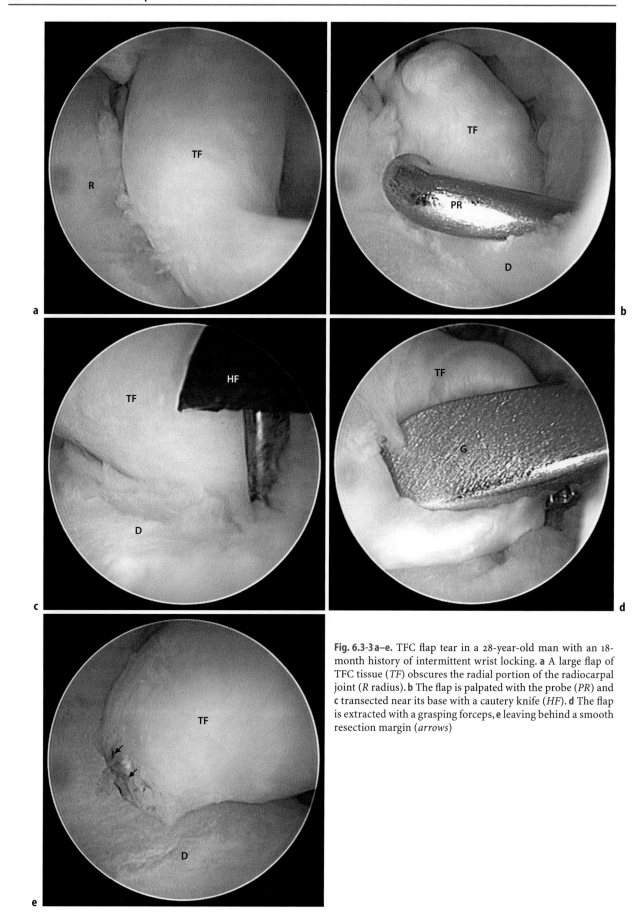

Fig. 6.3-3 a–e. TFC flap tear in a 28-year-old man with an 18-month history of intermittent wrist locking. **a** A large flap of TFC tissue (*TF*) obscures the radial portion of the radiocarpal joint (*R* radius). **b** The flap is palpated with the probe (*PR*) and **c** transected near its base with a cautery knife (*HF*). **d** The flap is extracted with a grasping forceps, **e** leaving behind a smooth resection margin (*arrows*)

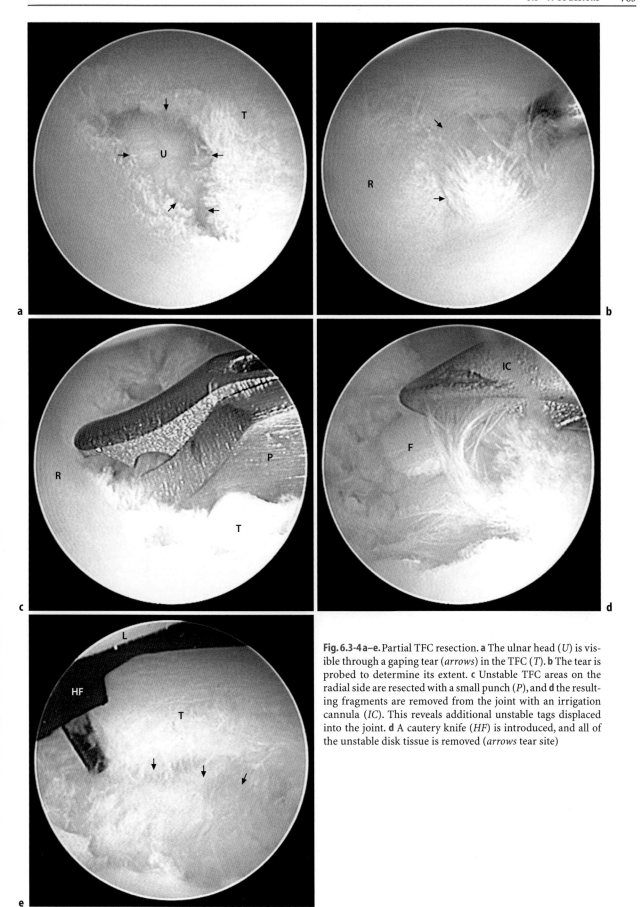

Fig. 6.3-4a–e. Partial TFC resection. **a** The ulnar head (*U*) is visible through a gaping tear (*arrows*) in the TFC (*T*). **b** The tear is probed to determine its extent. **c** Unstable TFC areas on the radial side are resected with a small punch (*P*), and **d** the resulting fragments are removed from the joint with an irrigation cannula (*IC*). This reveals additional unstable tags displaced into the joint. **d** A cautery knife (*HF*) is introduced, and all of the unstable disk tissue is removed (*arrows* tear site)

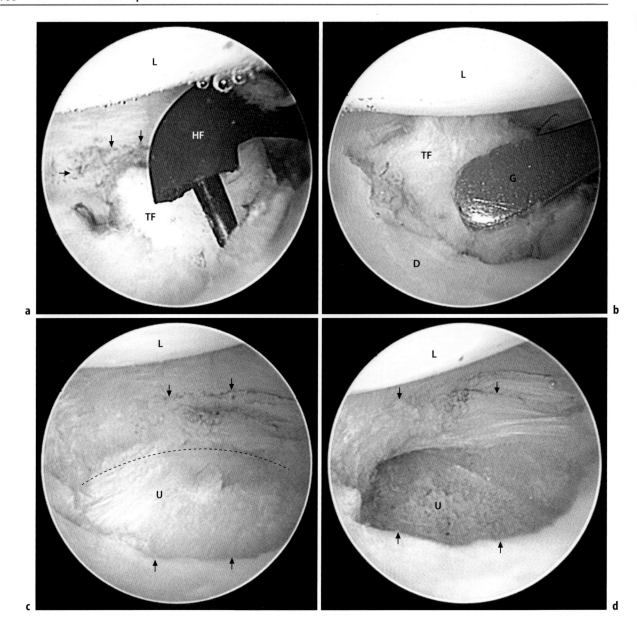

2. **Probing.** The extent of unstable disk areas is assessed by probing. Sometimes the tear patterns are similar to those found in meniscal tears of the knee joint. Unstable flaps may be displaced toward the joint capsule, making them inaccessible to probing and inspection.

3. **Resection.** Small, unstable disk fragments are removed with a small shaver (Fig. 6.3-3a). Because some of the TFC tissue is quite firm, the small meniscus cutter is recommended. Larger fragments cannot be removed with small-bore cutting attachments. Large radially based flaps are partially detached with a small basket forceps and extracted with a small grasping forceps (Fig. 6.3-3b). Ulnar-based flaps are

Fig. 6.3-5a–d. Partial TFCC resection (continued from Fig. 6.3-4). **a** The unstable TFC area (*TF*) is detached (*arrows*) with the cautery knife (*HF*) (*L* lunate). **b** The TFC fragment is extracted with a grasping forceps (*G*). **c** The ulnar head (*U*) bulges through the defect in the TFC (*dashed line*). **d** A wafer resection of the distal ulna is also performed to relieve ulnocarpal impingement

difficult to reach with a basket forceps, and an electrocautery probe (small hook electrode) makes a better resection instrument in this situation (see Fig. 5.3-2). The ability of the cautery knife to cut in all directions is a particular advantage in the wrist (Fig. 6.3-4). Multiple hard TFC fragments can be cut with the cautery knife into smaller fragments that can be removed piecemeal with a shaver. If only mechanical instruments are available, the portals will have to be interchanged. It is recommended that a 4-5 portal be established for this purpose.

4. **Probing.** The remaining disk is probed to exclude additional unstable fragments at the resection margins and check for proximally displaced flaps.

5. **Impingement testing.** While the distraction is released, the wrist is pronated and supinated to check for impingement of the ulnar head on the lunate (ulnocarpal impingement, Figs. 6.3-3 c, 6.3-5 d). If impingement occurs, an arthroscopic wafer procedure or ulnar shortening osteotomy should be performed (see Sect. 6.7).

Repair
(Figs. 6.3-6 and 6.3-7)

1. **Inspection.** A peripheral tear is easy to detect when no more than 2–3 weeks old. Older tears are covered by synovium and are more difficult to evaluate.

2. **Probing.** Often a partial synovectomy must be performed before the peripheral portions of the TFC can be probed. The extent of a fresh tear is easily determined. With an older tear, the probe will slip through the synovial covering into the softened tear site (Fig. 6.3-6 a). The TFC can be markedly displaced from the periphery with the probe. (This can also be done if the TFC or ligaments are hyperlax.) If clinical symptoms are present, repair is indicated.

3. **Freshening the tear.** The tear site is freshened with a small synovial resector, meniscus cutter, or rasp. Needling is also performed, both to freshen the tear and to determine the optimum direction of suture needle insertion for the repair.

4. **Suturing the tear.** An outside-in technique is used. First a trial needle is inserted. Multiple needle insertions will do no harm, as they will freshen the tear while defining the optimum portal location.
Two suture needles are prepared. Each is threaded from the tip with 3-0 PDS. In one needle the free end of the suture is left protruding from the needle tip. In the second needle, the suture is passed through the needle and tied to itself or clamped to form a loop.

The repair is carried out in a specified sequence of steps:

- **Inserting the needle with the free suture end.** The first needle is inserted in the optimum direction previously determined with the trial needle. It is advanced just until the needle tip appears on the disk surface (Fig. 6.3-6 b). The needle is not overadvanced, as it could damage the lunate cartilage.

- **Skin incision.** A 2- to 3-mm skin incision is made at the needle insertion site.

- **Spreading the subcutaneous tissue.** The subcutaneous tissue is spread longitudinally and transversely with a fine blunt clamp. This ensures that subcutaneous nerve branches will not get caught in the suture.

- **Inserting the second needle.** The needle threaded with a looped suture is introduced through the same skin incision, and the needle tip enters the joint space under arthroscopic control. The needle is carefully retracted and advanced to enlarge the intraarticular suture loop (Fig. 6.3-6 c).

- **Grasping the free suture end.** A fine grasping forceps is passed through the 6 R portal and through the suture loop. If the loop is so large that it obstructs vision, its size should be reduced. This will not significantly limit the mobility of the grasping forceps. The free suture end is grasped, and both needles are retracted below the level of the TFC. The free end is brought out through the 6 R portal with the forceps (Fig. 6.3-6 d). Then both needles are completely withdrawn, and the suture loop is pulled, dragging the exteriorized suture back into the joint. After passing through the TFC tissue, the suture is again brought out the instrument portal, creating a mattress stitch (Fig. 6.3-7 a).

- **Checking suture placement.** The efficacy of the suture is checked by pulling on both ends while the tear is probed. The suture should reduce the disk securely to the capsule (Fig. 6.3-7). Two sutures may be necessary for an extensive tear.

- **Tying the sutures.** After any associated intraarticular lesions have been identified and treated, wrist traction is reduced and the sutures are tied together. The knots are buried on the joint capsule. Since the suture material is PDS, multiple knots (at least 4, preferably 5) should be tied. The skin is mobilized if retracted by the suture.

▶ **Tip:** If the suture is volar to the extensor carpi ulnaris tendon, make the skin incision slightly larger to avoid injuring the dorsal branch of the ulnar nerve.

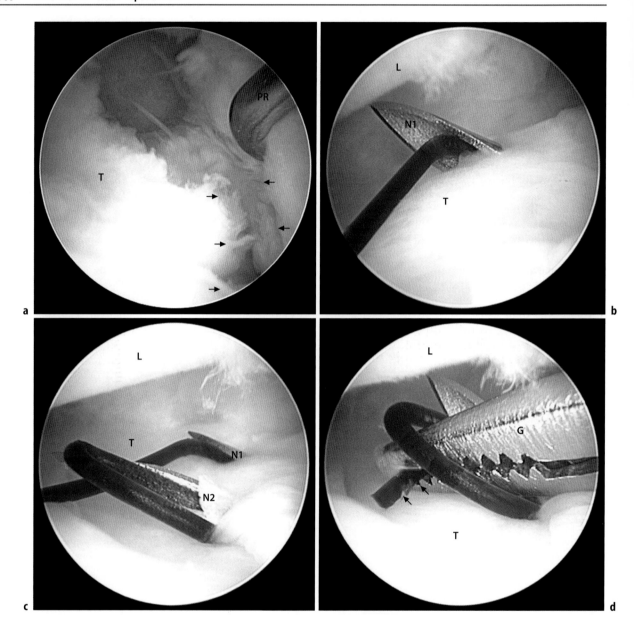

Postoperative Care

The wrist is immobilized for 6 weeks in a forearm splint. It may then be gradually mobilized, depending on associated injuries (e.g., ligament injury). Extreme wrist movements (maximum volar flexion and dorsiflexion) should be avoided for 3 months. Axial loading of the dorsiflexed wrist (e.g., pushups) should be avoided for at least 4–5 months, depending on the extent of the tear.

Resection and Repair

First the unstable portions of the disk are resected, and then the remaining portion is repaired using the technique described above.

Fig. 6.3-6a–d. TFC repair in a 28-year-old professional athlete (hockey player) with a 6-month history of wrist complaints after a fall onto the hand. The patient had a positive hammer test and severe dorsoulnar tenderness. **a** Arthroscopy reveals an extensive dorsoulnar tear (*arrows*) of the TFC (*T*) (*PR* probe). **b** After the tear is freshened with a meniscus cutter, a needle (*N1*) with a free suture end is introduced, taking care not to touch the lunate cartilage with the needle tip. **c** Next a second needle (*N2*) threaded with a looped suture is inserted. **d** The free end of the first suture (*arrows*) is grasped through the loop with a very small grasping forceps (*G*)

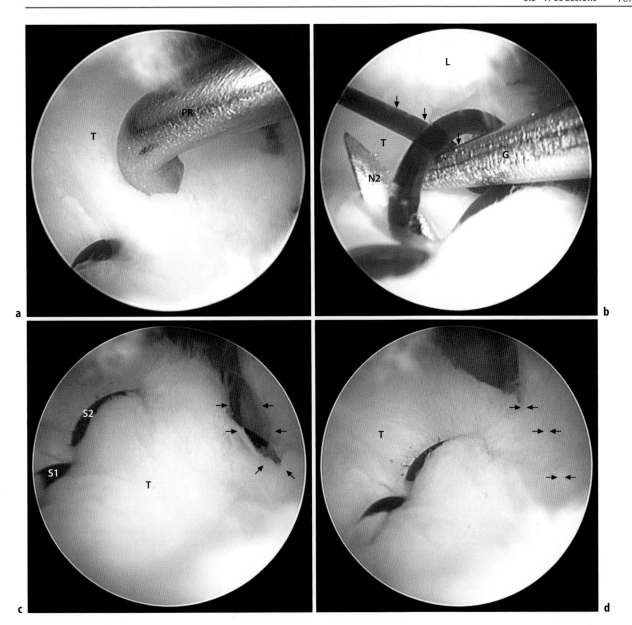

Fig. 6.3-7 a–d. TFC repair (continued from Fig. 6.3-6). **a** While tension is placed on the repair suture, the TFC (*T*) is probed to assess the quality of the coaptation (*PR* probe). If the tear is still dehiscent, a second suture is placed. **b** The two needles are reinserted, and the free suture end (*arrows*) is grasped and pulled through the suture loop with a grasping forceps (*G*) (*L* lunate). **c** At this stage both sutures (*S1, S2*) have been placed but not tightened, and the tear site (*arrows*) is still dehiscent. **d** Tightening the sutures produces complete coaptation of the tear (*arrows*)

6.4 Loose Bodies

Cause

Loose bodies in the wrist may result from chondral flake fractures or degenerative joint changes. Other potential causes are intraarticular fractures, a disturbance of cartilage nutrition, or infection.

Symptoms

Pain, locking, and a snapping sensation may be present. Some loose bodies cause intermittent limitation of wrist motion.

Clinical Diagnosis

The wrist is examined for areas of tenderness and to exclude a ligamentous lesion. No specific tests are available for detecting free loose bodies.

Radiographs

Large, partially calcified loose bodies are visible on radiographs, but most small loose bodies cannot be seen. As a result, radiographs are usually unrevealing in the absence of associated injuries.

MRI

MRI can be helpful in detecting chondral flake fractures and small osteochondral fragments. If MRI is negative but symptoms persist, arthroscopy should still be performed. This limits the role of MRI in loose body diagnosis.

Arthroscopic Findings

The arthroscopic features of loose bodies are the same as described in other joints (see Sect. 2.9). Associated lesions may be detectable, depending on the etiology.

Therapeutic Management

Treatment consists of arthroscopic removal of the loose body. Multiple loose bodies (rare) should be counted prior to removal and the smaller bodies removed before the larger ones. Preliminary fixation with a percutaneous needle can be helpful.

Operative Technique

Removal of Free Loose Bodies
(Fig. 6.4-1)

1. **Inspection.** The loose body is inspected to determine its location and extent (Fig. 6.4-1 a). Reactive synovitis is not an uncommon finding. The loose body also may be adherent to the synovium, creating a fixed loose body. If the loose body is engulfed in scar tissue (rare) or embedded in inflamed synovium, the scar tissue should be removed or a partial synovectomy performed so that the extent of the loose body can be defined.
   Preliminary fixation of the loose body with a percutaneous needle is recommended to keep the object from slipping into hard-to-reach volar joint areas.

2. **Removal.** Small loose bodies are grasped and extracted with a small grasping forceps (Fig. 6.4-1). Larger loose bodies can be extracted with a small, sharp mosquito clamp.
   When the object has been securely grasped, it is extracted from the joint under arthroscopic control.

Postoperative Care

Generally the wrist should be rested for several days following loose body removal. In other respects, the postoperative regimen is determined by the associated lesions and the surgical measures used to treat them.

6.5 Ligamentous Lesions

Ligamentous injuries are undoubtedly among the most common missed intraarticular injuries. Tears of the interosseous (SL and LT) ligaments are difficult to diagnose clinically and also difficult to treat.

Cause

Ligamentous lesions often have a traumatic etiology (e. g., a fall onto the hand) and often occur in association with TFC lesions and fractures. Viegas (1987) found that tears of the LT ligament correlated with age. In experimental cadaver studies, he found a 27.6 % incidence of LT tears at age 60 or older, compared with a zero incidence under age 45. LT lesions also correlated with TFC lesions and positive ulnar variance. These findings support a degenerative etiology and suggest that even normal wrist loads or minor trauma can cause ligament tears in older patients.

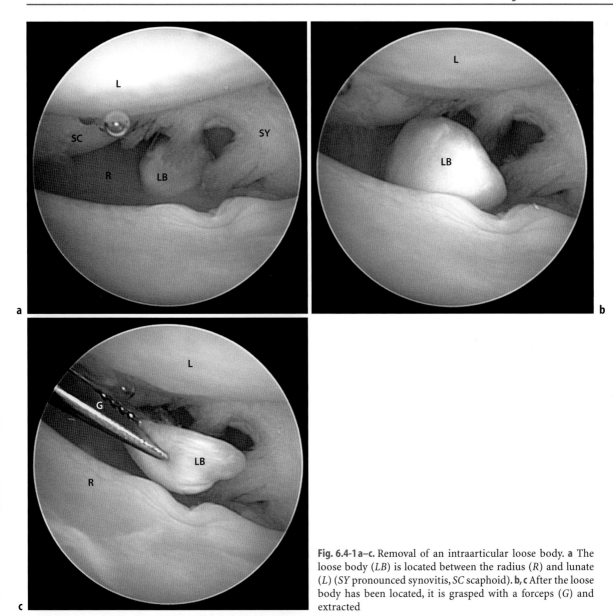

Fig. 6.4-1 a–c. Removal of an intraarticular loose body. **a** The loose body (*LB*) is located between the radius (*R*) and lunate (*L*) (*SY* pronounced synovitis, *SC* scaphoid). **b, c** After the loose body has been located, it is grasped with a forceps (*G*) and extracted

North and Meier found ligamentous and cartilage lesions in 96.3% of patients with chronic wrist pain. They detected an average of 2.6 ligament lesions per wrist, the central ligaments showing a higher frequency of involvement than the peripheral ligaments.

Symptoms

Loading of the wrist causes pain. Rest pain and painful motion loss are characteristic of advanced cases. A feeling of instability, snapping, and intermittent locking may be present and can be debilitating.

Clinical Diagnosis

Areas of pain and tenderness are palpated, and active and passive range of motion are assessed. Maximal movements may elicit a painful click or snap. Various ligament tests are also performed (Fig. 6.5-1):

- **Watson test (for scapholunate instability).** The examiner presses on the distal pole of the scaphoid from the volar side. The wrist is then radially and ulnarly deviated. Pain or clicking signifies a lesion of the SL ligament.

- **Shuck test (for lunotriquetral instability).** The pisiform is fixed with the examiner's thumb and the dorsal side

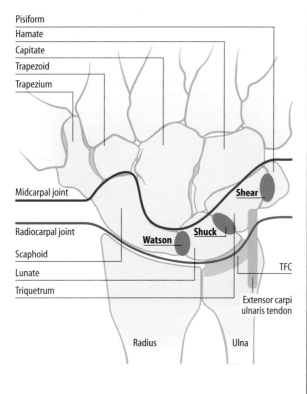

Fig. 6.5-1. Clinical tests for carpal instabilities (see text for explanation)

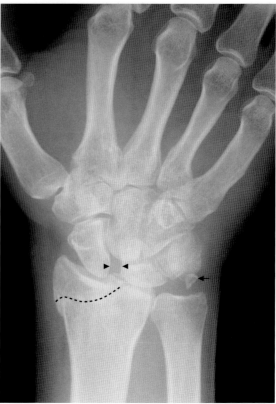

Fig. 6.5-2. Scapholunate diastasis (*arrowheads*) ("Terry Thomas sign") secondary to an old SL lesion. The patient, a 42-year-old man, sustained a distal radial fracture 6 years ago with articular involvement (*dashed line*) and an avulsion of the styloid process (*arrow*)

of the lunate with the fingers, and the wrist is radially and ulnarly deviated. Dorsal wrist pain in the area of the lunate or LT joint space indicates a ligament injury.

- **Shear test (for pisotriquetral instability).** The radial part of the pisiform is palpated, fixed, and pressed ulnarly with the examiner's thumb. Pain or instability indicates ligament injury.

- **Scapholunate squeeze test.** This is accomplished by grasping the volar and dorsal aspects of the lunate with one hand, grasping the scaphoid with the other hand, and pressing the two bones together. Pain and/or instability indicates an SL lesion, which may be accompanied by reactive synovitis.

- **Lunotriquetral squeeze test.** As in the previous test, the lunate and triquetrum are fixed and pressed together. Pain and/or instability signifies instability.

In patients with chronic wrist pain, careful palpation will very often show maximum tenderness in the SL interval, consistent with a lax or deficient ligament. The differential diagnosis should include irritation of the distal radioulnar joint and TFCC and tendinopathies.

Radiographs

Widening of the SL interval on the PA radiograph (the "Terry Thomas sign") is pathognomonic for a torn SL ligament (Fig. 6.5-2). Maximum ulnar deviation or joint distraction causes further widening of the gap.

▶ **Tip:** Always assess the width of the SL and LT intervals on wrist radiographs.

It is common to find associated lesions such as a distal radial fracture or scaphoid fracture (Fig. 6.5-3). In many cases these are old injuries that are considered "re-

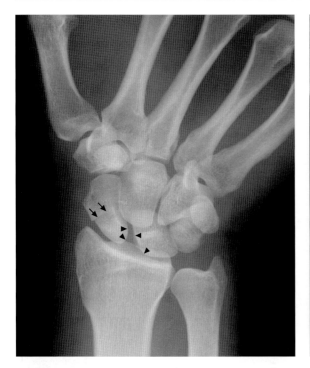

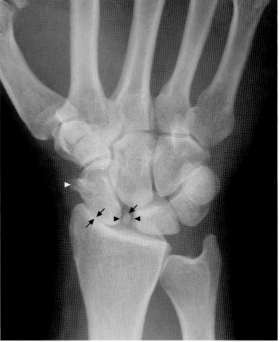

Fig. 6.5-3. Scapholunate diastasis (*arrowheads*) 5 months after the patient sustained a scaphoid fracture (*arrows*)

Fig. 6.5-4. Old SL lesion in a 67-year-old man with chronic wrist complaints. The patient fell onto the hand 8 years before. Afterward he had intermittent complaints, which his family doctor treated first as a sprain and then as chronic tendovaginitis. The widened SL interval (*arrowheads*) contains a local calcification (*arrow*). The radial drift of the scaphoid has almost completely obliterated the joint space between the scaphoid and radius (*arrows*). A marginal osteophyte (*arrowhead*) is visible on the scaphoid. The osteoarthritic changes between the scaphoid and trapezium are also a result of the SL lesion (see also Fig. 5.18-2)

solved" from a clinical standpoint. The widened SL interval may also contain calcifications (Fig. 6.5-4).

With an SL lesion of long standing, the following secondary changes may be found in adjacent joint areas:

- **Spurring of the radial styloid process**
- **Joint space narrowing between the radius and scaphoid**
- **Varying grades of degenerative change between the scaphoid and trapezium** (see Fig. 5.18-2)
- **Marginal spurring of the scaphoid** (Fig. 6.5-4)

If an SL or LT lesion is suspected despite a negative PA radiograph, function views of the wrist should be obtained (Fig. 6.5-5).

Ostermann (1995) notes that arthrography is helpful in detecting a tear of the LT ligament. The radiographic contrast medium should be injected into the midcarpal joint to demonstrate a communication between the midcarpal and radiocarpal joints through the LT lesion.

MRI

MRI can demonstrate elongated ligaments, ligament irregularities, or the complete absence of ligaments. Arthroscopy is better for evaluating the interosseous ligaments, however.

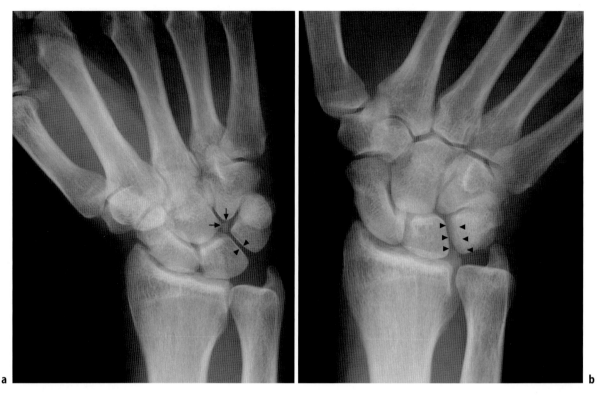

Fig. 6.5.5 a, b. LT lesion in a 42-year-old professional tennis player with severe pain following a hyperextension-ulnar deviation injury. Positive shuck test. **a** AP radiograph shows a normal LT interval (*arrowheads*) and a calcification between the capitate and triquetrum (*arrows*). **b** Function view in ulnar deviation shows marked widening of the LT interval (*arrowheads*) consistent with an LT lesion

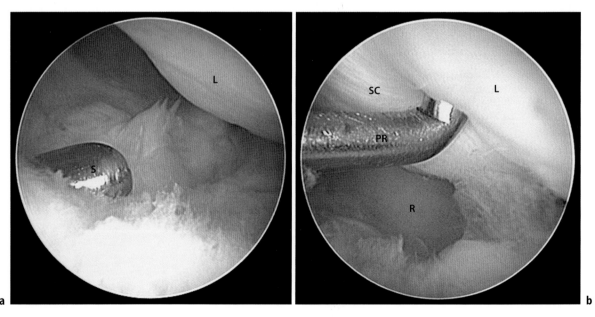

Fig. 6.5-6 a, b. Probing of the SL ligament. **a** Partial synovectomy is performed with a shaver (*S*) inserted through the 3-4 portal. The arthroscope is in the 6R portal (*L* lunate). **b** The junction of the scaphoid (*SC*) and lunate is palpated with the probe (*PR*). The slight depression indicates laxity of the SL ligament, but a complete tear is not present (*R* radius)

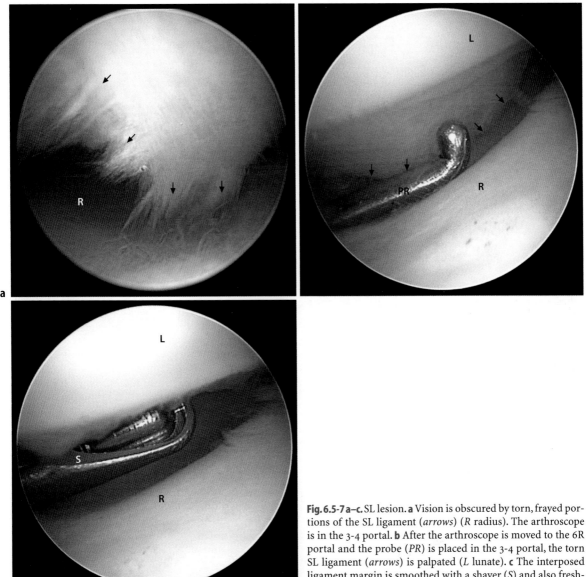

Fig. 6.5-7 a–c. SL lesion. **a** Vision is obscured by torn, frayed portions of the SL ligament (*arrows*) (*R* radius). The arthroscope is in the 3-4 portal. **b** After the arthroscope is moved to the 6R portal and the probe (*PR*) is placed in the 3-4 portal, the torn SL ligament (*arrows*) is palpated (*L* lunate). **c** The interposed ligament margin is smoothed with a shaver (*S*) and also freshened to induce scar formation

Arthroscopic Findings

SL Ligament

Findings range from a fully intact ligament surface to the complete absence of the ligament (Fig. 6.5-6). With a torn SL ligament, a flap may be displaced into the joint and may obscure the adjacent compartment (Fig. 6.5-7). With a severe deficiency, the arthroscope can be passed from the radiocarpal joint into the midcarpal joint through the expanded SL interval (Fig. 6.5-8).

LT Ligament

LT lesions are less common than SL lesions. They present similar features, but it is rare to find a complete deficiency with pronounced joint space widening. Associated lesions include lunate and triquetral cartilage damage and TFC lesions (see Fig. 5.14-3).

The LT ligament is difficult to evaluate with the arthroscope in the 3-4 portal, and therefore the scope should be moved to an ulnar portal (6R portal). A communication between the radiocarpal and midcarpal joints can also be demonstrated intraoperatively. This is done by passing a needle into the midcarpal joint and watching for outflow of fluid instilled into the radiocarpal joint. Another option is to carefully inject air into the midcarpal joint and watch for air bubbles entering the radiocarpal joint through the tear.

The midcarpal joint should be inspected in all cases of suspected LT pathology, because tears are easier to identify from the midcarpal side.

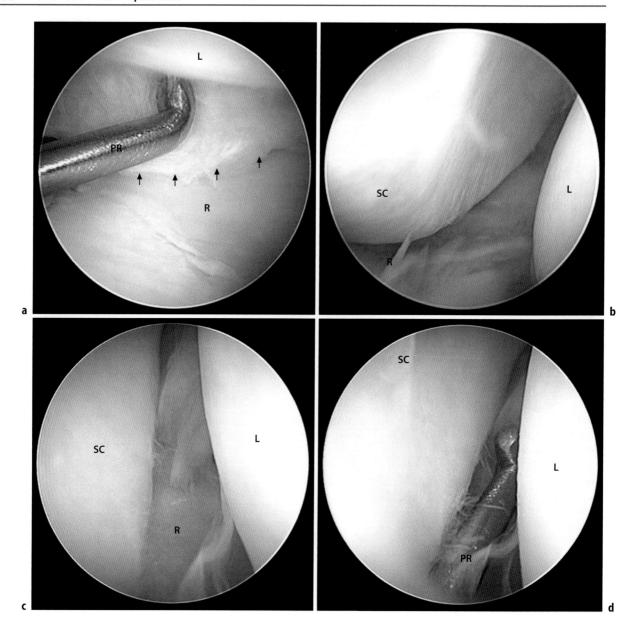

Fig. 6.5-8a–d. SL lesion. **a** The SL ligament (*arrows*) is palpated with the probe. The torn ligament extends down to the radial articular surface (*R*) (*L* lunate). **b** When the arthroscope is moved to the 3-4 portal and swept distally, the wide gap between the scaphoid (*SC*) and lunate (*L*) comes into view. **c** The lesion can be evaluated even more clearly from the mid-carpal joint by moving the arthroscope to the MCR portal. The radial articular surface (*R*) is visible in the deep portion of the field. **d** When the probe (*PR*) is passed through the 3-4 portal, it can be seen between the scaphoid and lunate

▶ **Note:** A cartilage lesion on the triquetrum or lunate, a TFCC lesion, or any positive ulnar variance should raise suspicion of an LT lesion.

Therapeutic Management

SL Ligament Lesions

The treatment of an SL lesion, which is the most common severe interosseous ligament injury, is still a matter of controversy. Authors have described ligament reconstructions, ligament repairs, dorsal capsulodesis, midcarpal fusions (scapholunate fusion, STT fusion), and temporary pinning with Kirschner wires. Cast immobilization is also an option, but only for acute lesions and only if the relative anatomic alignment of the carpal bones is corrected.

Bearing in mind that the prolonged immobilization of a joint leads to stiffness or ankylosis, immobilization is still appropriate for an acute SL lesion. Care should be taken, however, that the SL joint is immobilized in a position of perfect anatomic reduction. This led Whipple (1992) to advocate placing Kirschner wires across the SL interspace under arthroscopic control, followed by casting. He obtained better results in more recent injuries: K-wire pinning improved SL dissociation and reduced symptoms in 83% of patients whose instability was less than 3 months old and who had less than a 3-mm side-to-side difference in the scapholunate interval. By contrast, SL dissociation was improved and symptoms reduced in just 53% of patients whose instability was more than 3 months old and who had more than a 3-mm SL interval difference between the sides. Follow-up studies at 2–7 years showed that 85% of the patients in the first group had acceptable stability and no complaints.

In deciding among treatment options, one should consider not only the end result but also the complexity of the operation and the potential risks. Many patients with intercarpal fusions have unsatisfactory functional results with persistent pain and limitation of motion. Thus, this type of treatment is advised only in cases where all conservative options and arthroscopic measures have been unsuccessful.

Acute SL Lesion

- **Temporary pinning.** A Kirschner wire is placed across the SL joint space under arthroscopic and fluoroscopic control. The wire is removed at 8 weeks.

- **Conservative treatment with immobilization.** If the ligament shows only a partial tear with hemorrhagic changes and if widening of the SL interval is seen only in maximum radial and ulnar deviation, it is sufficient to immobilize the wrist (for 6 weeks) in the absence of severe associated injuries.

Chronic SL Lesion

- **Debridement of a deficient SL ligament, followed by immobilization.** This is appropriate if clinical symptoms are present but mild and the SL ligament is elongated.

- **Temporary pinning.** Temporary cross-pinning is appropriate for a complete tear or widened SL interval in a patient who is symptomatic. This treatment has a lower success rate than in acute tears, however.

It should be emphasized that a treatment of choice for these injuries does not yet exist. A technique should be chosen that combines low morbidity with the greatest possible efficacy.

LT Ligament Lesions

Because the LT ligament consists of three anatomic components, precise arthroscopic evaluation is of particular importance. The dorsal and volar components are firm and fibrous, while the central component is thin and membranous (Ostermann 1995).

Treatment options consist of immobilization, transosseous sutures, intercarpal fusion, and ligament reconstruction. Intercarpal fusions often result in significant limitation of motion and an altered pattern of wrist movements. Two arthroscopic treatment options are available:

- **Debridement.** Freshening the ligament to induce scarring is appropriate for acute partial tears after associated injuries have been excluded. After surgery the wrist is immobilized in a scaphoid splint for six weeks.

- **Temporary pinning.** The technique is the same as in the SL joint.

Associated injuries of the ulnocarpal ligaments or TFCC and cartilage lesions on adjacent bones should be excluded or treated as required.

Operative Technique

Debridement – Freshening the SL Ligament
(Fig. 6.5-9)

1. **Inspection.** The 3-4 portal can be used for viewing, but the very tight joint space limits visualization of the ligament, which is located just distal to the portal. The SL ligament can be viewed more clearly through the 6R portal (Fig. 6.5-9).

2. **Probing.** The arthroscope is in the 6R portal, the probe in the 3-4 portal. Ligament laxity is a common condition marked by an elongated SL ligament that can be pushed into the SL interval with the probe. With a ruptured ligament, torn fibers may be displaced into the joint and should be removed (Fig. 6.5-9). The lunate and scaphoid are pushed distally with the probe in alternating fashion. The ability to move the scaphoid and lunate in isolation ("piano-key" phenomenon) is typical of a ligament lesion. The superficial part of the ligament is carefully abraded with a small synovial resector to induce scarring. Meanwhile a synovectomy is performed on the dorsal capsule to further increase scarring. The ligament

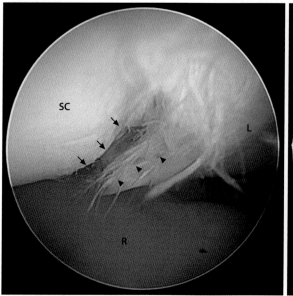 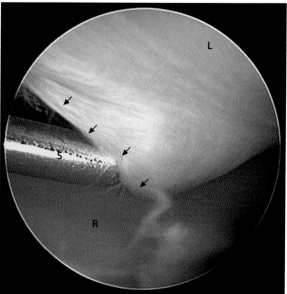

a

b

Fig. 6.5-9 a, b. Freshening the SL ligament. **a** Inspection through the 3-4 portal demonstrates the SL tear. The ligament (*arrowheads*) has been avulsed from its insertion on the scaphoid (*SC, arrows*) (*L* lunate, *R* radius). **b** After the arthroscope and instrument portals are switched, a shaver (*S*) is passed through the 3-4 portal, and the SL ligament (*arrows*) is freshened to induce scarring

can also be "pinned" by placing a Kirschner wire through the lunate and scaphoid. It is better to view and treat the ligament through the midcarpal joint, however.

3. **Associated lesions.** Associated lesions such as cartilage damage on the lunate or scaphoid and opposing radial articular surface and TFC lesions are also treated.

Postoperative care. The wrist is immobilized in a forearm splint for 6 weeks, followed by graded mobilization (physical therapy is indicated only in very unmotivated patients). Maximum flexion and extension should not be achieved for 3–4 months.

▶ **Note:** It is not the goal of physical therapy to achieve maximum wrist motion as soon as possible.

Temporary K-Wire Pinning
(Fig. 6.5-10)

1. **Inspection.** The tear site and SL joint space are arthroscopically inspected. In some patients with a complete SL tear or old deficiency, the arthroscope can be

advanced through the SL interspace to the midcarpal joint. When reactive synovitis is present, a partial synovectomy is necessary to evaluate the pathology.

2. **Probing.** The portals are switched to facilitate inspection and especially probing of the SL lesion (arthroscope in the 6R portal, instruments in the 3-4 portal). The scaphoid and lunate are probed to assess their mobility (piano-key phenomenon). Fibers that have slipped into the joint are debrided (see Fig. 6.5-9).

3. **Inspecting the SL joint from the midcarpal joint.** The SL interval is inspected through the MCR portal. With a complete tear or complex deficiency, the radiocarpal joint can also be viewed through this approach.

4. **Arthrodesis.** With the arthroscope still in the MCR portal, a Kirschner wire is drilled through the scaphoid and into the lunate under fluoroscopic control. Care is taken to protect the radial artery, which is very close to the radial surface of the scaphoid. With an acute tear of the SL ligament, it is sufficient to freshen the ligament and pin the bones in position with one or two carefully placed Kirschner wires. With a chronic ligament deficiency, two or three Kirschner wires should be used (Fig. 6.5-7).

▶ **Tip:** The joy-stick technique is helpful in cases where the scaphoid and lunate cannot be anatomically aligned. This is done by drilling K-wires into the scaphoid and lunate from the dorsal side and using the percutaneous wires like joy sticks to manipulate the bones into the desired position and hold them there before cross-pinning the joint space with another Kirschner wire.

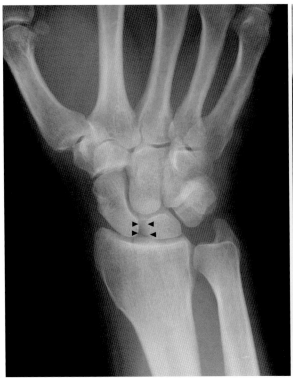 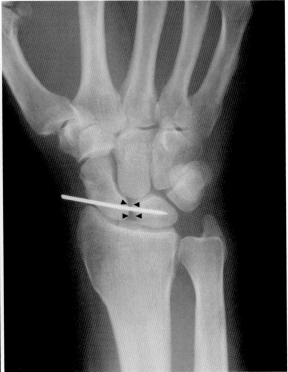

a   b

Fig. 6.5-10 a, b. Temporary pinning of the SL joint space. The patient, a 42-year-old man, presented with severe wrist pain 6 days after a fall onto the hand. **a** Widening of the SL interval (*arrowheads*) is consistent with an SL ligament tear. **b** Radiograph after Kirschner wire insertion shows narrowing of the SL interval

The Kirschner wire is buried beneath the skin, after first confirming the reduced position fluoroscopically in two planes. All K-wire joy sticks are removed.

Postoperative care. The wrist is immobilized in a forearm splint for 6 weeks. The Kirschner wires are removed at 8–9 weeks, and rehabilitation is begun. The goal is not to achieve immediate full range of motion but to increase wrist motion in gradual increments. The final range of motion should be achieved at about 4–5 months, or at about 6 months in patients with chronic instability. Forcible physical therapy to expedite functional recovery is contraindicated.

Temporary Pinning of the LT Joint

The technique is analogous to SL pinning but uses an ulnar-sided approach. The procedure is done under fluoroscopic control.

6.6 Hyperlaxity

Ligament hyperlaxity, while not classified as a ligament injury, is still a debilitating condition that frequently affects young patients.

Cause

The cause is constitutional ligamentous laxity or recurrent trauma.

Symptoms

The cardinal symptoms are pain, compromise of wrist function (in sports, on the job, or recreationally), and increased range of motion. Not infrequently, these symptoms are combined with chronic tenosynovitis and wrist ganglia.

Clinical Diagnosis

Common physical findings are diffuse tenderness and increased relative mobility of the carpal bones, with motion-dependent pain. The general impression is that of a "floppy" wrist, often with positive ligament tests (see Sect. 6.5).

Radiographs

No specific changes are found.

MRI

MRI is unrevealing in terms of specific signs. It may show incidental findings, but usually these cannot account for the hyperlax condition of the wrist.

Arthroscopic Findings

Arthroscopy may reveal a reactive synovitis with otherwise normal intraarticular findings. The intercarpal ligaments appear lax. The arthroscopic evaluation proceeds without difficulty, since the lax ligaments permit wide distraction of the joint spaces.

Therapeutic Management

Treatment should be carefully considered, weighing the potential risks against the pain and suffering of the patient. Many of these young patients, most of whom are women, are in considerable distress. The pain and disability are often sufficient to create a workplace hazard or prompt a change of occupation. Conservative treatments such as splinting and bracing are of only transient benefit. Occasionally patients are forced to consider early retirement, and some are suspected of feigning or exaggerating their symptoms for monetary gain.

Given the very significant pain and suffering that may occur, alternative treatment options must be considered. The goal is to stabilize the wrist without introducing new biomechanical parameters into the articular system as a whole.

In many patients who undergo a partial synovectomy or even diagnostic arthroscopy, a fibrotic reaction of the joint capsule occurs in response to the surgical trauma. Generally this reaction is not desired, but it can be beneficial in patients with hyperlax ligaments. We performed a partial synovectomy in 11 patients who had hyperlax ligaments and no apparent intraarticular pathology. When the initial results were evaluated after an average of 18 months, 8 of the patients showed marked improvement ranging to a complete absence of complaints. Four patients with an average history of 26 months were completely free of complaints and were able to return to work after several months of disability. Three of the patients experienced no improvement.

This basic concept (controlled capsular fibrosis by arthroscopy) should therefore be considered a valid treatment option in this patient group, although more precise scientific studies are still needed. The biological capacity of ligamentous and capsular tissue to scar and shorten (= shorter distance from origin to insertion) in response to an external stimulus is still given too little attention in the treatment of ligament instabilities. In the case of elongated ligaments and general ligamentous laxity, the possibilities of this concept are particularly intriguing. It is quite conceivable that a specific, surgeon-induced ligament lesion will produce effective tightening (shortening) of an elongated or partially deficient ligament. The means by which the lesion is induced, whether mechanically (shaver, rasp) or with a laser or electrocautery device, requires additional study. Tissue shrinkage is already being used in the knee and shoulder joints. It is reasonable to expect that many new discoveries will be made in this area during the next few years.

Operative Technique

Partial Synovectomy
See Sect. 6.1.

Postoperative Care

The wrist is immobilized postoperatively in a forearm splint for 5–6 weeks. It is then mobilized gradually, achieving full range of motion at 3–5 months.

6.7 Ulnocarpal Impingement Syndrome (UCIS)

Cause

UCIS results from increased pressure on the ulnar structures caused by a relative or absolute lengthening of the ulna. The ulnar head exerts a chronic pressure on the TFC, and the pressure is transmitted to the ulnar carpal bones (Fig. 6.7-1).

A relative or absolute lengthening of the ulna can have various causes:

- **Congenital positive ulnar variance**
- **Previous radial head resection**
- **Premature closure of the distal radial epiphysis**
- **Chronic overloading of the wrist**
- **Previous distal radial fracture**

The pathomechanical results of this length discrepancy are superficial TFC lesions (Palmer Class 2A and 2B) and large central disk tears, possibly accompanied by lunate and triquetral cartilage lesions. Tears of the LT ligament can also occur.

UCIS should be excluded whenever degenerative TFC lesions are found (see Sect. 6.3). Most patients are over 30 years of age and do not give a history of trauma.

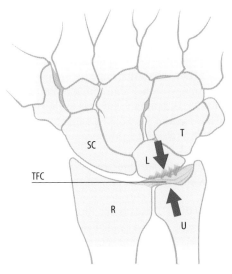

Fig. 6.7-1. Ulnocarpal impingement syndrome (UCIS). The ulnar head (*lower arrow*) exerts pressure on the TFC complex. The lunate (*L*) compresses the articular disk from the distal side (*upper arrow*) (*R* radius, *U* ulna, *SC* scaphoid, *T* triquetrum)

Symptoms

Patients typically present with ulnar-sided pain, swelling, painful limitation of motion, and occasional snapping on the ulnar side of the wrist. Locking (TFC lesions) may also occur.

Clinical Diagnosis

Areas of pain and tenderness are found in the ulnar portion of the wrist. The pain may be aggravated by axial loading of the TFC (ulnar deviation, pronation, supination) and by axial loading of the wrist. The LT ligament and SL ligament are also examined (see p. 789 for techniques).

The differential diagnosis includes distal radioulnar joint abnormalities (ulnar impingement syndrome, osteoarthritis, subluxation), tendinopathies of the extensor muscles or flexor carpi ulnaris, and pisiform or triquetral osteoarthritis.

Radiographs

Ulnar lengthening is relatively easy to detect on the PA film (Fig. 6.7-2). Contour irregularities and/or cystic changes in the ulnar head or ulnar circumference of the lunate provide indirect signs of increased pressure in the ulnocarpal joint. Radiographs should exclude distal radial deformity (e.g., secondary to a radial fracture) and subluxation of the distal radioulnar joint (lateral view).

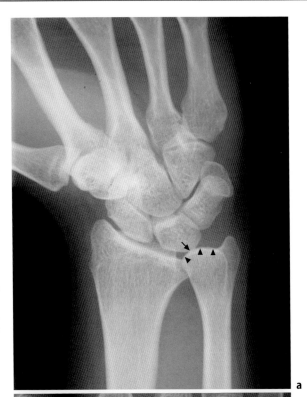

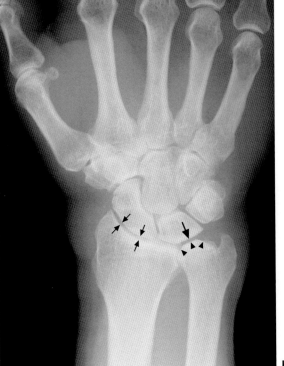

Fig. 6.7-2 a, b. Ulnocarpal impingement syndrome (UCIS). **a** The disk is literally crushed between the ulnar head (*arrowheads*) and lunate (*arrow*). **b** Note the flattening of the opposing surfaces of the ulnar head (*arrowheads*) and lunate (*arrow*) and increased subchondral sclerosis in chronic UCIS. The radiocarpal joint space is narrowed (*arrows*)

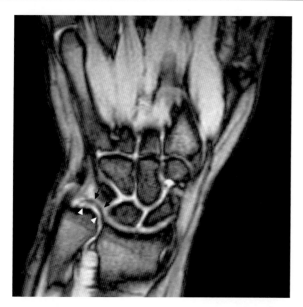

Fig. 6.7-3. MRI appearance of UCIS. The disk (*arrow*) is compressed from the proximal side by the elongated ulnar head (*arrowheads*) and from the distal side by the triquetrum (*arrows*) and lunate

MRI

Although MRI does not influence treatment planning when typical clinical and radiographic findings are present, it can vividly demonstrate the problems associated with UCIS and the compression of the disk tissue (Fig. 6.7-3).

Arthroscopic Findings

Arthroscopy is the only means of accurately evaluating the condition of the ulnocarpal joint. Superficial areas of TFC degeneration are found. Inspection of the distal radioulnar joint also shows degenerative wear on the undersurface of the TFC.

Advanced cases feature central TFC perforations of varying size, sometimes accompanied by cartilage damage on the lunate and less commonly on the triquetrum.

Therapeutic Management

Two important factors should be clarified before treatment is planned:

1. **The condition of the TFC.** If the TFC is intact, an arthroscopic wafer procedure will require the creation of a central TFC perforation. This is contraindicated, however, by the functional importance of the TFC. In

these cases we recommend superficial smoothing of the TFC (see p. 781), if necessary combined with a partial synovectomy in the ulnocarpal joint. If subsequent immobilization, supported by oral anti-inflammatory agents, does not improve the patient's complaints, an open ulnar shortening osteotomy should be considered. Another option is to shorten only the ulnar head via an arthrotomy while leaving the TFC intact.

2. **Primary or secondary ulnocarpal impingement syndrome.**

- **Secondary UCIS.** This is based on a relative lengthening of the ulna caused by changes in the radius, such as:
  - a distal radial fracture with marked dorsoradial angulation,
  - excision of the radial head, or
  - injury to the distal radial epiphysis (absolute radial shortening).

- **Primary UCIS.** This is caused by a lengthening of the ulna relative to the radius.

Treatment of the syndrome is directed by its cause (primary or secondary). With secondary UCIS, an arthroscopic wafer procedure is of limited benefit in the presence of a TFC lesion, because the root cause of the condition is radial deformity. An exception is a distal radial fracture that has healed in an anatomic position with shortening. This essentially preserves the anatomic relationships while producing an "absolute shortening" of the ulna.

If the TFC is intact in secondary UCIS, corrective bone surgery is advised (corrective osteotomy or shortening osteotomy). If pronounced degenerative changes are present in the distal radioulnar joint, arthroplastic measures or arthrodesis (Sauve-Kapandji operation) should be considered.

Shortening of the ulnar head is an established treatment for primary UCIS. Mechanical studies have shown that 18% of axial wrist loads are transmitted to the ulna. Lengthening the ulna by 2.5 mm increases this proportion to 42%, while shortening the ulna by 2.5 mm reduces it to just 4% of the total axial load (Palmer 1984). Thus, only a slight reduction in ulnar length can greatly reduce the pressure loads that are transmitted across the ulnocarpal joint.

Arthroscopic shortening of the ulnar head by 2–3 mm, utilizing an existing TFC lesion for gaining access to the ulnar head, is an effective and appropriate treatment.

Treatment should include associated lesions of the TFC (removing unstable areas) as well as cartilage lesions, which are most commonly found on the lunate.

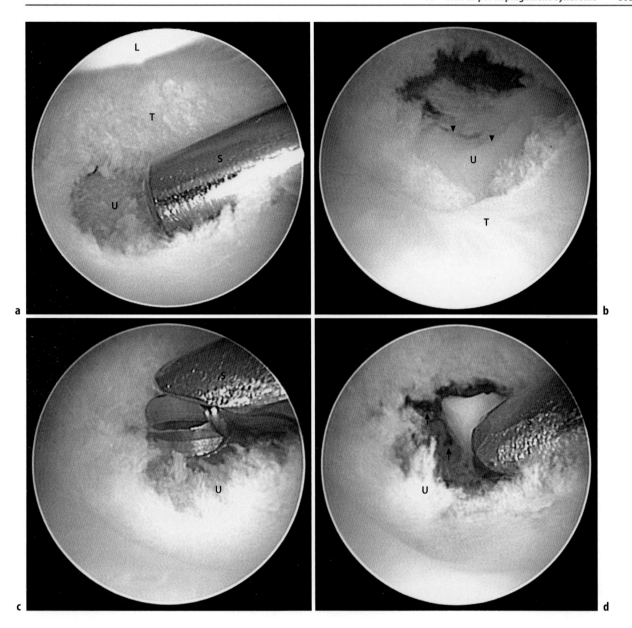

Operative Technique

Arthroscopic Wafer Procedure
(Figs. 6.7-4 and 6.7-5)

1. **Inspection.** When a large central TFC lesion is present, the cartilage on the ulnar head is visible through the tear. Anatomic identification can be difficult if the cartilage exactly fills the perforation, and an inexperienced surgeon may interpret it as an "intact TFC."

2. **Probing and removing unstable disk tissue.** The disk is probed through the 6R portal. Unstable portions of the TFC are resected (see Sect. 6.3, p. 781) (Fig. 6.7-4).

Fig. 6.7-4a–d. Arthroscopic wafer procedure in UCIS. **a** The articular cartilage is removed from the ulnar head (*U*) (*S* shaver, *T* TFC, *L* lunate). **b** The peripheral portions of the ulnar head (*U*) are demonstrated by pronation and supination (*arrowheads* extent of cartilage resection). **c** The ulnar head is shortened by 2–4 mm with a spherical bur (*S*). **d** Bleeding cancellous bone (*arrows*) in the ulnar head

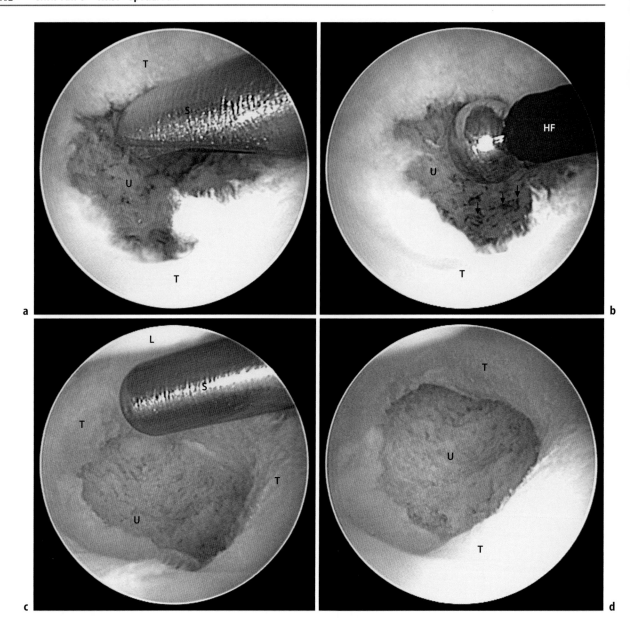

3. **Impingement testing.** Pronation and supination of the wrist will often show intrusion of the ulnar head into the radiocarpal joint. This test demonstrates the impaction mechanism.

▶ **Tip:** When evaluating the ulnocarpal joint arthroscopically, keep in mind that the joint is in a distracted condition. The normal state can be approximated by decreasing the distraction force. This limits vision but more clearly demonstrates the ulnar abutment. This technique is unnecessary, however, in patients with unequivocal clinical and radiographic findings.

Fig. 6.7-5a–d. Arthroscopic wafer procedure in UCIS (continued from Fig. 6.7-4). **a** The margins of the central disk tear are trimmed with a shaver (*S*) (*T* remaining peripheral TFC, *U* ulnar head). **b** Local bleeding sites are coagulated with a ball-tipped electrocautery probe (*HF*). **c** The free margin of the disk is smoothed (*L* lunate). **d** Final appearance of the shortened and smoothed ulnar head. All unstable TFC tissue has been removed

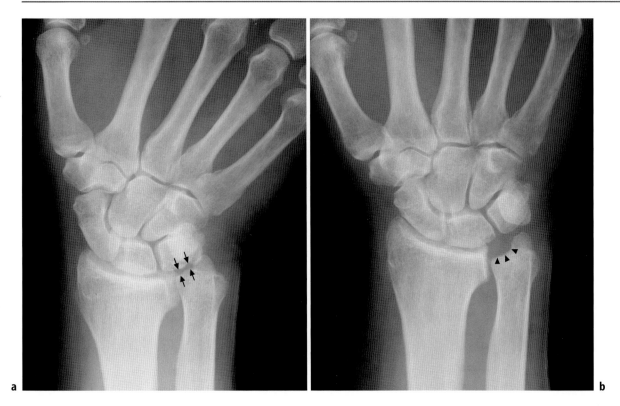

a   b

Fig. 6.7-6. a UCIS in a 39-year-old woman who sustained a distal radial fracture 5 years before. **b** Arthroscopic wafer resection of the distal ulna (*arrowheads*) has markedly widened the space between the lunate, triquetrum, and ulnar head

4. **Wafer resection.** A small round bur (round abrader from the small joint set) is used to remove the cartilage from the ulnar head (Fig. 6.7-4). Because the joint space is very narrow, the suction should be carefully adjusted; continuous suction could collapse the joint. When the accessible portions of the ulnar head cartilage have been removed, the wrist is supinated at the radioulnar joint. This brings into view the dorsal portions of the cartilage in the TFC defect, which are resected. Next the forearm is pronated for removing the cartilage on the volar side. Normally the ulnar head is shortened by 2–3 mm. A 3–3.5 mm wafer resection is recommended if advanced degenerative changes are present (massive fibrillation of the TFC, lunate cartilage lesions). The small probe is used to estimate the depth of the resection.

▶ **Caution:** Be sure to leave an adequate bony bridge connecting the ulnar styloid process to the ulna. Removing too much bone from the middle and ulnar thirds of the ulnar head can lead to intra- or postoperative avulsion of the styloid process, resulting in disintegration of the distal radioulnar joint.

When the wafer resection is completed, the resection site is smoothed with a fine rasp or bur. The site can be inspected by passing a small mirror or the arthroscope itself through the 6R portal.

Final smoothing of the shortened ulnar head is accomplished with a ball-tipped electrode, which also provides hemostasis (Fig. 6.7-5 b, c).

5. **Impingement testing.** The impingement test is repeated. No portion of the ulnar head should enter the TFC perforation. Doubts are resolved by decreasing the traction force and repeating pronation/supination of the wrist (Fig. 6.7-5 d).

Postoperative Care

The wrist is immobilized in a splint for 2–3 weeks postoperatively, followed by gradual mobilization by the patient. Vigorous physical therapy is contraindicated.

Postoperative radiographs are obtained to document the extent of the wafer resection (Fig. 6.7-6).

6.8 Fractures

Cause

A fall onto the hand.

Symptoms

Definite and equivocal fracture signs are present. The symptoms of scaphoid fractures range from an absence of complaints to severe pain.

Clinical Diagnosis

In patients with acute trauma and severe pain, a detailed workup is performed (if necessary) after radiographs have been obtained.

Radiographs

Distal radial fracture. The AP film is useful for defining the fracture pattern. Displacement is usually present and is evident on clinical examination. The fracture pattern and number of fragments are determined. Doubts can be resolved by additional imaging studies such as CT or MRI plus oblique radiographic views.

Avulsion of the ulnar styloid process. This is frequently but not always associated with a distal radial fracture.

Scaphoid fracture. The fracture line is not always defined on initial radiographs. If the history and clinical examination raise suspicion of a scaphoid fracture but a definite fracture line is not seen, the arm should be immobilized for 7 days. Repeat radiographs at this time will usually demonstrate the fracture line. MRI is helpful in doubtful cases, after first obtaining a Stecher projection of the scaphoid.

MRI

MRI can be helpful if radiographs are unrevealing.

Arthroscopic Findings

Arthroscopy will demonstrate the fracture lines along with ligamentous injuries and chondral flake fractures. The intraarticular findings are usually more severe than X-rays would suggest.

Therapeutic Management

Whether a fracture is amenable to arthroscopic stabilization depends basically on the fracture type and the surgeon's experience.

Because arthroscopic fracture treatment is still in its early stages and wrist fractures vary greatly in their extent, pattern, and associated injuries, a specific operative technique cannot be recommended at this time. In principle, the fractures could be stabilized with the Whipple modification of the Herbert screw (Herbert-Whipple screw). Because the screw is cannulated, it is inserted over a preplaced Kirschner wire that holds the fracture in the reduced position. Reduction can be aided by using percutaneous dorsal Kirschner wires as joy sticks to manipulate the fragments into position. Besides the modified Herbert screw, Kirschner wires or small cannulated screws can be used to stabilize distal radial fractures (e.g., fix an isolated avulsion of the radial styloid process).

More specific data will become available during the next few years as researchers review large series of patients whose fractures have been treated by internal fixation under arthroscopic control.

6.9 Scarring and Arthrofibrosis

Cause

Trauma, fractures, intraarticular hemorrhage, or prolonged immobilization after an injury.

Symptoms

The dominant features are limited motion and pain.

Clinical Diagnosis

The wrist is examined for areas of tenderness and for range of motion. Associated injuries (TFC, LT ligament, SL ligament) should be excluded.

Radiographs

Associated injuries determine the radiographic findings. There are no typical signs of intraarticular scarring and adhesions.

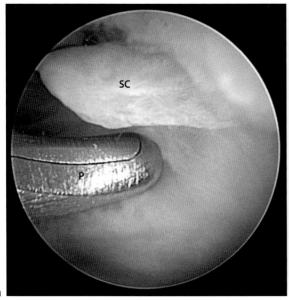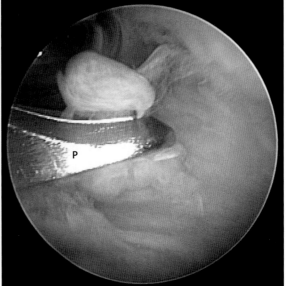

a   b

MRI

MRI is rewarding only if generalized arthrofibrosis is present.

Arthroscopic Findings

Findings range from isolated adhesions and scar plaques that partly or completely subdivide the radiocarpal joint to complete arthrofibrosis (Fig. 6.9-1).

Therapeutic Management

Resection or division of the scar tissue is the treatment of choice in patients with load-dependent pain and normal-appearing radiographs. There are no other therapeutic options. Conservative measures (physical therapy, braces, immobilization, etc.) are of no benefit.

Operative Technique
(Figs. 6.9-1 and 6.9-2)

1. **Arthroscope portal.** Intraarticular scarring can significantly reduce the capacity of the joint, allowing only 1–2 mL of fluid to be injected during joint distention. The joint space may be compartmentalized by scar plaques or largely obliterated by scar tissue. The surgeon should proceed very carefully when introducing the sheath. Adequate muscular relaxation and optimum distraction should be provided.

Fig. 6.9-1 a, b. Lysis of adhesions in the radiocarpal joint. A scar-tissue band (*SC*) (**a**) is resected with a punch (*P*) (**b**)

2. **Inspection.** The areas of intraarticular scarring are inspected. If scar tissue subdivides the joint into multiple compartments, it will be difficult to establish an instrument portal. It may be necessary to use a different portal site (e.g., the 4-5 portal), but it is better to insert a trial needle at the 6R site and try to reach the arthroscope tip with the tip of the needle. If this is possible, the 6R portal is carefully established.
▶ **Caution:** Avoid iatrogenic injury to the TFC.

3. **Lysis of adhesions.** Individual adhesive bands or scar plaques are divided with a small basket forceps or shaver (Fig. 6.9-2). Another option is to use a small cautery knife (with small hook electrode). Diffuse scar tissue can be resected with the shaver. Sometimes it is helpful to cut the scar tissue into smaller fragments with a basket forceps or cautery knife for piecemeal removal.

4. **Range of motion testing.** After all adhesions have been lysed, the range of wrist motion is tested and documented. Any associated injuries (TFC lesion, chondral lesions, loose bodies) are identified and treated in the same sitting.

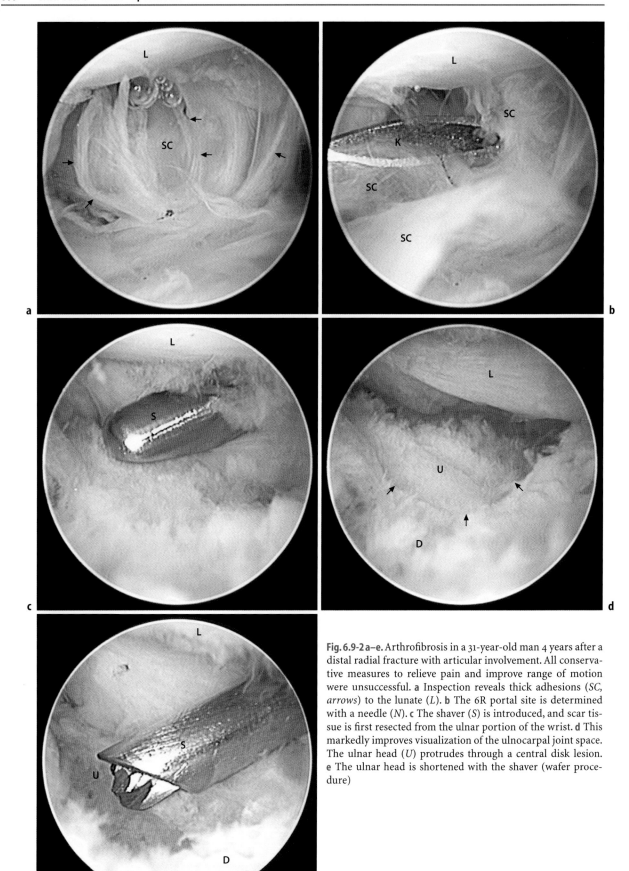

Fig. 6.9-2 a–e. Arthrofibrosis in a 31-year-old man 4 years after a distal radial fracture with articular involvement. All conservative measures to relieve pain and improve range of motion were unsuccessful. **a** Inspection reveals thick adhesions (*SC, arrows*) to the lunate (*L*). **b** The 6R portal site is determined with a needle (*N*). **c** The shaver (*S*) is introduced, and scar tissue is first resected from the ulnar portion of the wrist. **d** This markedly improves visualization of the ulnocarpal joint space. The ulnar head (*U*) protrudes through a central disk lesion. **e** The ulnar head is shortened with the shaver (wafer procedure)

Postoperative Care

Gentle therapeutic exercises are started on the first post-operative day. All exercises are kept strictly below the pain threshold. Forcible, painful exercises predispose to reflex sympathetic dystrophy.

▶ **Note:** The success of arthroscopic lysis is not measured by range of motion alone. The primary goal is to reduce pain; motion improvement is a secondary concern.

6.10 Ganglia

The wrist is the most common site of occurrence of ganglia. Most of these lesions (60%–70%) involve the dorsal, medial portion of the wrist.

Cause

Despite numerous studies, the causes of wrist ganglia are not fully understood. A communication with the joint space is often postulated and confirmed by injection techniques. A valve mechanism has also been suggested, analogous to Baker cysts in the knee. Acute or chronic loads on the scapholunate joint space have been implicated as the cause of dorsal wrist ganglia. It has also been suggested that volar ganglia are caused by loads acting chiefly on the scaphotrapezial-trapezoid (STT) joint (Angelides 1988). The trauma theory of ganglia is supported by the fact that 10% to 50% of patients give a history of wrist trauma. Thus, the development of wrist ganglia is considered a manifestation of carpal instability. This led Watson (1989) to advocate a selective examination of the ligaments in patients whose complaints persist following excision.

Angelides (1988) found that dorsal ganglia originated from the SL ligament and claimed that without surgical removal of the ganglion attachment to the ligament, 30% to 80% of these lesions would recur.

Symptoms

The complaints are determined by the structures that are close to the ganglion and are compressed by it. The symptoms also depend strongly on the size of the ganglion, which may develop swiftly or gradually. Pain and cosmetic deformity are the principal complaints. Very small ganglia can lead to severe pain.

Clinical Diagnosis

The size of the ganglion is assessed along with its mobility relative to adjacent structures. Associated lesions are excluded (instability, nerve compression). The dorsal wrist ganglion is most easily palpated in a position of volar flexion.

Radiographs

The radiographic findings are determined by associated lesions (e.g., widening of the SL interval).

MRI

MRI can show evidence of associated injuries but is rarely necessary.

Arthroscopic Findings

Arthroscopy shows a localized bulging of the joint capsule into the joint. Ostermann (1995) described finding a bead-like structure arising from the dorsal part of the SL ligament and representing the origin of a ganglion. Accompanying the ganglion was a reactive synovitis.

Ganglia can be arthroscopically visualized through an ulnar approach.

Fifty percent of the patients in Ostermann's series had associated intraarticular lesions such as SL ligament tears, TFCC tears, and radial and triquetral cartilage lesions.

Therapeutic Management

An important consideration in treatment planning is that 20%–50% of wrist ganglia spontaneously recur. Simple needle aspiration, with or without cortisone injection, has a success rate of about 35%–50% (Ostermann 1995). The open excision of a ganglion may lead to motion loss if the wrist is immobilized for a prolonged period, and the recurrence rate is up to 40% or more. An essential part of surgical treatment is to excise the attachment or root of the ganglion on the SL ligament or dorsal capsule. Thus, open surgery leaves a capsular defect of 10–15 mm that must be treated and requires postoperative immobilization of the wrist.

Initially, surgeons did not consider arthroscopy for the treatment of ganglia. In 1987, Ostermann treated a woman for a TFC lesion that was accompanied by an asymptomatic wrist ganglion. The patient asked the surgeon if her dorsal wrist ganglion could also be treated during the arthroscopic treatment of the TFC lesion. The ganglion was opened during creation of the 3-4 portal and apparently drained into the joint. The lesion did not recur. This observation has directed attention toward arthroscopy as a modality for the treatment of wrist ganglia.

Arthroscopic treatment involves removing the origin of the ganglion from the SL ligament and releasing it from its attachment to the dorsal capsule.

Given the high incidence of concomitant lesions (50%), ganglia and especially recurrent ganglia should prompt a detailed workup that includes arthroscopic inspection and any necessary treatment (ganglion drainage, excision of the ganglion origin).

Operative Technique

1. **Inspection.** For a dorsal ganglion, the arthroscope is introduced through an ulnar portal (6R portal). The dorsal capsule in the area of the 3-4 portal, which is opposite the SL ligament, is inspected first. The base of the ganglion appears as a bead-like structure arising from the SL ligament. Associated lesions, such as an SL ligament tear and cartilage damage, are also identified.

2. **Creation of the 3–4 portal.** A needle is advanced through the ganglion at the 3-4 portal site until it appears within the joint. After making the skin incision and spreading the subcutaneous tissue, the surgeon passes a small synovial resector through the 3-4 portal to the base of the ganglion. The ganglion base and portions of the dorsal capsule attached to the SL ligament are arthroscopically resected.

▶ **Caution:** Avoid injury to the extensor tendons that directly overlie the capsule.

Following the capsular resection, the extensor pollicis longus or extensor digitorum communis tendons can be seen.

3. **Arthroscopy of the midcarpal joint.** The midcarpal joint is also scrutinized for ganglion-like lesions in the area of the SL ligament.

Postoperative Care

A forearm splint is worn for 1–2 weeks after surgery.

PART IV

Elbow Joint

CHAPTER 7

Elbow Joint – General Part

7.1 Historical Development

As early as 1931, Michael Burman described arthroscopic examination of the elbow joint in cadavers using a 3-mm telescope. He concluded, however, that the elbow was poorly suited for arthroscopic examination and that it was not possible to establish access portals to the anterior compartment of the joint. This became possible, however, when Watanabe (1971) and others succeeded in developing smaller optical systems.

In 1978, Johnson reported on the first successful arthroscopic examinations in patients. He described the portal sites and the intraarticular structures that could be seen. He was able to visualize the humeral capitellum, the radial head, and the ulnar portion of the elbow with the coronoid process. He also identified intraarticular fractures not seen on radiographs, degenerative changes, intraarticular loose bodies, and changes in the humeroradial joint due to lateral epicondylitis (cartilage lesions on the radial head with accompanying synovitis).

Since 1985, arthroscopic surgery of the elbow joint has become more widely practiced. While Andrews reported on 24 patients in 1985, Watanabe described his experience with 201 patients in the same year. By 1994, Hempfling had performed elbow arthroscopy in 339 patients.

7.2 Instrumentation (Arthroscopy System)

As in other joints, a standard 4-mm 30° wide-angle arthroscope can be used. We recommended a shortened barrel to facilitate handling and permit the more accurate visualization of pathologic findings. This shortened version of the 4-mm arthroscope is also used in the ankle joint (see Sect. 3.2, Fig. 3.2-1).

When elbow arthroscopy is performed in the prone position (see below), care is taken to provide a sufficiently long light cord.

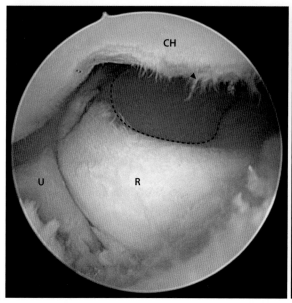
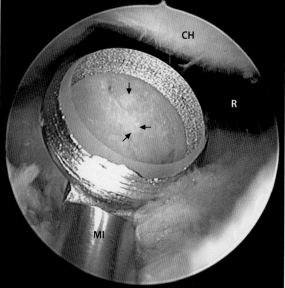

a   b

7.3 Video System

The arthroscopic video system must satisfy the same requirements as in other joints (see Sect. 1.3).

7.4 Probe

As in other joints, the surgeon uses the probe as a "palpating finger" in the elbow joint (see Sect. 1.4 for details).

7.5 Mirror

A mirror is a helpful tool in elbow arthroscopy. It has proven especially useful for the following applications:

- **Inspection of the capitellum.** A mirror is passed through a low posterolateral portal to inspect chondral lesions on the capitellum (Fig. 7.5-1).

- **Inspection of the olecranon.** A mirror is used to inspect the olecranon and evaluate degenerative spurs on the olecranon tip during elbow flexion and extension. The mirror is inserted through the posterocentral portal.

- **Loose body removal.** When multiple loose bodies are removed, some of the fragments may slip into areas where there is very little fluid turbulence. A loose body that slips under the sheath and toward the camera cannot be seen arthroscopically. In this case a mirror can be passed through the opposite portal to look for "strays" (see Fig. 8.3-4).

Fig. 7.5-1 a, b. Use of a mirror in the elbow joint. **a** Only a small portion of the humeral capitellum (*CH*) can be viewed directly. Note the superficial fibrillated cartilage lesions (*arrowheads*) and the large cartilage defect (*dashed line*) on the radial head (*R*) (*U* ulna). **b** A mirror (*MI*) passed through a low posterolateral portal shows more of the capitellum and reveals deep cartilage lesions with exposed bone areas (*arrows*)

7.6 Operating Instruments

7.6.1 Mechanical Instruments

Elbow arthroscopy requires the same mechanical instruments that are used in other joints (see Sect. 1.6.1). Basket forceps are used essentially for dividing intraarticular scar tissue. A small grasping forceps and small basket forceps are needed to retrieve small loose bodies that slip into tight spaces (see Sect. 5.6.1, Fig. 5.6-1).

A standard Kocher clamp and large grasping forceps should be available for extracting large loose bodies.

7.6.2 Motorized Instruments (Shaver)

The shaver is very useful in the elbow joint (see Sect. 1.6.2). Because of the tightly confined spaces and thin joint capsule, small blades from the small-joint set should be used (see Sect. 5.6.2, Fig. 5.6-2). Large blades like those used in the knee joint can be difficult to handle in the elbow, and larger access portals are required.

7.6.3 Electrosurgical Instruments

Electrocautery is useful for dividing adhesive bands in the elbow and for local hemostasis (see Sect. 1.6.3).

7.6.4 Lasers

There are situations in which laser ablation is a useful option for osteophytes in the elbow. Some osteophytes occur in hard-to-reach joint areas that require the use of a small, high-precision ablation device.

7.6.5 Switching Sticks

In contrast to other joints, two switching sticks are an absolute necessity for interchanging the instrument and viewing portals in elbow arthroscopy.

7.7 Anesthesia

General anesthesia or regional techniques (plexus block, i.v. regional anesthesia) can be used. General anesthesia is preferred for two reasons: (1) optimum muscular relaxation is helpful in achieving joint distraction, and (2) the prone position, which is standard for elbow arthroscopy, is easier to tolerate when the patient is asleep.

7.8 Positioning

Two positioning options are available:

1. **Supine position.** The shoulder is abducted 90° with the elbow flexed 90°. The hand is connected through finger traps or an elastic bandage to an overhead traction device like that used in shoulder arthroscopy (Fig. 7.8-1). Usually a counterweight is attached to the upper arm.

▶ **Disadvantages**
- **Difficult access to posterior joint areas**
- **Difficulty with distraction;** an assistant must set up the arm holder or apply manual distraction
- **Difficult to adjust the traction force**
- **Difficult to adjust the flexion angle** (but necessary in many operations)
- **Risk of traction injury to the hand and fingers**
- **Elbow suspended in an unstable position** (can "swing back and forth")

2. **Prone position.** The patient is positioned face down

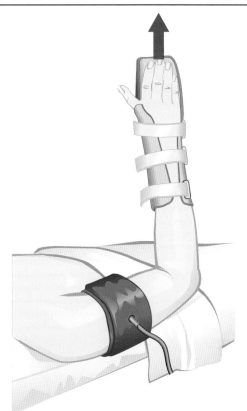

Fig. 7.8-1. Supine position with an overhead traction device. The hand and forearm are fixed in a holder

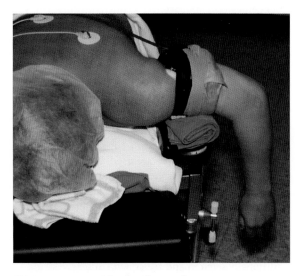

Fig. 7.8-2. Prone position for elbow arthroscopy

with the shoulder abducted 90° and the upper arm resting on a well-padded support on the side of the operating table (Fig. 7.8-2).

▶ **Caution:** It is essential to avoid neurovascular pressure injuries in the upper arm.

▶ The prone position offers several advantages:
- **Ease of access to posterior joint areas**
- **Good distraction provided by the intrinsic weight of the forearm** (no traction device on the hand)
- **Ease of adjusting flexion and extension**
- **Stable position for arthroscopy** (no "swinging elbow")
- **Easy access for draping**

One disadvantage is the necessity of moving the anesthetized patient to the prone position. The anesthesiologist must consider this when selecting the endotracheal tube (flexible tube).

With its preponderance of advantages, the prone position has become the standard position for elbow arthroscopy.

7.9 Tourniquet

When the anesthetized patient has been moved to the prone position, the arm is exsanguinated by wrapping it with an Esmarch bandage and inflating the pneumatic tourniquet on the upper arm (250–300 mm Hg). A lower pressure should be used in frail patients.

7.10 Draping

Following sterile preparation of the hand, forearm, and elbow region, the elbow is extended with the upper arm abducted and a surgical drape is wrapped around the elbow and secured on the posterior side of the upper arm.

▶ **Caution:** Avoid skin injury.

Next the patient is completely covered posteriorly with towel drapes. Since elbow arthroscopy employs fluid distention, waterproof drapes are used. The hand and distal half of the forearm are wrapped in a waterproof drape, and all drapes are secured with adhesive tape. Next a waterproof extremity sheet (like that used in knee arthroscopy) is placed over the forearm and pulled toward the upper arm until just above the elbow joint. If the upper arm is thin, the aperture in the sheet should be additionally secured and sealed with adhesive strips.

7.11 Distension Medium

Since electrocautery will be used, the joint is distended with a nonelectrolytic medium. A different solution (Ringer's lactate) is acceptable if it is certain that electrocautery will not be used. In the elbow as in other joints, gas distention is not commonly used.

7.12 Setup and Preparations for Arthroscopy

The surgeon sits in front of the elbow, with the arthroscopy cart on the opposite side of the table. This setup requires adequate cable lengths (shaver cable, light cord), especially when operating on an obese patient. The scrub nurse stands next to the instrument table toward the foot end of the operating table.

7.13 Portal Placement

7.13.1 Anatomic Landmarks

Since many neurovascular structures run anterior and posterior to the elbow joint, accurate positioning of the portals is essential to avoid neurovascular complications. The first step is to palpate and identify the anatomic landmarks on which the portal sites are based.

First the landmarks are palpated while the patient is awake. The lateral and medial epicondyles and the olecranon are palpable even in obese patients. Palpation of the radial head is more difficult in these patients but is facilitated by alternately pronating and supinating the forearm. The sulcus for the ulnar nerve is also palpated and evaluated for scars from any previous operations. Particular attention is given to scars in the ulnar region of the elbow, as they may signify a previous ulnar nerve transposition procedure. If doubt exists, the patient can be asked specifically about this type of surgery.

Palpation of the elbow is repeated after the patient has been positioned and draped and before the portals are established. Key anatomic landmarks should be outlined on the skin with a marker.

7.13.2 Anterior Portals

Anterior portals are necessary to gain access to the anterior compartment. Two standard anterior portals are available: anterolateral and anteromedial. A high anterolateral portal (superomedial portal) has also been described.

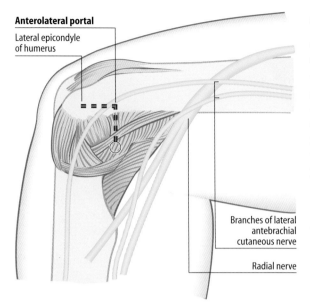

Fig. 7.13-1. Location of the anterolateral portal (lateral view)

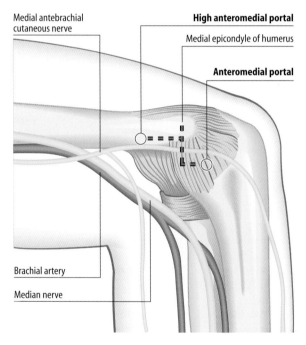

Fig. 7.13-2. Location of the anteromedial and high anteromedial portals (medial view)

Anterolateral Portal

This portal serves as the primary arthroscope portal. The key landmark is the palpable lateral epicondyle of the humerus. The portal is placed 2 cm distal and 2 cm anterior to the epicondyle (Fig. 7.13-1). The radial head can be palpated slightly posterior and distal to the lateral epicondyle during pronation and supination of the forearm. The anterolateral portal often passes through the extensor carpi radialis brevis muscle. Care is taken to protect the radial nerve, which runs an average of 4 mm anterior to this portal when the elbow is not distended. Distention increases this distance to an average of 11 mm, and therefore the radial nerve is at minimal risk when the joint is adequately distended. The posterior antebrachial cutaneous nerve and its side branches are subcutaneous and at risk.

Anteromedial Portal

This portal is created under arthroscopic control and is used for instrumentation (see Instrument Portal, Sect. 7.13.6). It is placed 2 cm anterior and 2 cm distal to the palpable medial epicondyle of the humerus (Fig. 7.13-2). The medial antebrachial cutaneous nerve is at risk. The portal also traverses parts of the flexor carpi radialis and flexor digitorum superficialis muscles. Deeper structures at risk are the median nerve and brachial artery. Luensch et al. (1986) found that the neurovascular bundle was located between 4 and 6 mm from the anteromedial portal in the undistended joint. The median nerve was 3–10 mm from the portal, the brachial artery 8–13 mm. When the joint is distended, however, the neurovascular bundle is located more than 10 mm from the anteromedial portal. It should be noted that placing the portal too close to the humerus significantly limits the maneuverability of the arthroscope and instruments (Fig. 7.13-3).

High Anteromedial Portal

Lindenfeld (1990) described this portal, which is located 1 cm proximal and 1 cm anterior to the medial epicondyle (see Fig. 7.13-2). The portal is anterior to the medial intermuscular septum and does not jeopardize the ulnar nerve. Lindenfeld found that the average distance of the median nerve from the portal was 22 mm when the elbow was distended. The brachial artery is also located a safe distance away (approximately 20 mm).

The most accurate technique for creating the high anteromedial portal is to use a percutaneous needle to locate the optimum portal site under arthroscopic control.

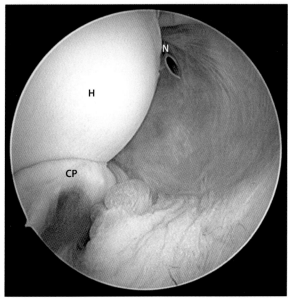
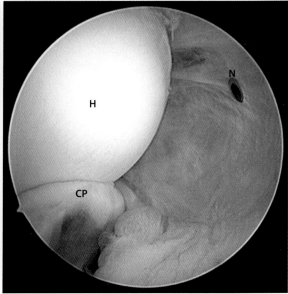

a   b

Fig. 7.13-3 a, b. Determining the location of the anteromedial portal with a trial needle. **a** If the needle (*N*) is introduced just anterior to the humeral anterior surface (*H*), it will be deflected toward the anterior capsule. The same will happen with instruments inserted at that site (*CP* coronoid process). **b** The portal should be placed far enough anteriorly to ensure adequate instrument clearance

7.13.3 Posterior Portals

Four portals are available for accessing the posterior compartment of the elbow:

- Low posterolateral portal
- High posterolateral portal
- Posterocentral portal
- High posteromedial portal

Low Posterolateral Portal (Distal Posterolateral Portal)

This portal is located at a palpable soft spot in the triangle between the radial head, olecranon, and medial epicondyle (Fig. 7.13-4). It is strongly recommended that this portal, whether used for instrumentation or viewing, be established under arthroscopic control. It initially provides needle access for joint distention before the arthroscope portal is created.

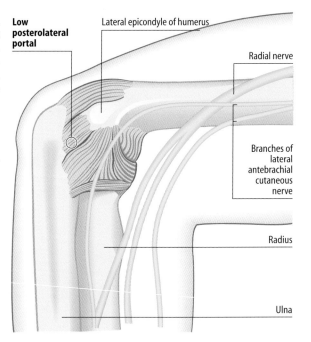

Fig. 7.13-4. Location of the low posterolateral portal (posterolateral view)

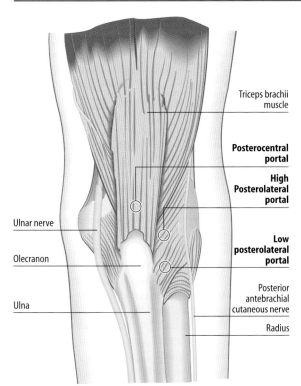

Fig. 7.13-5. Location of the high posterolateral and posterocentral portals (posterior view)

Labels on figure:
Triceps brachii muscle
Posterocentral portal
High Posterolateral portal
Low posterolateral portal
Ulnar nerve
Olecranon
Ulna
Posterior antebrachial cutaneous nerve
Radius

High Posterolateral Portal (Proximal Posterolateral Portal)

This portal is placed at the level of the olecranon tip, radial to the triceps tendon (Fig. 7.13-5). It is the primary arthroscope portal for viewing the posterior compartment.

▶ **Note:** If the high posterolateral portal is placed more than 10 mm proximal to the olecranon tip, it will be difficult later to advance the arthroscope distally toward the proximal radioulnar joint. If the portal is placed more than 5 mm distal to the olecranon tip, it cannot be used for viewing the posteromedial recess.

Posterocentral Portal

This portal is placed directly through the triceps tendon about 1 cm proximal to the olecranon tip (see Fig. 7.13-5). It is analogous to the transtendinous portal in the knee (Gillquist portal, see Sect. 1.13.1.2) and the transtendinous portal for accessing the posterior ankle joint (see p. 679).

Posteromedial Portal

The posteromedial portal is placed on the ulnar side of the triceps tendon and olecranon. Though it is described in the Anglo-American literature, we do not use this portal and consider it obsolete. It offers no significant advantages and carries an exorbitant risk of ulnar nerve injury.

7.13.4 Portal Principles

The elbow is a relatively small joint whose capsule is located relatively far from the skin surface, depending on the thickness of the subcutaneous tissue layer. Additionally, the anterior and posterior compartments are equivalent in their diagnostic and therapeutic importance, and each may harbor an equal number of lesions that require arthroscopic treatment.

▶ **Note:** Simple inspection of the anterior compartment is completely inadequate.

The surgeon must consider these circumstances when carrying out the tactical aspects of the operation, i.e., creating the instrument portals and treating the lesions. Many authors favor a set routine for elbow arthroscopy that starts with joint distention and the creation of an arthroscope portal. The anterolateral portal is usually recommended. If the scope is inadvertently retracted into the subcutaneous tissue during inspection or because of technical problems (e.g., adhesions), the subcutaneous tissue will become distended with fluid. When adhesions are present, the surgeon may be unable to determine whether the tip of the scope is embedded in scar tissue or has already exited the joint. If it has left the joint, often the sheath cannot be reinserted to reestablish entry. Forcible insertion is very risky:

- **Risk of second capsule perforation.** When the joint is reentered, fluid will leak through the first capsule opening, and the extravasation can hamper the rest of the procedure.
- **Risk of capsular fibrosis.**
- **Increased risk of synovial fistulae.**

If the joint cannot be reentered, it is first necessary to redistend the joint with fluid.

Another problem arises when it becomes necessary to move the arthroscope and instruments to posterior portals after two anterior portals have already been established. Extravasation occurs through the existing portals, causing loss of joint distention and making it risky or even impossible to insert the sheath into a posterior portal.

▶ **Tip:** Always have a portal available for accessing the anterior and posterior compartments, regardless of which compartment you are working in.

If the surgeon retracts the arthroscope out the front of the joint or is having visualization problems, the joint should be continuously distended through an inflow cannula in the posterior portal. If the arthroscope is retracted out the back of the elbow, the inflow should be placed in an anterior portal.

▶ **Note:** Having an "inflow portal" in a non-instrumented compartment provides a safety reserve and is particularly advantageous when problems arise.

7.13.5 Creating the Arthroscope Portal: Technique

A standard routine is followed in creating the arthroscope portal:

1. **Marking the anatomic landmarks.** The olecranon, the lateral and medial epicondyles, and if possible the radial head are palpated and marked on the skin with a sterile marker.

2. **Needle test.** First a needle is inserted at the prospective site of the low posterolateral portal (soft spot). When the needle has entered the joint, it is easily moved in the lateral and medial directions (Fig. 7.13-6).

3. **Distending the joint.** Sometimes it is remarkable how much fluid the elbow joint can hold. In some cases 40–50 mL is sufficient to fully distend the joint (Fig. 7.13-7). After the first 10 mL has been injected, the syringe is detached from the needle to check for backflow. Fluid backflow from the needle hub confirms that the needle has entered the joint. Complete joint distention is manifested by a marked bulging of the posterior joint spaces, creating a "horseshoe-shaped" prominence around the olecranon. When the joint is fully distended, the needle is withdrawn while pressure is kept on the plunger. Fluid outflow through the needle should be avoided, as it compromises joint distention.

4. **High posterolateral portal (inflow portal).** An "inflow portal" is established before the arthroscope portal is created. The high posterolateral portal is recommended for inflow, as it can be established quickly and safely.

- **Skin incision.** A longitudinal skin incision about 4–5 mm long is made just proximal and radial to the olecranon tip. Only the skin is incised.

- **Spreading the subcutaneous tissue.** The subcutaneous tissue, fascial and distal portions of the triceps muscle are spread with a clamp.

▶ **Tip:** Do not enter the joint with the clamp at this time, as this would cause sudden fluid outflow with loss of joint distention.

- **Inserting the inflow cannula.** A large-bore cannula (5 mm in diameter) with a blunt obturator is inserted into the olecranon fossa. This should be done at a relatively steep angle, since the olecranon fossa is located lower than one might suppose. Thus, the inflow cannula should be advanced in the direction of the distal humeral shaft. A more tangential insertion angle would cause the cannula to enter the distal portion of the triceps brachii muscle.
Loss of resistance is felt when the cannula enters the joint. The obturator is carefully loosened, and the high intraarticular pressure will tend to push it out of the cannula. If this "pushing" effect is not felt, the insertion direction and position of the inflow cannula should be rechecked, as it may have not yet entered the olecranon fossa.
A coupler is used to connect the fluid inflow line to the inflow cannula. This ensures that constant, adequate joint distention will be maintained throughout the procedure.

5. **Anterolateral portal.** Again, it is helpful to follow a set routine in creating this portal.

- **Needle test.** A needle is inserted approximately 2 cm anterior and 2 cm distal to the lateral epicondyle of the humerus (Fig. 7.13-8). Fluid outflow confirms adequate distention of the anterior compartment. Anterior scarring can significantly reduce joint distention, and the needle test will safely exclude inadequate distention of the anterior compartment. The needle should be advanced in the direction of the medial epicondyle. A more tangential angle will hit the anterior capsule too far on the ulnar side, making it difficult to insert the sheath.

- **Skin incision.** An incision 4–5 mm long is made through the skin only.

- **Spreading the subcutaneous tissue.** The subcutaneous tissue and muscle are carefully spread open with a fine, blunt clamp (Fig. 7.13-9). The clamp should not yet pierce the capsule.

- **Inserting the sheath.** With a spigot open and the blunt obturator in place, the sheath is inserted into the joint (Fig. 7.13-10). The tip of the sheath is directed toward the medial epicondyle. If inserted at too flat an angle, the sheath will be deflected anteriorly by the capsule,

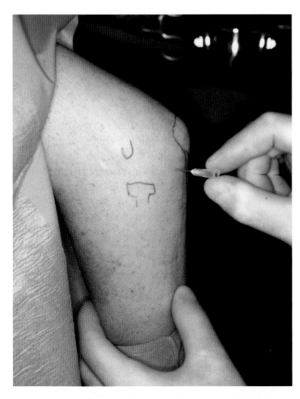

Fig. 7.13-6. Needle test. The needle is inserted into the low posterolateral portal prior to joint distention

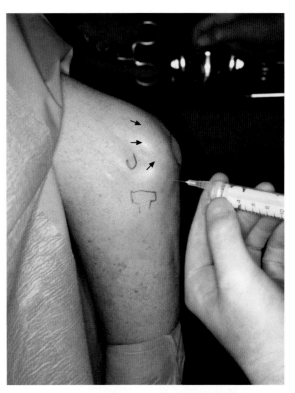

Fig. 7.13-7. Irrigating fluid is injected into the joint. Note the horseshoe-shaped distention of the posterior compartment around the olecranon (*arrows*)

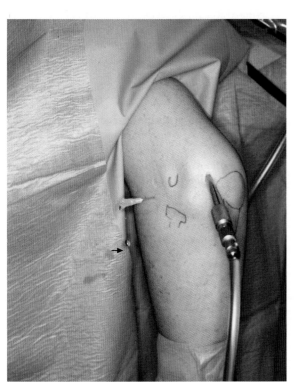

Fig. 7.13-8. Needle test in the anterolateral portal. After the inflow cannula has been placed in the high posterolateral portal (inflow portal), a needle is inserted at the anterolateral portal site. Fluid outflow (*arrow*) confirms that the anterior compartment is adequately distended

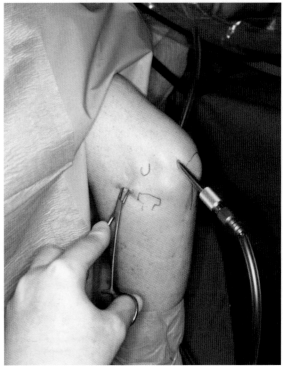

Fig. 7.13-9. Spreading the subcutaneous tissue with a clamp

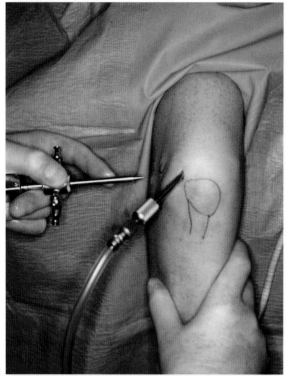

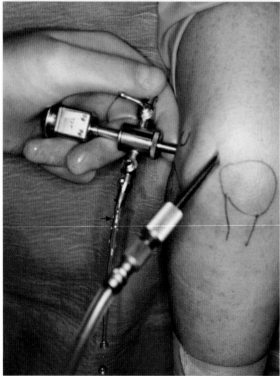

Fig. 7.13-10a,b. Insertion of the sheath. **a** The index finger is placed about 2–3 cm from the tip of the sheath. **b** Fluid outflow through the open spigot (*arrow*) confirms that the sheath has entered the joint

which may be quite firm. Either the sheath will not enter the joint or will perforate the capsule in its central third.

▶ **Note:** Perforating the capsule too far medially can have several consequences:

Limited arthroscope mobility due to the large distance from the skin to the site of capsule entry.

Difficulty inspecting the radial head. When the scope is retracted, it may slip rapidly from the joint, making it difficult to visualize the radial head.

Limited ability to maneuver instruments when the portal is used as an instrument portal (due to relative shifting of tissue layers).

Joint entry is confirmed by fluid outflow from the open spigot. Next the obturator is removed and the arthroscope is inserted. The ulnar half of the anterior compartment is inspected.

The rest of the procedure depends on local findings and is described fully in the sections dealing with operative technique.

7.13.6 Creating the Instrument Portal: Technique

After the primary anterolateral portal has been established, the anteromedial portal can be created under arthroscopic control. The portal can also be placed by inserting a switching rod over the sheath in the anterolateral portal. The low posterolateral portal used for instrumentation of the posterior compartment (proximal radioulnar joint) and the posterocentral portal for accessing the olecranon fossa are also placed under arthroscopic control.

Technique for Creating the Anteromedial Portal
(Fig. 7.13-11)

1. **Palpation.** The approximate portal location is determined by finger palpation. This is easily accomplished in thin patients. The portal is located 2 cm anterior and 2 cm distal to the medial epicondyle, but it may be placed slightly higher if necessary (e.g., to reach osteophytes on the coronoid process).

2. **Trial needle.** A percutaneous needle is inserted at the prospective portal site and advanced through the capsule (Fig. 7.13-11a,b). The needle is used to determine whether an instrument in that portal can reach the target lesion, such as an osteophyte on the coronoid process or in the coronoid fossa. With osteophytes or large loose bodies, the portal should not be placed too close to the humeral shaft, as this could interfere with instrumentation (e.g., loose body extraction).

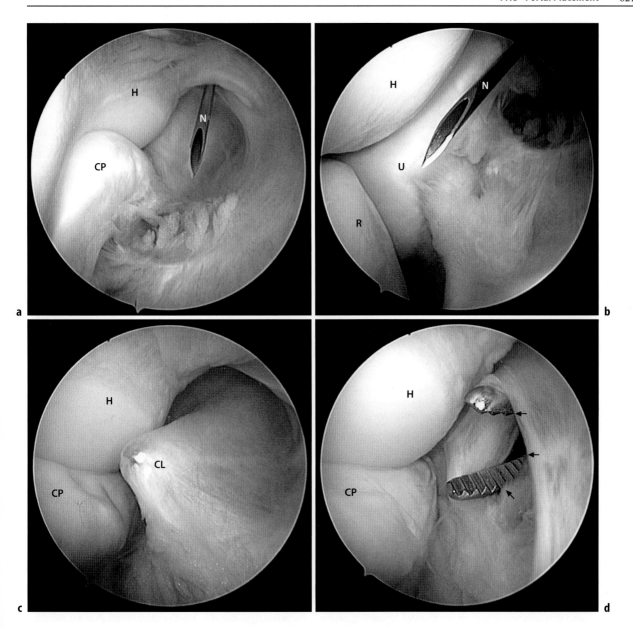

Fig. 7.13-11 a–d. Creating the anteromedial portal. a A trial needle (N) is used to determine optimum portal location. The needle should not enter the joint directly anterior to the humeral anterior surface (H), as this would deflect instruments toward the anterior joint capsule (CP coronoid process). b The trial needle confirms access to the radial head (R). c After spreading the subcutaneous tissue, a small clamp (CL) is advanced to the medial capsule. Arthroscopy confirms tenting of the capsule by the closed clamp. d After perforating the capsule, the clamp is opened to create a capsular incision (arrows)

3. **Skin incision.** A 3–5 mm incision is made through the skin only.

4. **Spreading the subcutaneous tissue and capsule.** First the subcutaneous tissue is spread with a blunt mosquito clamp, and then the closed clamp is advanced through the medial capsule into the joint under arthroscopic control. When the clamp has entered the joint space, the jaws of the instrument are opened to spread the capsular incision (Fig. 7.13-11 d).

▶ **Tip:** If there are small loose bodies in the anterior compartment, spread the capsule very carefully to prevent loose body spillage through the capsular incision into the subcutaneous tissue.

The probe, operating instruments, or irrigation cannula are inserted next. A switching rod is used to interchange portals (Fig. 7.13-12).

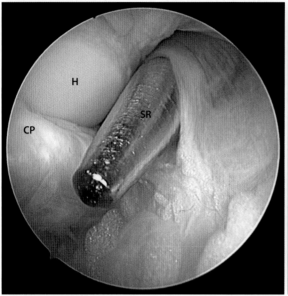 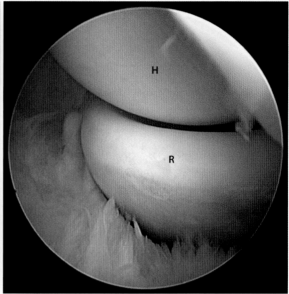

a   b

Fig. 7.13-12a,b. Switching portals. **a** A switching rod (*SR*) is introduced through the anteromedial portal (*H* humeral anterior surface, *CP* coronoid process). **b** The sheath is advanced over the switching rod, and the arthroscope is inserted to inspect the anterolateral corner with the radial head (*R*)

Switching Rod (Inside-Out) Technique for Creating the Anteromedial Portal

1. **Inspecting the anteromedial capsule.** The anteromedial capsule is inspected arthroscopically.

2. **Removing the arthroscope.** While the sheath is held in a constant position, the scope is withdrawn.

3. **Inserting the switching rod.** A switching rod is advanced through the sheath to the medial (ulnar) capsule. It then perforates the capsule and is advanced further until its tip is palpable beneath the skin. Vulnerable structures are safely pushed aside by the blunt tip.

4. **Skin incision.** The skin over the tip of the switching rod is carefully incised (3–4 mm), and the tip is advanced through the incision.

5. **Removing the switching rod.** The switching rod is withdrawn if the anteromedial portal is needed for instrumentation. To inspect the lateral compartment, the sheath is removed from the anterolateral portal and introduced over the switching rod into the anteromedial portal.

6. **Inserting the scope into the sheath and inserting instruments.** Of the two techniques described for creating the anteromedial portal, we favor the arthroscopically controlled needle technique because it is more precise and permits individual tailoring of portal placement. If necessary, the portal can be placed higher or more anteriorly to facilitate access (e.g., for removing osteophytes from the coronoid process).

Technique for Creating the Low Posterolateral Portal
(Fig. 7.13-13)

1. **Visualizing the proximal radioulnar joint.** From the high posterolateral portal, the arthroscope is advanced distally to visualize the proximal radioulnar joint. This may meet with resistance if degenerative changes are present, and it may be necessary to maneuver the scope distally via the posteromedial recess. The radial head, ulna, and capitellum can be identified unless obscured by synovitis.

2. **Inserting the trial needle.** The needle is inserted at the soft spot until it appears within the joint (Fig. 7.13-13a). Synovitis can make it difficult to locate the needle, but this should not deter creation of the low posterolateral portal, since the presence of synovitis may suggest a lesion of the capitellum or radial head or loose bodies in the proximal radioulnar joint.

3. **Skin incision.** A 2–4 mm skin incision is made at the needle insertion site.

4. **Spreading the subcutaneous tissue and penetrating the capsule.** The subcutaneous tissue is spread with a

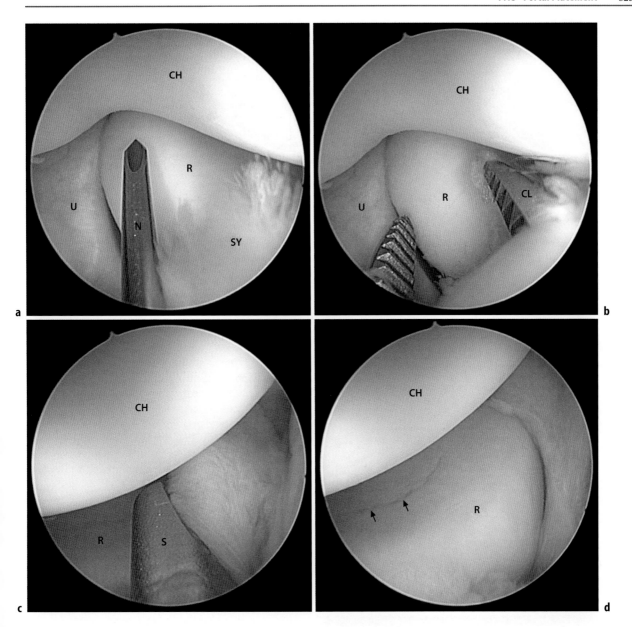

Fig. 7.13-13 a–d. Creating the low posterolateral portal. **a** The trial needle (*N*) reaches the posterior compartment just proximal to the proximal radioulnar joint. Local synovitis (SY) obscures a portion of the radial head (*R*) (*CH* capitellum, *U* ulna). **b** A clamp (*CL*) is passed through the joint capsule and spread open. **c** Synovectomy is performed with a shaver (*S*) to improve visualization of the radial head. **d** Inspection now reveals a fine chondral fissure (*arrows*) in the radial head blunt clamp. The clamp then perforates the capsule and is opened to make an adequate capsular incision (Fig. 7.13-13 b). If the structures are markedly obscured by synovitis, we recommend inserting a small synovial resector (shaver) and performing a partial synovectomy until the posterolateral structures can be adequately evaluated (Fig. 7.13-13 c, d).

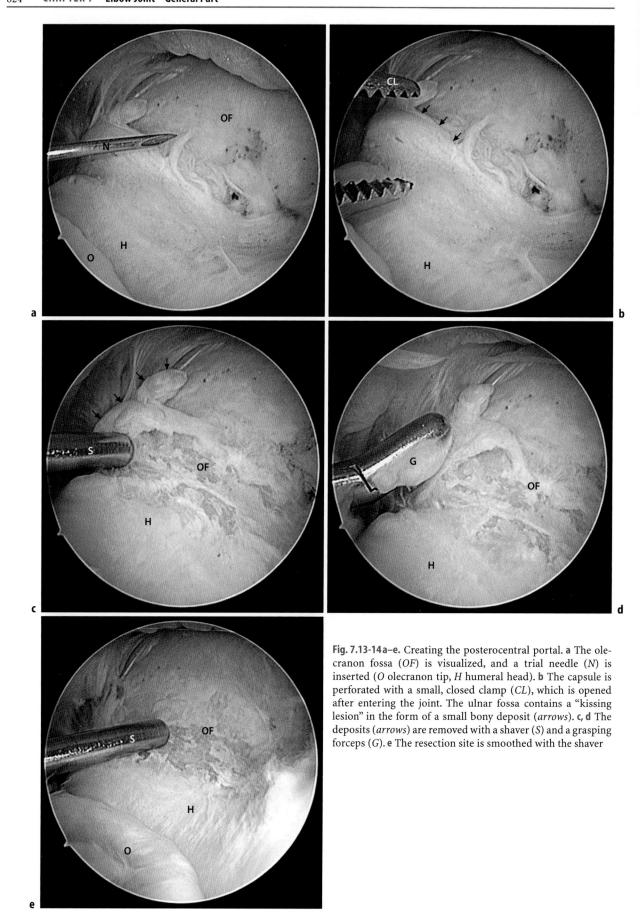

Fig. 7.13-14a–e. Creating the posterocentral portal. **a** The olecranon fossa (*OF*) is visualized, and a trial needle (*N*) is inserted (*O* olecranon tip, *H* humeral head). **b** The capsule is perforated with a small, closed clamp (*CL*), which is opened after entering the joint. The ulnar fossa contains a "kissing lesion" in the form of a small bony deposit (*arrows*). **c, d** The deposits (*arrows*) are removed with a shaver (*S*) and a grasping forceps (*G*). **e** The resection site is smoothed with the shaver

Technique for Creating the Posterocentral Portal
(Fig. 7.13-14)

1. **Visualizing the olecranon fossa.** The olecranon fossa is visualized with the arthroscope, and its extent is defined. The tip of the olecranon should be visible.

2. **Trial needle.** A needle is inserted percutaneously and advanced to the olecranon fossa (Fig. 7.13-14 a). Any osteophytes on the olecranon tip or calcifications at the triceps tendon insertion may obstruct access to the olecranon fossa, making it necessary to reposition the needle.

3. **Skin incision.** A 2–4 mm skin incision is made at the needle insertion site.

4. **Spreading the subcutaneous tissue and entering the joint.** The subcutaneous tissue and tendons are spread with a blunt clamp, which is then advanced through the joint capsule (Fig. 7.13-14 b). An alternative technique is to place a pointed knife blade in the skin incision and deepen the longitudinal incision through the subcutaneous tissue, tendon, and capsule until the blade appears within the joint. This ensures that the tendon will be incised in line with its fibers.
▶ **Caution:** Never cut across the triceps tendon; always cut longitudinally in the direction of its fibers.

7.13.7 Switching Portals

Two switching rods are needed so that portals can be switched within one compartment (e.g., between the anterolateral and anteromedial portals) and also between compartments (anterior and posterior). A standard routine is followed.

1. **Inserting the switching rod into the arthroscope compartment.** A switching rod is inserted into the compartment where the scope is positioned (see Fig. 7.13-12). The switching rod may be passed through an existing instrument portal or through the sheath after the scope is withdrawn. The sheath and arthroscope are removed from the compartment.

2. **Inserting a switching rod into the inflow compartment.** The switching stick is inserted through the inflow cannula, which is then removed. Care is taken to match the diameters of the switching stick and inflow cannula.

3. **Reinserting the inflow cannula.** The inflow cannula is inserted over the first switching stick into the compartment formerly occupied by the arthroscope. The switching rod is removed, and inflow is started to reestablish joint distention.

4. **Inserting the sheath.** Fluid extravasation along the switching rod will usually confirm that the joint has been redistended. The sheath is passed into the joint over the switching rod, and outflow from the open spigot confirms joint entry. The switching rod is removed, the arthroscope is inserted, and arthroscopy is continued.
▶ **Tip:** If adequate distention is not obtained in the area to be inspected, connect the inflow line to the sheath. Leave the inflow cannula in the other compartment but occlude it with a blunt obturator.
▶ **Caution:** Do not remove the inflow cannula. Besides providing a backup for redistention, it seals the portal and prevents fluid leakage into the subcutaneous tissues.

7.14 Examination Sequence

A standard examination sequence is followed in the elbow as in other joints, although some lesions (e.g., loose bodies) may require a modified routine. First it is important to consider the structures that can be visualized from the various portals.

7.14.1 Anterolateral Portal

The ulnar joint capsule, the ulnar half of the anterior joint capsule, the coronoid process, and the humeral anterior surface with the coronoid fossa can be viewed from the anterolateral portal (Fig. 7.14-1). The scope can be retracted to view the ulnar portion of the proximal radioulnar joint. The radial head is easily identified by pronation and supination.

▶ **Problem:** If the anterolateral portal pierces the joint capsule in its central third, it may be difficult or impossible to visualize the radial head.

The radial articular cartilage can be evaluated by further retracting the scope and pronating and supinating the forearm. If the radial annular ligament is lax or torn, the distal synovial fold of the proximal radioulnar joint and the sacciform recess can be inspected.

7.14.2 Anteromedial Portal

The radial joint capsule, the radial half of the anterior joint capsule, and the humeral anterior surface and radial head can be seen. Pronation and supination are helpful in identifying the radial head and detecting possible cartilage lesions. Flexion/extension helps to demonstrate cartilage lesions on the capitellum.

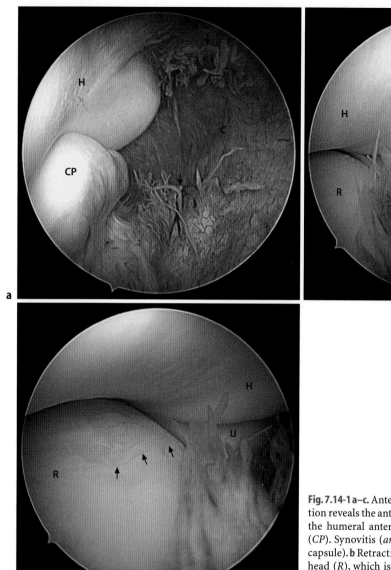

Fig. 7.14-1 a–c. Anterolateral corner of the elbow joint. **a** Inspection reveals the anteromedial joint capsule, the ulnar portion of the humeral anterior surface (*H*), and the coronoid process (*CP*). Synovitis (*arrows*) is commonly found (*C* anteromedial capsule). **b** Retracting the scope demonstrates part of the radial head (*R*), which is partially obscured by synovitis (*arrows*). **c** Pronation/supination reveals cartilage lesions (*arrows*) on the radial head

Retracting the arthroscope demonstrates the lateral portions of the ulna, followed by the coronoid process, the humeral anterior surface, and medial portions of the anterior joint capsule.

7.14.3 High Posterolateral Portal

This portal affords a view of the olecranon fossa and olecranon, along with any osteophytes that are present (Fig. 7.14-2). When the scope is advanced in the ulnar direction, the posteromedial recess can be seen from above. Inspection of this area may reveal cartilage lesions on the humeral posterior surface or loose bodies. The scope is then retracted for inspecting the radial portion of the olecranon.

The proximal radioulnar joint can also be inspected from this portal. This is done by passing the scope distally through the posteromedial recess (if it is not obstructed by adhesions) or advancing it directly along the radial side of the ulna (Fig. 7.14-2). The latter route may prove difficult due to degenerative changes or adhesions. When the scope is swept distally through the posterolateral recess, fine synovial folds can be seen that are similar to those in the lateral recess of the knee (Fig. 7.14-3). The radial portion of the proximal radioulnar joint is reached from the proximal side. The radial head is identified by pronation and supination (Fig. 7.14-3). Synovitis and adhesions can make this part of the examination difficult. Sometimes the radial head is obscured by a synovial plica interposed between the humerus and radial head.

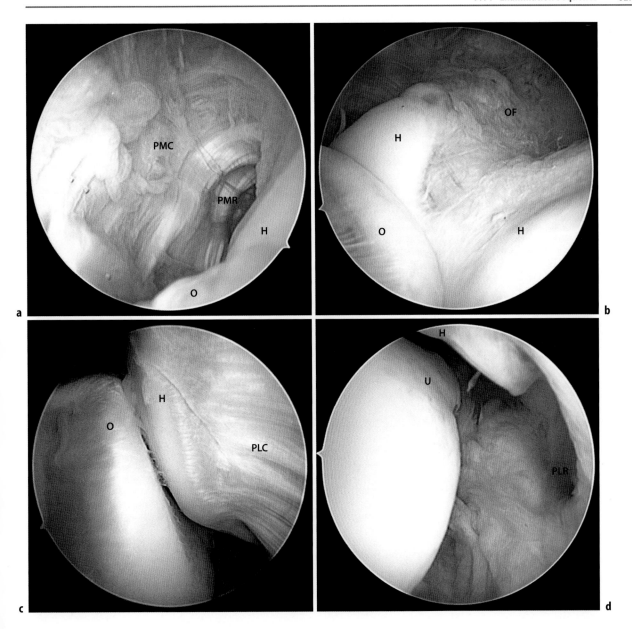

Fig. 7.14-2 a–d. Inspection of posterior joint structures through the high posterolateral portal. **a** *PMC* Posteromedial capsule, *PMR* posteromedial recess, *O* olecranon, *H* humeral posterior surface). **b** Retracting the scope brings the olecranon fossa (*OF*), humeral posterior surface (*H*), and olecranon (*O*) into view. **c** Sweeping the scope distally shows the radial part of the olecranon (*O*) and humeral posterior surface (*H*) in a well-distended joint (*PLC* posterolateral capsule, *U* ulna). **d** The proximal radioulnar joint is viewed by advancing the scope farther distally through the posterolateral recess (*PLR*)

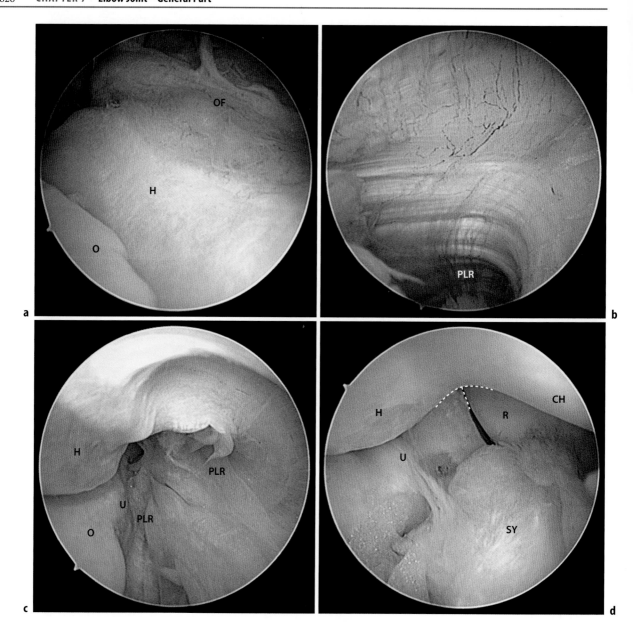

Fig. 7.14-3 a–d. Visualization of the proximal radioulnar joint. **a** Arthroscope in the high posterolateral portal demonstrates the olecranon fossa (*OF*), humeral posterior surface (*H*), and olecranon tip (*O*). **b** The scope is advanced distally through the posterolateral recess (*PLR*). **c** The recess is bounded on the ulnar side by the humerus (*H*) and ulna (*U*). **d** Farther distally is a T-shaped structure (*dashed line*) corresponding to the proximal radioulnar joint and the posterior part of the humeroradial joint. Vision is frequently obscured by synovitis (*SY*) (*R* radial head, *CH* capitellum, *U* ulna)

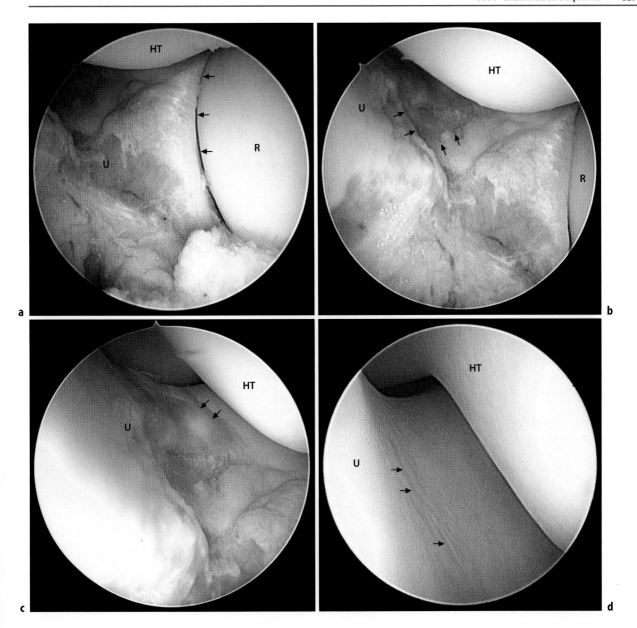

Fig. 7.14-4a–d. Inspection of the humeroulnar joint. **a** The humeroulnar joint is identified adjacent to the proximal radioulnar joint (*arrows*) (*R* radial head, *HT* humeral trochlea, *U* ulna). **b, c** Cartilage-free areas (*arrows*) on the ulnar surface do not represent chondral lesions but variable discontinuities in the cartilaginous zone (*arrows*). **d** Normal-appearing cartilage in a 7-year-old boy. Only mild superficial changes (*arrows*) are observed

When the arthroscope is advanced on the radial side of the ulna, the ulnar articular cartilage can be seen if the joint is adequately distended. The scope negotiates a narrow spot before entering the posterior compartment, which widens out like a funnel toward the proximal radioulnar joint. Often this field appears initially as whitish structures traversed by dark joint lines (Fig. 7.14-4). Pronation and supination help to identify the radial head as well as other anatomic structures. Alternating flexion/extension of the arm is also helpful. The posterior half of the radial head and the capitellum (cartilage lesions, osteochondritis dissecans) can be evaluated through this portal, and the ulnar portion of the posterior humeral surface can be examined.

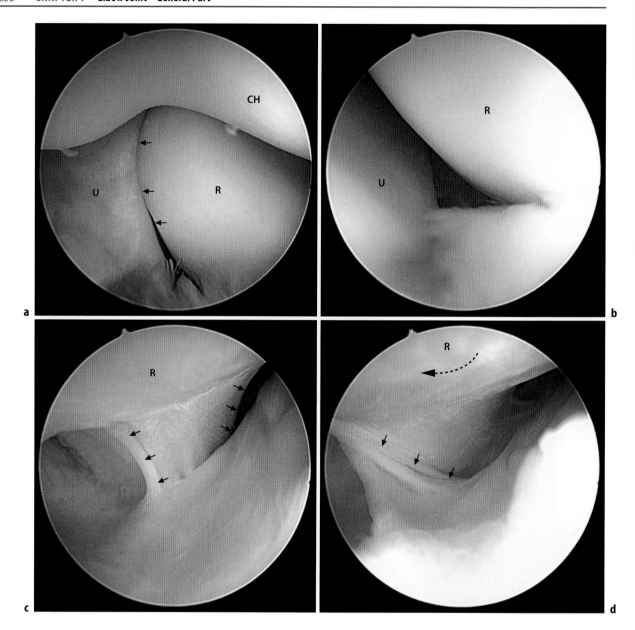

Fig. 7.14-5. a Inspection of the proximal radioulnar joint (*arrows*) with the radial head (*R*), capitellum (*CH*), and ulna (*U*) from the posterior side. **b** Advancing the scope farther distally in a lax joint demonstrates **c** the space below the radial head with the joint capsule (*arrows*). **d** Twisting of the joint capsule (*dashed arrow*) occurs with pronation and supination

In a lax elbow, the arthroscope can be advanced farther distally past the radial annular ligament to inspect the proximal humeroulnar joint with the superior sacciform recess (Fig. 7.14-5). The capsule in this area is easily identified by pronating and supinating the forearm.

7.14.4 Low Posterolateral Portal

This portal is rarely used as an arthroscope portal, because the high posterolateral portal is usually adequate for viewing (see above). The low posterolateral portal can be useful, however, for a detailed evaluation of the capitellum.

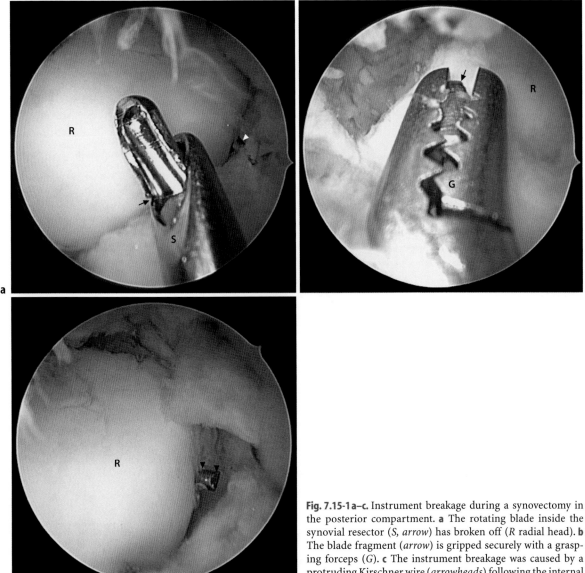

Fig. 7.15-1a–c. Instrument breakage during a synovectomy in the posterior compartment. **a** The rotating blade inside the synovial resector (*S, arrow*) has broken off (*R* radial head). **b** The blade fragment (*arrow*) is gripped securely with a grasping forceps (*G*). **c** The instrument breakage was caused by a protruding Kirschner wire (*arrowheads*) following the internal fixation of a radial head fracture

7.15 Complications

Besides general complications (infection, postoperative bleeding, effusion, instrument breakage, reflex sympathetic dystrophy) (Fig. 7.15-1), complications specific to elbow arthroscopy can also occur:

- **Nerve injuries.** The proximity of the nerves to the joint capsule was previously mentioned (see Sect. 7.13).

- **Vascular lesions** (brachial artery).

- **Position-related complications:** injury to the radial nerve or proximal arm muscles.

- **Losing track of loose bodies.** Because loose bodies are commonly found in the elbow, there is a risk of losing or flushing these bodies into the subcutaneous tissue.

In summary, we may say that a standardized technique of portal placement is the most effective way to avoid complications in elbow arthroscopy.

7.16 Documentation

Documentation in elbow arthroscopy should meet the same requirements as in any arthroscopic procedure (see Sect. 1.16).

7.17 Outpatient Arthroscopy

More than 95% of our elbow arthroscopies (n = 394 from 1992 to 2000) have been performed on an ambulatory basis. Certain procedures, such as the reattachment of a displaced osteochondral fragment or the treatment of a radial head fracture, require image intensification fluoroscopy. These techniques, as well as the arthroscopic treatment of empyema, should be performed in an inpatient setting.

7.18 Indications

Growing experience and improvements in arthroscopic instrumentation have significantly expanded the indications for elbow arthroscopy. As in other joints, no distinction is drawn between diagnostic and operative arthroscopy because the goal in every patient is to treat the lesion in the same sitting, if possible using arthroscopic technique.

7.18.1 Limitation of Motion

Limitation of motion is a common presenting symptom. It may be caused by dislocations, fractures, ligament injuries, immobilization, repetitive trauma (work, sports), osteochondritis dissecans, loose bodies, osteophytes, or previous surgery (Fig. 7.18-1).

Three causes are distinguished with respect to surgical planning:

- **Free or fixed loose bodies**
- **Osteophytes**
- **Adhesions**

For better operative planning, it is necessary to make a differential diagnostic analysis of the potential intra- and extraarticular causes of limited motion (Table 7.18-1).

Table 7.18-1. Causes of motion loss in the elbow joint

Causes of extension loss:
- Free or fixed loose body in the olecranon fossa
- Free or fixed loose body in the proximal radioulnar joint
- Fixed loose body on the olecranon tip
- Large, free loose body in the anterior compartment
- Osteophyte in the olecranon fossa
- Osteophyte on the olecranon
- Adhesions in the anterior compartment
- Osteochondritis dissecans (Panner disease)
- Posttraumatic bony deformity

Causes of flexion loss:
- Free or fixed loose body in the anterior compartment
- Free or fixed loose body in the proximal radioulnar joint
- Osteophyte in the coronoid fossa
- Osteophyte on the anterolateral humeral surface
- Adhesions in the posterior compartment
- Bony deformity

Fig. 7.18-1 a–f. Arthroscopy in a 26-year-old woman with intermittent, painful limitation of elbow motion and effusions. **a, b** Inspection through a high posterolateral portal shows wear tracks (*arrows*) on the humeral posterior surface (*H*) (*O* olecranon tip). **c** Advancing the scope toward the proximal radioulnar joint shows the wear track on the humeral posterior surface with associated chondral defects (*arrows*) (*U* ulna). **d** A fixed loose body (*arrows*) is discovered by probing the olecranon fossa (*OF*) (*PR* probe). **e** The loose body (*LB, arrows*) is grasped and extracted with a grasping forceps (*G*). **f** Then the olecranon fossa is debrided with a curette (*CU*)

7.18.2 Loose Bodies

Intermittent locking and radiologic evidence of loose bodies are a definite indication for arthroscopic removal.

7.18.3 Osteophytes

The limited motion may be caused by radiographically detectable osteophytes. Arthroscopic removal is usually feasible (Fig. 7.18-2), but the presence of multiple osteophytes or deep chondral lesions will compromise the prognosis.

7.18.4 Osteoarthritis

Besides pain, a common symptom of degenerative joint disease is limited motion (extension and/or flexion deficit). Pain is improved in most patients by loose body

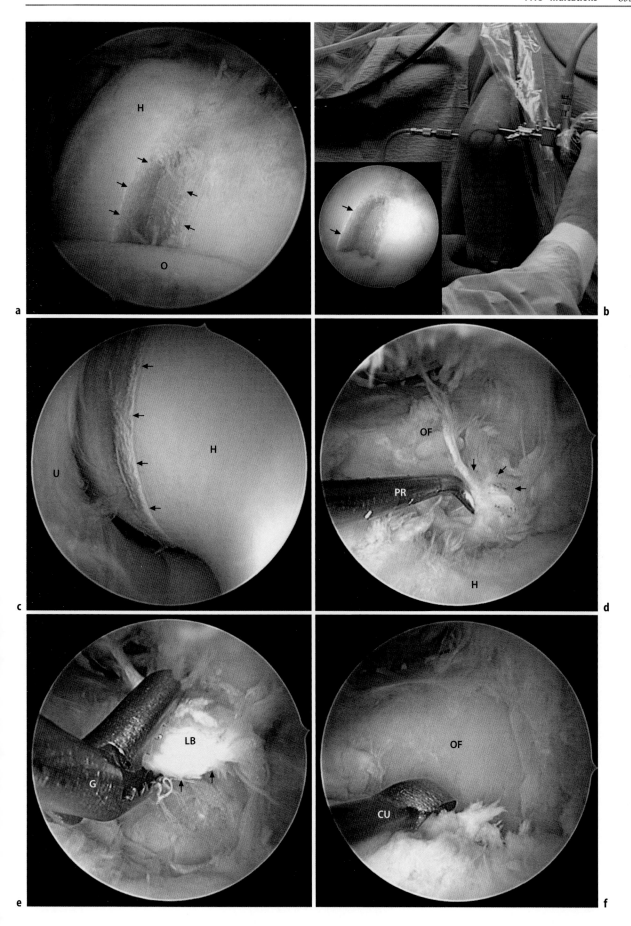

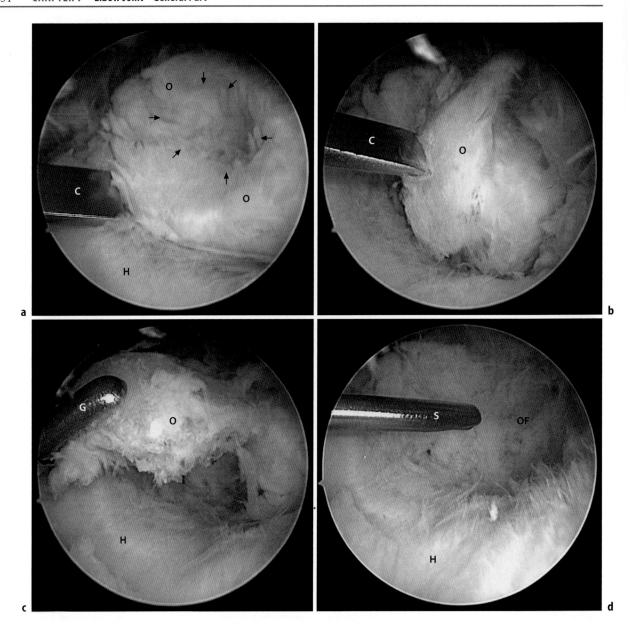

Fig. 7.18-2 a–d. Persistent extension deficit in a 47-year-old man. **a** A large osteophyte (*O*) fills the olecranon fossa. A chisel (*C*) is inserted through the posterocentral portal (*H* humeral posterior surface, *arrows* imprint of the olecranon tip in the osteo-phyte). **b, c** The osteophyte is partially detached with the chisel and extracted with a grasping forceps (*G*). **d** The olecranon fossa (*OF*) is debrided with a shaver (*S*) to remove unstable osteophyte remnants and scar tissue

removal, osteophyte excision, partial synovectomy, or by removing unstable cartilage fragments. Complaints will probably recur, however, especially if the patient resumes activities that stress the elbow (work, sports).

7.18.5 Chronic Pain

If the cause of chronic pain cannot be established by clinical examination and imaging studies, arthroscopy should be performed. If it is uncertain whether the pain really has an intraarticular cause, the intraarticular injection of a local anesthetic can be tried to differentiate between an intra- and extraarticular pain etiology. Extraarticular pain is frequently caused by insertional tendinopathies of the flexor and extensor muscles. Cervical spine lesions and neuropathies should also be excluded.

Chronic pain can also result from cartilage lesions that are not demonstrable with imaging studies and from impingement due to plicae or intraarticular scars and adhesions.

7.18.6 Recurrent Effusions

If the clinical examination and imaging studies do not show a morphologic cause for the effusions, arthroscopy should be performed. In addition to partial synovectomy, a synovial biopsy should always be obtained. Joint swelling can also result from small chondral loose bodies (e. g., in synovial chondromatosis). These fragments do not always cause catching or limited motion.

Arthroscopic synovectomy is a useful procedure in rheumatoid conditions. It permits a more radical excision than an open synovectomy, and the low morbidity of arthroscopic surgery is a particular advantage in the elbow.

7.18.7 Fractures

A few cases have been published describing the arthroscopically assisted treatment of radial head fractures. Minimally displaced humeral fractures would also be amenable to arthroscopically assisted treatment. The arthroscopically assisted internal fixation of elbow fractures is still in the developmental stage, and further experience is needed in large clinical series.

7.18.8 Osteochondritis Dissecans (Panner Disease)

Besides evaluating cartilage lesions, arthroscopy provides access for drilling osteochondral defects and reattaching loose fragments, depending on the stage of the process.

7.18.9 Infection

Arthroscopy is preferred over open surgery for the treatment of joint infections resulting from percutaneous aspiration, arthroscopy, intraarticular injection, or hematogenous spread.

7.19 Contraindications

Besides general contraindications (see Sect. 1.19), it is necessary to exclude local skin changes with redness and possible suppuration (pustules, pimples, onychitis) on the affected extremity. It may be necessary to reschedule arthroscopy for a later date.

Elbow Joint – Special Part

8.1 Synovitis

Cause

An inflammatory reaction of the synovial membrane can occur in response to trauma, degenerative changes, or rheumatoid disease (see Sect. 2.3 for details).

Symptoms

Swelling, pain, and terminal motion loss are the chief complaints. Because synovitis is often reactive in nature, the predominant symptoms are usually based on the causative disorder (e.g., loose bodies that cause intermittent locking).

Clinical Diagnosis

Tenderness, capsular thickening, and intraarticular effusion should be excluded. The extent of synovial changes cannot be determined clinically.

Radiographs

The radiographic findings are determined by associated pathology such as advanced degenerative changes or loose bodies.

MRI

MRI can demonstrate thickening of the synovial membrane and coexisting lesions. MRI is of minor importance, however, in its implications for synovial treatment.

Arthroscopic Findings

As in other joints, arthroscopy permits a detailed evaluation of the synovium (see Sect. 2.3 for details). Synovitis is usually a reactive process that has the following sites of predilection in the elbow:

- **Anterior joint capsule.** Synovitis can hamper or prevent evaluation of the radial head and loose body detection.

- **Olecranon fossa.** Loose bodies and osteophytes are also commonly found in this area.

- **Posterior to the humeroradial joint.** Synovitis occurs at this site in response to cartilage lesions on the radial head and/or the capitellum. Loose bodies in the humeroradial joint or the proximal ulnoradial joint are almost always associated with localized synovitis.

Therapeutic Management

Complete synovectomy is indicated for rheumatoid disease confirmed by synovial biopsy, but very often a partial synovectomy is necessary to permit the arthroscopic evaluation of anatomic structures and pathologic changes (loose bodies, osteophytes, etc.).

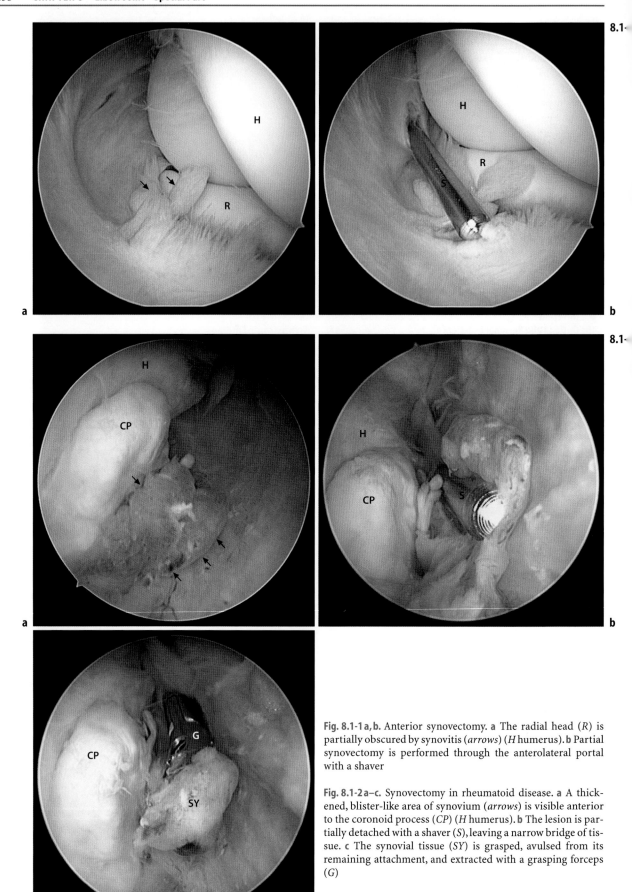

8.1-

8.1-

Fig. 8.1-1 a, b. Anterior synovectomy. **a** The radial head (*R*) is partially obscured by synovitis (*arrows*) (*H* humerus). **b** Partial synovectomy is performed through the anterolateral portal with a shaver

Fig. 8.1-2 a–c. Synovectomy in rheumatoid disease. **a** A thickened, blister-like area of synovium (*arrows*) is visible anterior to the coronoid process (*CP*) (*H* humerus). **b** The lesion is partially detached with a shaver (*S*), leaving a narrow bridge of tissue. **c** The synovial tissue (*SY*) is grasped, avulsed from its remaining attachment, and extracted with a grasping forceps (*G*)

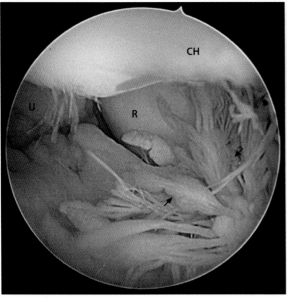
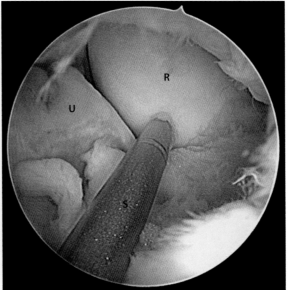

a   b

Fig. 8.1-3a,b. Synovectomy in the humeroradial joint (posterior). **a** The radial head (*R*) is mostly obscured by synovitis (*arrows*) (*CH* capitellum, *U* ulna). **b** Resecting the fronds with a shaver (*S*) greatly improves radial head visualization

Operative Technique

Synovectomy: Anterior Compartment
(Figs. 8.1-1 and 8.1-2)

With the arthroscope in the anterolateral portal, the synovectomy is performed through the anteromedial portal with a small synovial resector. If inspection raises suspicion of rheumatoid disease, a synovial biopsy is performed. The portals are switched (arthroscope to the anteromedial portal) to continue the synovectomy in the anterolateral part of the joint.

Synovectomy: Olecranon Fossa
The olecranon fossa is visualized through the high posterolateral portal. Then a posterocentral portal is established. Synovectomy is performed with a small synovial resector to define the extent of the olecranon fossa and confirm or exclude osteophytes and loose bodies in that area.

Synovectomy: Humeroradial Joint and Posterior Proximal Radioulnar Joint (Fig. 8.1-3)
This region is inspected through the high posterolateral portal. The low posterolateral portal is then established under arthroscopic vision (see Sect. 7.13.6, Fig. 7.13-13). Again, a small synovial resector is used to perform the synovectomy.

Postoperative Care

Full range of motion is allowed after swelling has subsided, but stresses on the elbow joint should be avoided for 2–3 weeks. In most cases the clinically predominant lesion will determine the postoperative protocol.

8.2 Cartilage Lesions

Cause

Traumatic and degenerative cartilage lesions can develop as a result of fractures or repetitive overloading of the elbow (work, sports).

Symptoms

Pain, intermittent snapping, locking, and occasional catching are described. Advanced cases with significant degenerative changes present with motion loss, effusions, and intraarticular crepitus.

Clinical Diagnosis

No specific tests are known. Areas of maximum tenderness and range of motion are determined.

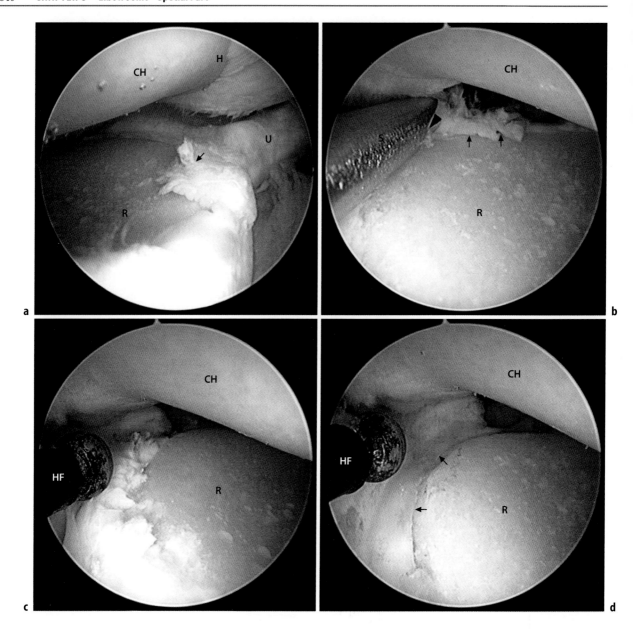

Radiographs

Localized cartilage lesions are almost never visible on radiographs, provided the lesions have not resulted from bone fractures. Increased subchondral sclerosis may be evident as an early sign of incipient degenerative change.

MRI

Images of acceptable quality can demonstrate local chondral defects extending to the bone. The actual lesions found at arthroscopy are usually more extensive than suggested by MRI.

Fig. 8.2-1 a–d. Osteoarthritis of the elbow. **a** The radial head (*R*) and capitellum (*CH*) are almost completely devoid of cartilage. Note the unstable cartilage remnant (*arrow*) on the anterior circumference of the radial head (*H* humerus, *U* ulna) (viewed through the anterolateral portal). **b** Viewing through the high posterolateral portal is advantageous for this type of lesion. The shaver (*S*) is inserted through the low posterolateral portal, and unstable cartilage fragments (*arrows*) are removed. The capitellum (*CH*) and radial head (*R*) are viewed from the posterior aspect. **c, d** Unstable cartilage areas are smoothed with a ball-tipped cautery probe (*HF*) to create a homogeneous surface (*arrows*)

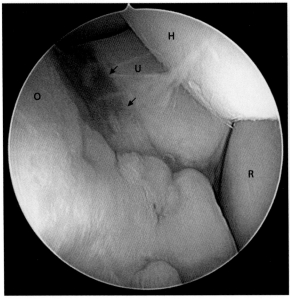
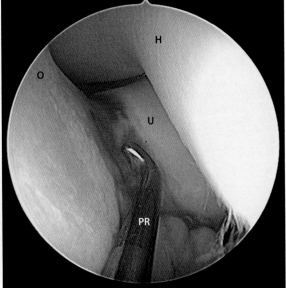

a   b

Arthroscopic Findings

The entire spectrum of traumatic and degenerative cartilage changes may be found in the elbow as in other joints (see Sect. 2.2 for details). The sites of predilection for cartilage lesions are as follows:

- **Radial head.** Findings range from localized grooves and superficial degenerative lesions to a complete loss of articular cartilage (Fig. 8.2-1).

- **Capitellum.** Areas of cartilage softening or fragmentation may be secondary to a previous axial compression injury, osteoarthritis of the humeroradial joint, or osteochondritis dissecans (Panner disease).

- **Humeral posterior surface (humeroulnar joint).** Besides superficial cartilage lesions, arthroscopy may show areas where the cartilage is softened but still superficially intact (stage II chondromalacia). This leads to snapping or pseudocatching of the unstable cartilage layer during flexion/extension despite the intact cartilage surface. More advanced stages present with varying degrees of surface disruption.

▶ **Note:** It is common to find a non-cartilage-bearing area on the ulna at the junction of the ulna and olecranon in the humeroulnar joint. This area, which has curvilinear boundaries with the olecranon and coronoid process, is not an advanced chondral lesion but a normal variant (Fig. 8.2-2). The size of this cartilage-free area is variable, and adjacent cartilage surfaces are intact.

Fig. 8.2-2a,b. Evaluating the ulnar cartilage. **a** An "apparent" cartilage lesion (*arrows*) is visible on the ulna (*U*) (*H* humerus, *O* olecranon, *R* radial head) (viewed through the high posterolateral portal). **b** Probing demonstrates a stable transition to surrounding cartilage (*PR* probe)

Therapeutic Management

Therapy is based on the general principles of arthroscopic cartilage treatment (see Sect. 2.2). Softened cartilage areas are left alone. If an area is severely softened, has an intact chondral surface, and is clinically symptomatic, arthroscopic debridement of the unstable cartilage should be considered. Fibrocartilage induction is appropriate for localized areas of exposed bone. More extensive cartilage defects, such as a completely "denuded" radial head, are not suitable for this type of treatment.

Operative Technique

Cartilage Debridement: Radial Head and Capitellum
(Fig. 8.2-3)

Cartilage fringe tags or rounded cartilage fragments may be found on the anterior or posterior aspects of the radial head and capitellum.

1. **Inspection.** The chondral lesion is optimally visualized arthroscopically, depending on whether it is best viewed through a posterior or anterior portal. A good general rule (with the arm in the neutral position) is

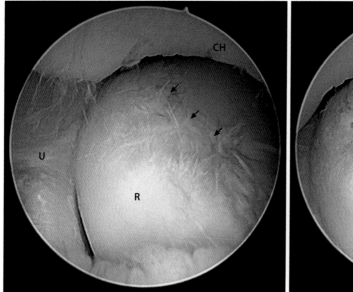
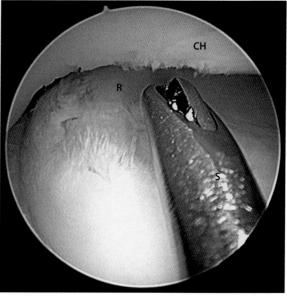

Fig. 8.2-3 a, b. Cartilage debridement on the radial head and capitellum. **a** Inspection through the high posterolateral portal shows fibrillated cartilage lesions (*arrows*) on the radial head (*R*) (*CH* capitellum, *U* ulna). **b** The fibrillations are debrided with a shaver (*S*) (synovial resector with a small-joint blade)

that cartilage lesions on the anterior half of the radial head are best treated from an anterior approach and posterior-half lesions from a posterior approach.

2. **Positioning the instrument portal.** The position of the instrument portal depends on the location of the lesion. Portal placement is more problematic for anterior compartment lesions, because cartilage lesions on the ulnar side of the radial head are more accessible through an anteromedial portal. This portal must be positioned so that the coronoid process will not deflect instruments anteriorly.

3. **Removing unstable cartilage.** Local fibrillations are removed with a small synovial resector or preferably with a small ronguer. A laser probe can also be used to resect an unstable cartilage fragment. Laser resection is helpful in cases of difficult portal placement.

Cartilage Debridement and Fibrocartilage Induction:
Humeral Posterior Surface and Capitellum
(Figs. 8.2-4 to 8.2-7)

1. **Inspection.** Unstable cartilage areas (which may be superficially intact) are inspected with the arthroscope in the high posterolateral portal.

2. **Probing.** The unstable cartilage areas are palpated with a probe through the low posterolateral portal. If instability is pronounced, probing of the unstable cartilage areas can reproduce the locking symptoms described by the patient.

3. **Abrasion.** If the cartilage surface is still intact, it may be possible to "melt down" the cartilage with a cautery probe (ball-tipped electrode). Generally this is not possible, however, and the unstable cartilage areas have to be removed. Usually it is difficult to reach these areas with ordinary operating instruments, and it may be necessary to use very small instruments or a laser fiber (Fig. 8.2-5).
The cartilage areas are extracted with a fine grasping forceps, or larger fragments can be removed with a small synovial resector.

4. **Fibrocartilage induction.** When the unstable cartilage has been debrided to bare bone, the bone is treated by subchondral abrasion or microfracturing to induce repair by fibrocartilage formation (Fig. 8.2-6 and 8.2-7).

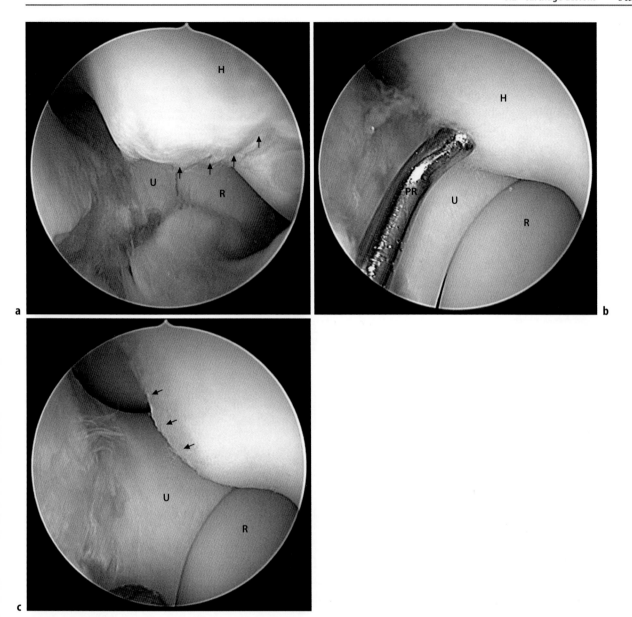

Postoperative Care

Range of motion exercises are started on the second postoperative day. Axial loading is prohibited for 6–8 weeks, depending on the size of the defects. Lymph-drainage is ordered to promote swelling control.

Fig. 8.2-4a–c. Elevated cartilage area on the humeral posterior surface in a 40-year-old man with intermittent locking and pain in the posterior elbow joint. **a** Arthroscopy shows marked cartilage elevation (*arrows*) on the humeral posterior surface (*H*) just proximal to the proximal radioulnar joint (*R* radial head, *U* ulna). **b** The unstable cartilage area is palpated with a probe (*PR*) through the low posterolateral portal. **c** The unstable cartilage areas (*arrows*) have been debrided with a laser

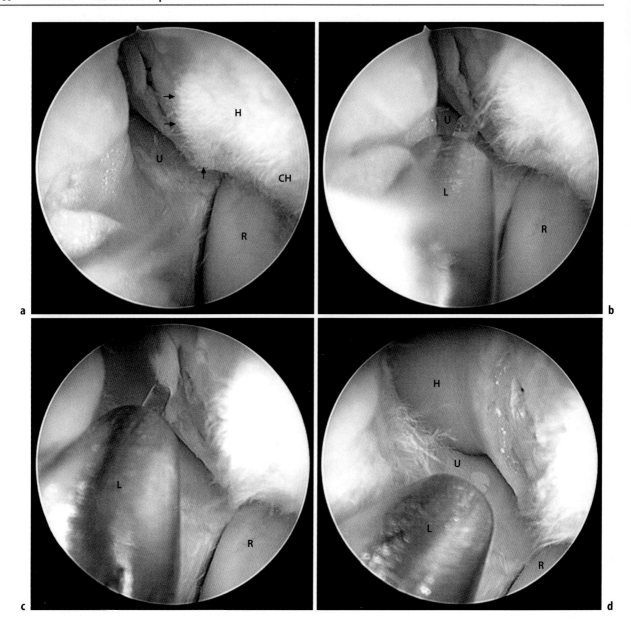

Fig. 8.2-5a–d. Cartilage lesions on the humeral posterior surface. **a** Fibrillated cartilage lesions (*arrows*) are visible on the humeral posterior surface (H). Note the elevated cartilage flaps with fibrillations (*arrowheads*) in the posterior part of the humeroulnar joint (*R* radial head, *U* ulna). **b** An ordinary shaver cannot fit into this area. Therefore a laser probe (*L*) is inserted through the low posterolateral portal, and **c, d** the unstable cartilage areas are ablated

Fig. 8.2-6a–e. Fibrocartilage induction on the capitellum. ▶ **a** Superficial inspection of the capitellum (*CH*) from the posterior side shows irregularities (*arrowhead*) in the cartilage surface (*R* radial head). **b** A mirror (*MI*) passed through the low posterolateral portal reveals deep chondral lesions (*arrows*) on the undersurface of the capitellum (*U* ulna). **c** Maximum flexion of the elbow exposes elevated cartilage fragments (*arrow*) on the capitellum. **d** After the unstable cartilage areas are removed, the base of the defect is treated with a microfracture chisel (*MC*) to induce fibrocartilage formation. **e** When the tourniquet is released, blood filaments emerge from the bleeding capitellum

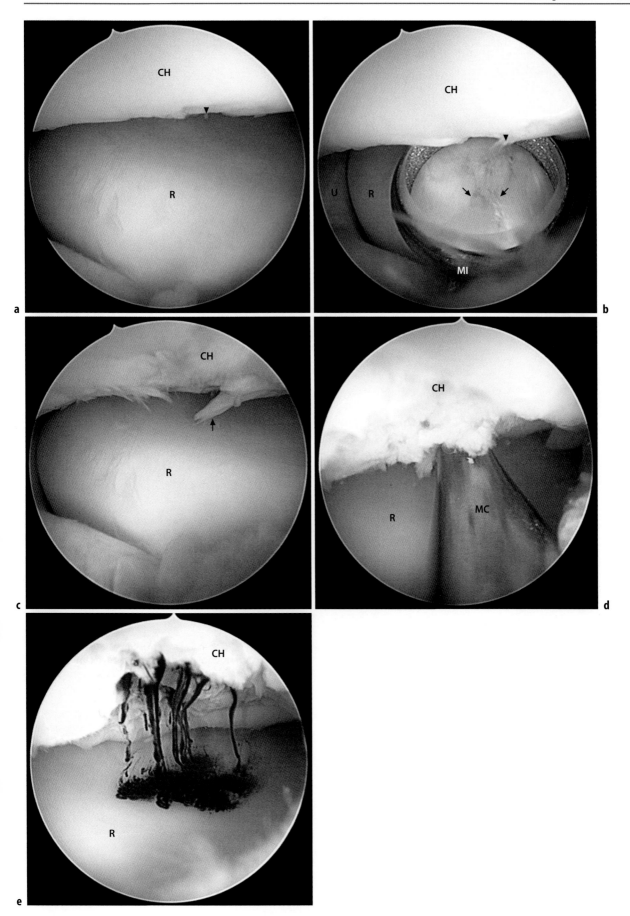

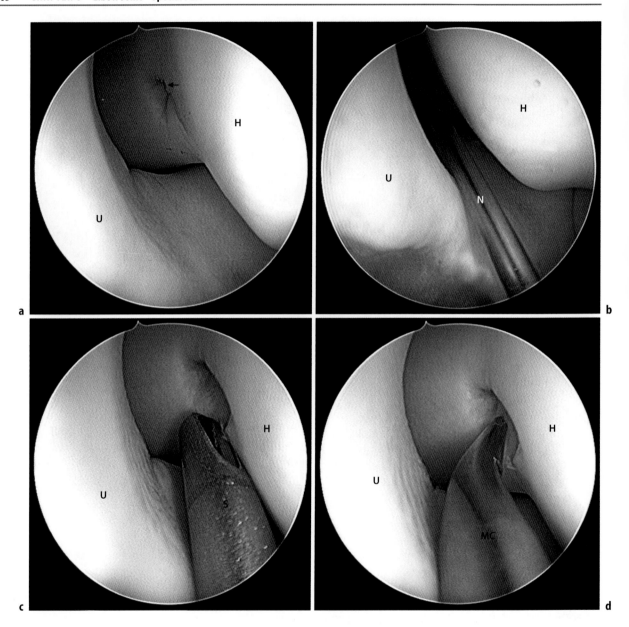

Fig. 8.2-7 a–d. Fibrocartilage induction. **a** A deep, circumscribed cartilage lesion (*arrow*) is found on the posterior surface of the humerus (*H*) (*U* ulna). **b** An optimum site for the instrument portal is located with a needle (*K*), and **c** unstable cartilage areas are removed with a shaver (*S*). **d** Next the microfracture chisel (*MC*) is introduced, and the cartilage defect is microfractured to induce fibrocartilage formation

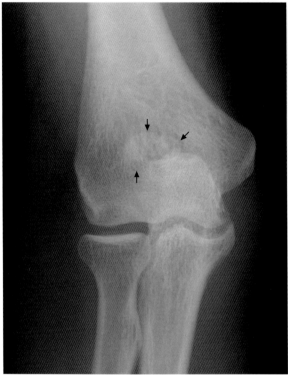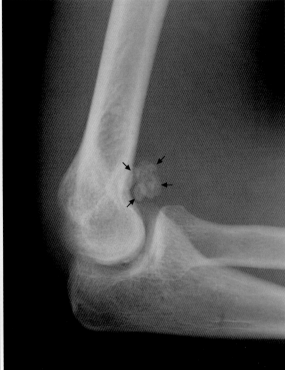

a   b

8.3 Loose Bodies

Cause

Loose bodies within the elbow joint may consist of chondral or, less frequently, osteochondral fragments resulting from a traumatic event (dislocation, fracture), chronic overuse (sports, job-related activity), or degenerative changes.

Symptoms

Symptoms consist of pain, swelling, and recurrent locking or limited joint motion (fixed loose body).

Clinical Diagnosis

The history and symptoms suggest the diagnosis. Larger loose bodies in the anterior compartment can be moved back and forth by external manipulation. Loose bodies in the posterior compartment may also be palpable in some cases.

Fig. 8.3-1 a, b. Loose bodies in the elbow joint. **a** AP radiograph shows a calcific density (*arrows*) projected over the olecranon fossa. **b** Lateral view demonstrates three loose bodies (*arrows*) in the anterior compartment

Radiographs

Intraarticular loose bodies often appear as rounded structures of calcific density on X-ray films. They are seen most clearly on lateral views, and AP films must be closely scrutinized (Fig. 8.3-1). Circumscribed densities in the area of the olecranon fossa or proximal radioulnar joint line may represent intraarticular loose bodies (Fig. 8.3-1). Multiple loose bodies in synovial chondromatosis are rare (Fig. 8.3-2).

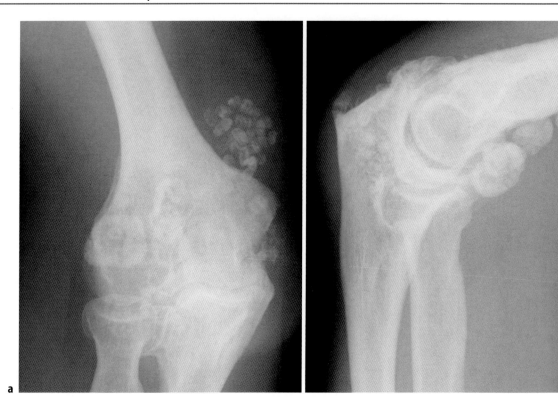

a   b

Fig. 8.3-2a, b. Multiple intraarticular loose bodies of varying size in synovial chondromatosis

Arthroscopic Findings

Free loose bodies may be found anywhere within the elbow joint. Sites of predilection are:

- **Anterior compartment**
- **Proximal radioulnar joint**
- **Humeroradial joint**
- **Olecranon fossa**

All loose bodies are not "loose," and the anterior capsule and olecranon fossa should be carefully searched for these fixed loose bodies.

A review of our own cases (88 patients) has shown that more than one loose body is present in over 60% of cases. We found that 48% of the loose bodies were located in the anterior compartment and 52% in the posterior compartment. This underscores the importance of arthroscopic visualization of the posterior joint areas. A partial synovectomy is nearly always necessary in order to determine the size and condition of the loose bodies (fixed or free).

Therapeutic Management

Tactical considerations in loose body removal are important for making the procedure safer and easier. A radiograph should be taken as soon before the operation as possible to recheck the exact location of the loose bodies.

Before removing loose bodies, the surgeon should understand that large loose bodies tend to cause limitation of motion while small loose bodies tend to cause intermittent locking.

A common tactical error is to remove a large loose body as soon as it is found. The large portal necessary for extracting the fragment causes significant fluid extravasation with loss of joint distention, making it difficult to inspect the remaining joint areas. This is of key importance, because these areas often contain smaller fragments that are responsible for the actual clinical symptoms. Without optimum distention, these fragments will be difficult to remove. Another problem is that the inflow may sweep smaller loose bodies through the large capsular incision into the subcutaneous tissue.

▶ **Tip:** In the elbow as in other joints, remove the smaller loose bodies before removing the larger ones.

The origin of any loose body should be determined, and a search should always be made for associated lesions that have been caused by intermittent loose body entrapment.

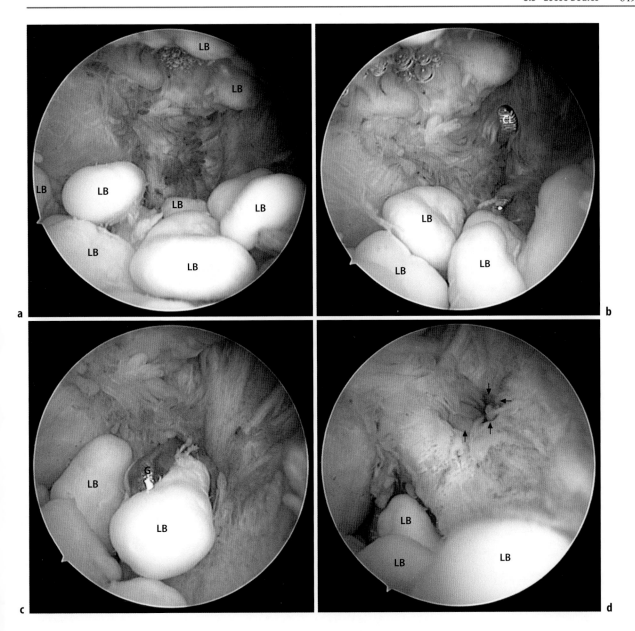

Operative Technique

Removal of Large or Multiple Loose Bodies: Anterior Compartment

(Figs. 8.3-3 and 8.3-4)

1. **Inspection.** The extent of the loose body is determined. A large anterior loose body is not probed right away to assess its consistency, as this would require an anteromedial portal. First it is necessary to exclude lesions (e.g., small loose bodies) in the posterior compartment.

2. **Switching portals (inflow to the anterolateral portal, arthroscope to the high posterolateral portal).** The ole-

Fig. 8.3-3 a–d. Removal of multiple loose bodies in synovial chondromatosis. **a** Arthroscopy demonstrates multiple loose bodies (*LB*) in the anterior compartment. **b** To create the anteromedial portal, a clamp (*CL*) is inserted and is spread after perforating the capsule. Care is taken not to make the capsular incision too large, as this might allow loose bodies to escape into the subcutaneous tissue. **c** The loose bodies are grasped with a forceps (*G*) and extracted under arthroscopic control. **d** The portal site is observed (*arrows*) to confirm passage of the loose body through the capsular incision and avoid (or promptly detect) the loss of smaller loose bodies in the subcutaneous tissue

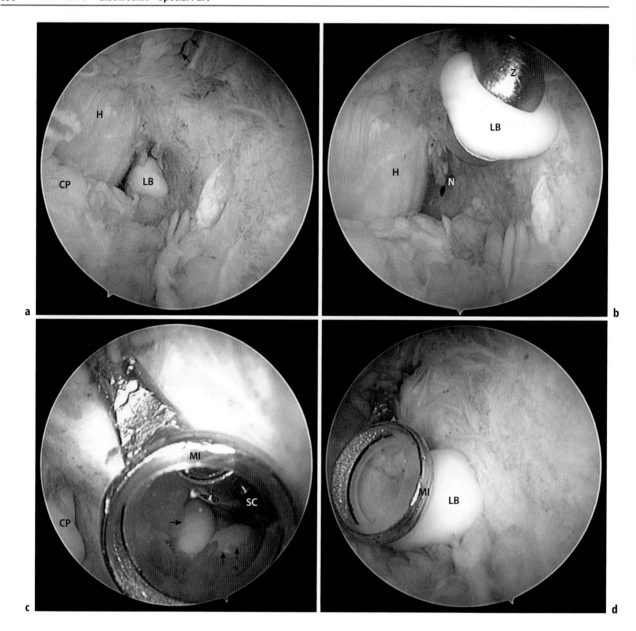

Fig. 8.3-4a–d. Removal of multiple loose bodies (continued from Fig. 8.3-3). **a** Most of the loose bodies have been removed. One loose body (*LB*) remains on the floor of the anteromedial recess (*H* humerus, *CP* coronoid process). The proximal level of the anteromedial portal (*arrows*) makes it difficult to reach the loose body with a grasper. **b** A percutaneous needle (*N*) is used to push the fragment to a more radial site, where it can be grasped and extracted with the forceps (*G*). **c** It is also necessary to check for loose bodies that have slipped beneath the arthroscope tip. An opposing mirror (*MI*) passed through the anteromedial portal demonstrates the scope tip (*SC*) and two loose bodies (*arrows*) lodged beneath it. **d** The surgeon tries to maneuver the loose body (*LB*) in an ulnar direction with the mirror so that the grasper can reach it

cranon fossa is inspected. If loose bodies or osteophytes are found there, they are removed through a posterocentral portal.

3. **Inspecting the proximal radioulnar joint.** Local synovitis may indicate the presence of a free loose body in the proximal radioulnar joint space.

4. **Creating the low posterolateral portal.** This portal is used for posterior synovectomy in the proximal radioulnar joint. If a free loose body is found, it is removed with a grasping forceps.

   It is not uncommon to find fixed loose bodies radial to the low posterolateral portal. The size of these bodies is assessed after partial synovectomy. They are partially detached and removed by avulsion and extraction.

5. **Switching portals.** After all lesions in the posterior compartment have been dealt with, the arthroscope is moved to the anterolateral portal and inflow to the high posterolateral portal.

6. **Anteromedial portal.** An anteromedial portal is created for probing and removing the loose body (see Fig. 8.3-3b). Degenerative osteophytes on the coronoid process and the size of the loose body should be considered in placing the portal. If the loose body is very large and there are degenerative spurs on the coronoid process, the portal should not be placed too close to the humeral anterior surface, as this could hamper the extraction. Even with a large loose body, a normal-size portal is created initially.

7. **Extracting the loose body.** The loose body is probed to assess its consistency. It is then pushed aside slightly to check for free or fixed loose bodies on the floor of the anterior compartment. This may necessitate a partial synovectomy. Small anterior loose bodies are grasped with a forceps or sharp mosquito clamp and extracted.

   Note: The controlled extraction of loose bodies is particularly important in the elbow, because loose bodies that become lost in the subcutaneous tissue are extremely difficult to retrieve due to the considerable thickness of the subcutaneous layer.

   Once smaller loose bodies have been excluded or removed, it is determined whether the primary loose body can be more easily extracted through the anterolateral or anteromedial portal, depending on the location of the body and the condition of the soft tissues. It may be necessary to switch the arthroscope and instrument portals.

   The extraction technique depends on the consistency of the loose body. Removing a soft loose body with a grasping forceps or Kocher clamp may break it into smaller pieces. The individual fragments are them removed as small or medium-size loose bodies.

   Tip: If it appears likely that a large loose body will break apart, consider a planned piecemeal extraction. The individual fragments are taken out separately as if they were small to medium-size loose bodies. Disadvantages are the need for frequent reinsertion of the grasping instrument and the potential for losing small pieces in the subcutaneous tissue. The advantage is that there is no need to enlarge the capsular incision.

   Extracting the loose body in one piece takes less time and offers higher confidence in a complete removal. Potential problems are losing the body in the subcutaneous tissue or, in the worst case, having it fragment within the subcutaneous tissue. It can be extremely difficult to retrieve the loose body or its fragments in this situation. Another disadvantage of one-piece removal is the need to enlarge the portal. The safest technique for removing a large, soft loose body is to fragment the loose body for piecemeal removal while it is still inside the joint, as this permits a more controlled extraction.

   Note: A controlled extraction is of critical importance in the removal of loose bodies. When multiple loose bodies are present, one or more of the fragments may "hide" beneath the arthroscope tip where they cannot be seen. An opposing mirror is useful for detecting these problem fragments (see Fig. 8.3-4).

8. **Switching portals.** The arthroscope is moved to the anteromedial or anterolateral portal to exclude broken-off fragments and any additional loose bodies that may be present.

Removal of Small and Medium-Size Loose Bodies
(Fig. 8.3-5)

The principles of removing these loose bodies are the same as described in the knee joint (see Sect. 2.9). With loose bodies in the posteromedial recess, the "rendezvous" technique can be used to maneuver the objects toward the olecranon fossa where they can be extracted with a grasping forceps passed through the posterocentral portal (see Fig. 2.9-4).

Removing Loose Bodies from the Olecranon Fossa
(Fig. 8.3-6)

Single or multiple loose bodies may be found in the olecranon fossa. When they are multiple, the smaller loose bodies are removed first. The posterocentral portal is convenient for extraction. Care is taken to grasp the smaller, softer loose bodies carefully but securely so that they are not fragmented and lost while passing through the subcutaneous tissue or the vertically split triceps

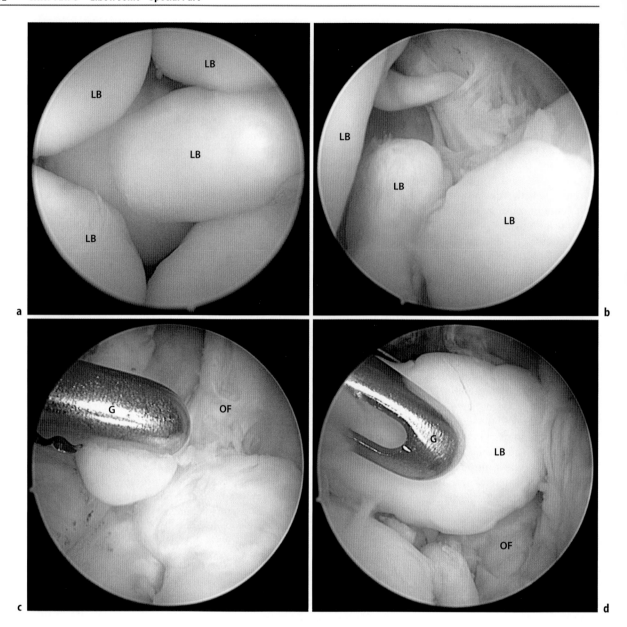

tendon. This is facilitated by using a sufficiently large grasping instrument. After all the loose bodies have been removed, the posterolateral and posteromedial recesses should be inspected for any residual debris. If a loose body has slipped into the posteromedial recess, the rendezvous technique is used to deliver it back toward the olecranon fossa where it can be grasped and extracted.

In the case of a large, isolated loose body, all other necessary intraarticular measures should be completed before the loose body is grasped with an appropriate-sized grasping forceps or Kocher clamp. The postero-central portal should be adequately enlarged prior to the extraction; otherwise the object may be stripped from the grasper while passing through the tendon and be-

Fig. 8.3-5 a–d. Multiple loose bodies in the olecranon fossa. **a, b** Loose bodies (*LB*) completely fill the olecranon fossa (*OF*). They are extracted through the posterocentral portal with a grasping forceps (*G*). **c** The smaller fragments are extracted first, **d** then the larger ones

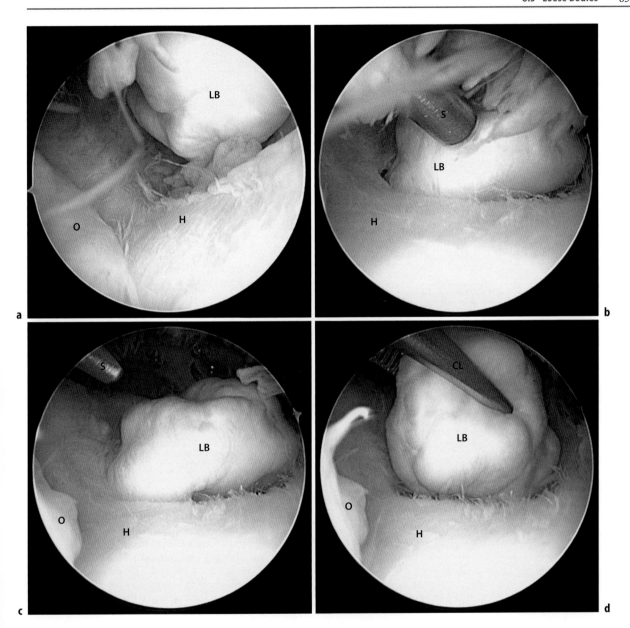

come lodged in the subcutaneous or peritendinous tissue.

▶ **Tip:** If extraction of the loose body encounters much resistance, pass the object back toward the olecranon fossa and enlarge the posterocentral portal. Another option is to switch portals, moving the scope to the posterocentral portal and extracting the loose body through the high posterolateral portal.

Fig. 8.3-6 a–d. Large loose body in the olecranon fossa. **a** A loose body (*LB*) completely fills the olecranon fossa (*H* humerus, *O* olecranon tip). **b, c** The surrounding synovium is debrided with a shaver (*S*) to obtain a clearer view. **d** The loose body is grasped and extracted with a clamp (*CL*)

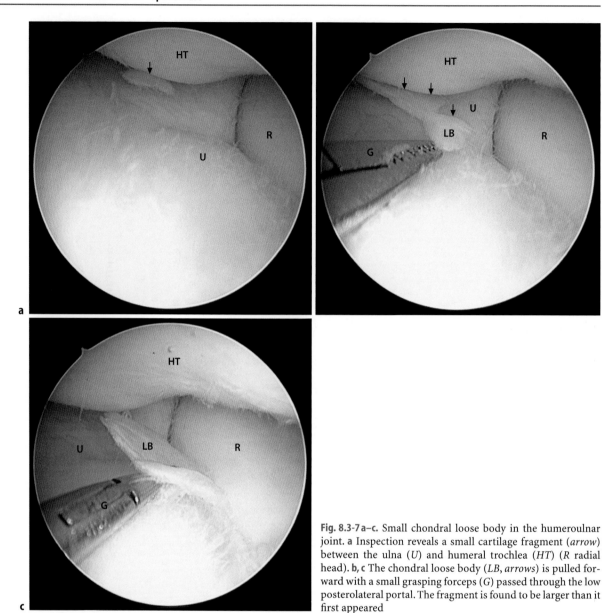

Fig. 8.3-7 a–c. Small chondral loose body in the humeroulnar joint. **a** Inspection reveals a small cartilage fragment (*arrow*) between the ulna (*U*) and humeral trochlea (*HT*) (*R* radial head). **b, c** The chondral loose body (*LB, arrows*) is pulled forward with a small grasping forceps (*G*) passed through the low posterolateral portal. The fragment is found to be larger than it first appeared

Removing Loose Bodies from the Posterior Humeroulnar and/or Humeroradial Joint
(Fig. 8.3-7)

This region tends to harbor small loose bodies that are not always evident on initial inspection. Local synovitis in this region should be considered an indirect sign of a free loose body. Synovectomy is performed to improve visualization of the proximal radioulnar and humeroradial joints. Even apparently small fiber remnants or tiny fragments may be part of a larger loose body and should therefore be maneuvered into the visible part of the proximal humeroulnar joint (Fig. 8.3-7). This should be done carefully to avoid fragmenting the loose body. Loose bodies occurring in this region are often responsible for intermittent locking of the elbow. Care is taken to grip the loose body securely during extraction.

Postoperative Care

When swelling has subsided, full range of motion is allowed below the pain threshold. If limitation of motion was an original presenting complaint, graded capsular stretching exercises should be performed. Vigorous exercises past the pain threshold are contraindicated.

▶ **Caution:** Reflex sympathetic dystrophy, capsular fibrosis.

8.4 Osteophytes

Cause

Degenerative joint changes due to trauma, fractures, or overuse in job- or sports-related activities (pitchers, javelin throwers, bowlers, tennis players) can lead to osteophyte formation.

Symptoms

The cardinal symptoms are pain and limitation of motion. Intermittent locking and joint swelling with local warmth may also be present.

Clinical Diagnosis

The range of elbow motion is assessed in relation to the opposite side. Flexion and extension are often decreased, with little or no limitation of pronation and supination. Large osteophytes are sometimes palpable in thin patients.

The differential diagnosis includes a range of conditions that can limit elbow motion (see Sect. 7.18.1).

Radiographs

Apparent osteophyte formation should always be differentiated from superimposed structures. It can be very difficult to confirm osteophytes in the olecranon fossa, except in pronounced cases where the fossa is filled in with osteophytes.

MRI

MRI has a supportive role in the evaluation of osteophytes, particularly in the olecranon fossa (Fig. 8.4-1). It adds very little, however, in cases with unequivocal clinical symptoms and findings.

Arthroscopic Findings

The following are sites of predilection for osteophytes of varying size:

- **Coronoid process**
- **Radial portion of the humeral anterior surface**
- **Coronoid fossa**
- **Olecranon tip**
- **Olecranon fossa**

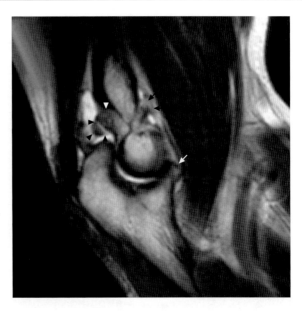

Fig. 8.4-1. MRI of an elbow with a flexion and extension deficit. The image shows a large osteophyte in the olecranon fossa (*arrowheads*) and small osteophytes in the coronoid process (*arrow*) and coronoid fossa (*arrows*)

When osteophytes are accompanied by synovitis, a partial synovectomy is necessary so that the true size of the osteophytes can be assessed.

Function testing under arthroscopic control will show whether an osteophyte is actually causing a block to elbow motion. Maximum flexion of the joint tests for osteophyte impingement in the anterior compartment, while maximum extension tests for impingement in the olecranon fossa (Fig. 8.4-2).

Therapeutic Management

The treatment of choice for isolated osteophytes is surgical removal. The presence of osteophytes in both the anterior and posterior compartments is a sign of advanced joint wear. Resected osteophytes are likely to recur, especially if the patient resumes his or her former physical activity or continues it at an increased level. The potential for osteophyte recurrence should be explained to the patient before surgery.

Isolated osteophytes have a relatively favorable prognosis. Repetitive trauma to the olecranon fossa in throwing sports (javelin, handball) or sports that involve forced extension or hyperextension of the elbow (bowling, tennis) predispose to osteophyte formation. Because the osteophyte is caused by contact between the olecranon and olecranon fossa, it is also termed a "kissing lesion." It has been reported that most of these osteophytes occur in the ulnar portion of the olecranon fossa.

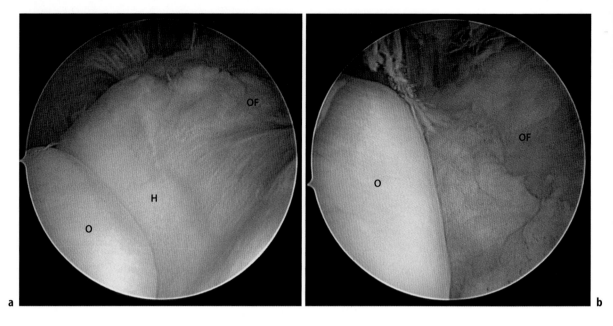

Fig. 8.4-2a, b. Function testing to exclude posterior bony impingement. **a** With the arm hanging freely, the olecranon tip (*O*), humeral posterior surface (*H*), and olecranon fossa (*OF*) are visualized with the arthroscope. **b** When the elbow is maximally extended, the tip of the olecranon should not impinge on the olecranon fossa

We have not seen this in our own cases, finding instead that isolated osteophytes are about equally distributed between the ulnar, central, and radial portions of the olecranon fossa.

The primary treatment goal with isolated osteophytes is to restore joint motion. This contrasts with the primary goal for multiple osteophytes, which is to improve joint function (reduce pain and irritation) before attempting to increase the range of motion.

Operative Technique

The general operative technique for osteophyte removal is basically the same, regardless of the site of occurrence.

1. **Determining size.** Usually the true size of an osteophyte is appreciated only after performing a partial synovectomy and then moving the joint through a range of motion.

2. **Partially detaching the osteophyte.** The osteophyte is partially detached with a fine chisel. Often it is necessary to cut around the base of an osteophyte in the olecranon fossa and then pry it loose. Another method is to remove the osteophyte with a shaver (small or large round bur) or laser. Because the pos-

terior joint space can be quite small, it can be very tedious and time-consuming to grind down a large osteophyte with a bur, since the joint tends to lose distention as the resected particles are suctioned out.

3. **Extracting the osteophyte.** The partially detached osteophyte is grasped, avulsed, and extracted with a grasping forceps under arthroscopic control.

4. **Smoothing the resection site.** The resection site is smoothed with a bur or fine rasp. An electrocautery probe (ball-tipped electrode) can provide simultaneous fine smoothing and hemostasis.

5. **Function testing** (see Fig. 8.4-2). The joint is moved through maximum flexion and extension to check for residual impingement at the resection site. Osteophytes on the opposing articular surface are excluded or removed if necessary.

Fig. 8.4-3 a–f. Osteophyte on the coronoid process. **a** Inspection ▶ of the anteromedial corner of the elbow reveals a large osteophyte (*O*) on the coronoid process (*CP*). The osteophyte impinges on the humerus (*H*) even at 90° of flexion. Marked synovitis (*SY*) is present. A trial needle (*N*) is used to determine the optimum position for the anteromedial portal. **b, c** Partial synovectomy is performed with a shaver (*S*) before the chisel (*C*) is introduced. **d, e** The osteophyte is partially detached with the chisel, then grasped and extracted with a grasping forceps (*G*). **f** The resection site on the coronoid process is smoothed with a shaver

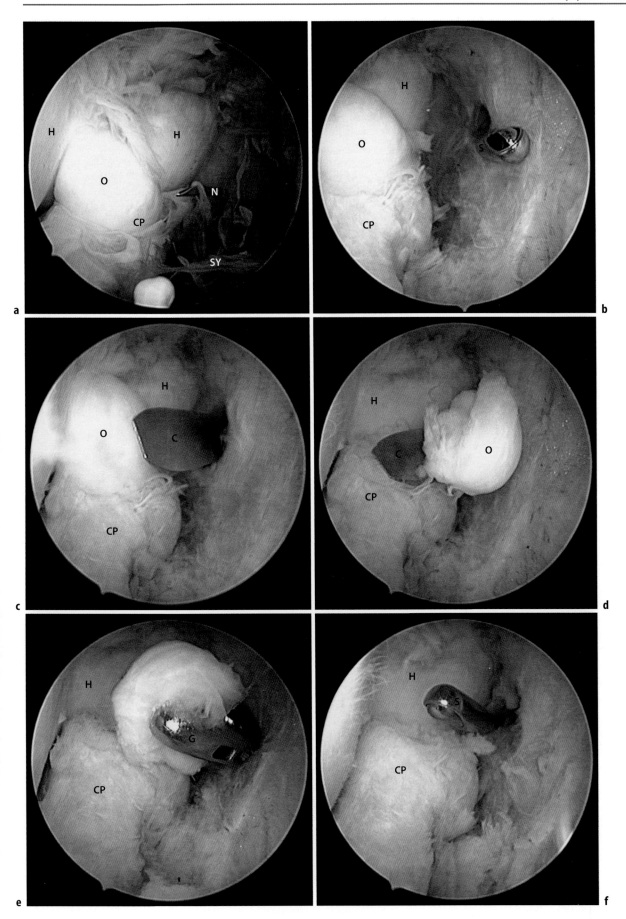

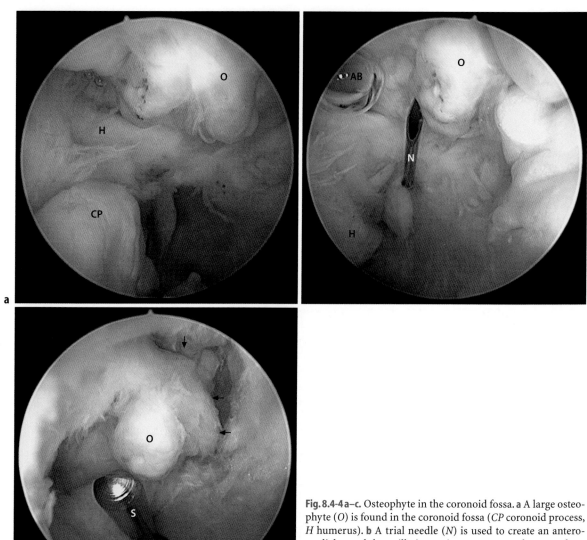

Fig. 8.4-4 a–c. Osteophyte in the coronoid fossa. **a** A large osteophyte (*O*) is found in the coronoid fossa (*CP* coronoid process, *H* humerus). **b** A trial needle (*N*) is used to create an anteromedial portal that will give optimum access to the osteophyte (*AB* air bubble). **c** The osteophyte has been partially detached (*arrows*) with a chisel. If vision is obscured, a synovectomy should be performed with a shaver (*S*) before the osteophyte is extracted with a grasping forceps

Osteophyte Removal from the Coronoid Process
(Fig. 8.4-3)

With the arthroscope in the anterolateral portal, the elbow is maximally flexed to check for osteophyte impingement on the coronoid fossa. If bony impingement occurs, the coronoid process is partially resected. This requires accurate positioning of the anteromedial portal. If the portal is placed too far posteriorly (i.e., just anterior to the humeral surface), it will not be possible to reach the coronoid process with a straight instrument. The portal must be very accurately positioned, therefore.

Osteophyte Removal from the Coronoid Fossa
(Fig. 8.4-4)

Osteophytes may fill the coronoid fossa so extensively that they completely cover the coronoid process during flexion. Even if osteophytes are resected from the coronoid process, bony impingement can still occur. Therefore the caudal portions of the osteophyte are removed while viewing the site from the anterolateral portal. Optimum placement of the anteromedial instrument portal is essential for successful removal.

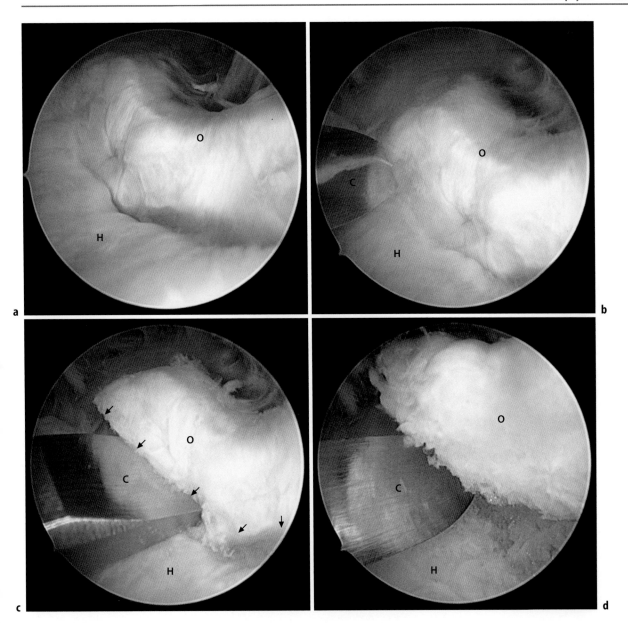

Osteophyte Removal from the Olecranon Tip

The osteophyte is visualized through the high posterolateral portal. The instrument portal is posterocentral. A mirror can also be passed through this portal to determine the size of the osteophyte and evaluate its contact with the olecranon fossa. A small chisel makes a good resection instrument.

Osteophyte Removal from the Olecranon Fossa
(Figs. 8.4-5 and 8.4-6)

The osteophyte is visualized through the high posterolateral portal and instrumented through a posterocentral portal. After impingement is assessed, large osteo-

Fig. 8.4-5 a–d. Osteophyte in the olecranon fossa. The patient, a 51-year-old man, had an extension deficit of 20°. **a** The osteophyte (*O*) completely fills the olecranon fossa (*H* humeral posterior surface). **b** A chisel (*C*) is inserted through the posterocentral portal. **c, d** The osteophyte is partially detached from the humerus (*arrows*)

phytes are circumscribed at their base with a chisel or osteotome to create a breakpoint for subsequent removal. Smaller osteophytes are partially detached and extracted.

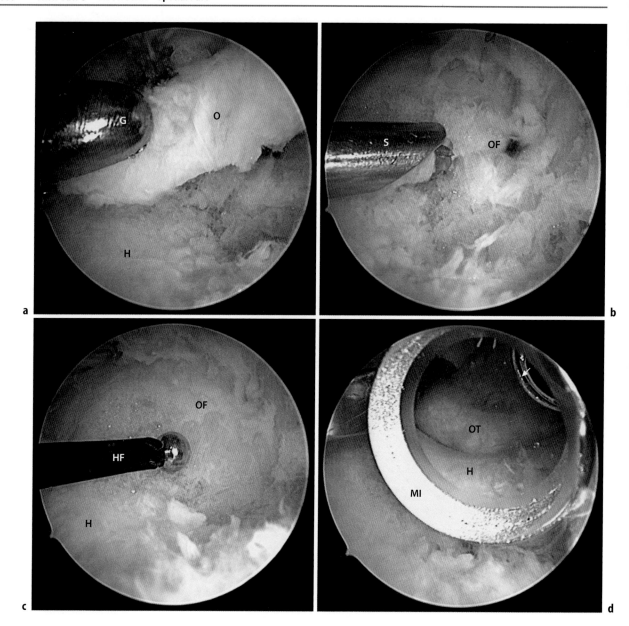

Fig. 8.4-6 a–d. Osteophyte removal from the olecranon fossa (continued from Fig. 8.4-5). **a** The osteophyte is grasped with a forceps (*G*) and extracted (*H* humerus). **b** The olecranon fossa (*OF*) is smoothed with a round burr (*S*). **c** Final smoothing is performed with a file and ball-tipped cautery probe (*HF*). **d** Inspection of the olecranon tip (*OT*) with a mirror (*MI*) (*arrow* tip of scope) confirms that the olecranon tip and olecranon fossa are free of significant osteophytes

Postoperative Care

Osteophyte removal is followed by gentle physical therapy that is below the patient's pain threshold. Traction exercises and careful passive mobilization are beneficial.

▶ **Caution:** Painful exercises and manipulations can incite a painful capsular reaction (capsular fibrosis) leading to elbow stiffness or even reflex sympathetic dystrophy. A gentle program is especially important when multiple osteophytes have been removed, since improved range of motion is not the primary goal of treatment in these patients.

8.5 Scarring and Adhesions

Cause

Elbow adhesions most commonly result from trauma (fractures, dislocations, etc.) or prolonged immobilization.

Symptoms

The predominant complaints are pain and limitation of motion (extension and/or flexion deficit).

Mild degrees of contracture are troublesome only if they interfere with personal, occupational, or athletic activities or are accompanied by significant pain. More severe motion loss can seriously compromise personal hygiene and other activities of daily living.

Clinical Diagnosis

Areas of pain and tenderness and elbow range of motion are assessed clinically. The motion loss may affect pronation and supination in addition to flexion/extension. The differential diagnosis should include all conditions that can cause limitation of elbow motion (see Sect. 7.18.1).

Radiographs

Calcifications in ligaments signify an extraarticular component of the motion loss. If films demonstrate pronounced periarticular calcifications, arthroscopy should not be performed. If the motion loss is the result of a fracture, attention must be given to the bony configuration and position of the joint. If bony deformity is responsible for the motion loss, arthroscopic treatment is unlikely to be of benefit.

MRI

MRI is useful for demonstrating associated lesions. It can also show a decreased intraarticular volume and fibrotic thickening of the joint capsule.

Arthroscopic Findings

Adhesive bands may be found in the anterior and posterior compartments, and scar tissue may fill the olecranon fossa. If range of motion is severely limited, arthroscopy may show extensive scarring that almost obliterates the joint cavity in some cases. It can be extremely difficult to perform elbow arthroscopy under these conditions.

Therapeutic Management

The main goal of surgical treatment is to improve the range of elbow motion. In patients with terminal motion loss that is causing minimal functional debilitation, the main goal of treatment is to relieve pain.

A preoperative prognostic evaluation is not only helpful to the surgeon but also helps the patient to maintain a realistic level of expectations.

Favorable prognostic factors are:
- **Extension deficit only (<20°)**
- **Flexion deficit only (<20°)**
- **No degenerative changes**
- **No extraarticular calcifications**
- **No osseous changes**

Unfavorable prognostic factors are:
- **Motion loss of long standing**
- **Motion loss following an infection**
- **Manipulation under anesthesia following an infection**
- **Several months of painful physical therapy**
- **Reflex sympathetic dystrophy**
- **Periarticular calcifications**
- **Several weeks' immobilization following a dislocation**
- **Bony deformity**

Because it can be extremely difficult to establish the arthroscope portal and perform surgical manipulations, this type of surgery is best reserved for experienced arthroscopists.

Operative Technique

The operative technique is basically the same as when treating adhesions in the knee. Isolated adhesive bands are divided, and plaquelike scars are divided or resected if at all possible (see Sect. 2.12.5).

Anterior Adhesions
(Fig. 8.5-1)

1. **Arthroscope portal.** After the joint has been distended and the inflow placed in the high posterolateral portal, the distention of the anterior capsule is tested with a needle (see Fig. 7.13-8). If the needle test does not confirm adequate anterior joint distention, the surgeon must proceed very carefully. The arthroscope sheath is advanced directly toward the humeral anterior surface with a slight twisting motion.

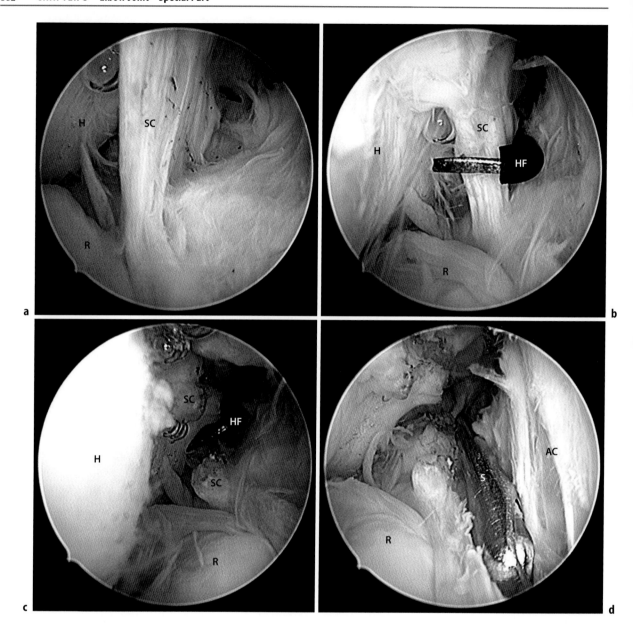

2. **Inspection.** It may be possible to see very little of the joint interior. The rest is obscured by whitish structures representing scar tissue (Fig. 8.5-1 a). The next step in this situation is to establish an anteromedial portal despite the poor visibility.

3. **Removal of adhesions.** The joint cavity is enlarged by resecting the scar tissue with a small synovial resector, or a small meniscus cutter should be used if the adhesions are very firm (Fig. 8.5-1 c). The proximal radioulnar joint next to the coronoid process is also cleared of scar-tissue bands; usually this requires interchanging the viewing and instrument portals.

Fig. 8.5-1 a–d. Adhesions in the anterior compartment following a radial head fracture. **a** Much of the anterior compartment is obscured by adhesive bands (*SC*) (*H* humerus). **b** Often it is difficult to create an anteromedial portal under arthroscopic control. The cautery device (hook electrode) (*HF*) is inserted through the anteroradial portal. (*H* humeral anterior surface, *R* radial head) **c** Vision is greatly improved after cutting the adhesive bands (*SC*) and **d** resection with the shaver (*S*) (*AC* anterior capsule)

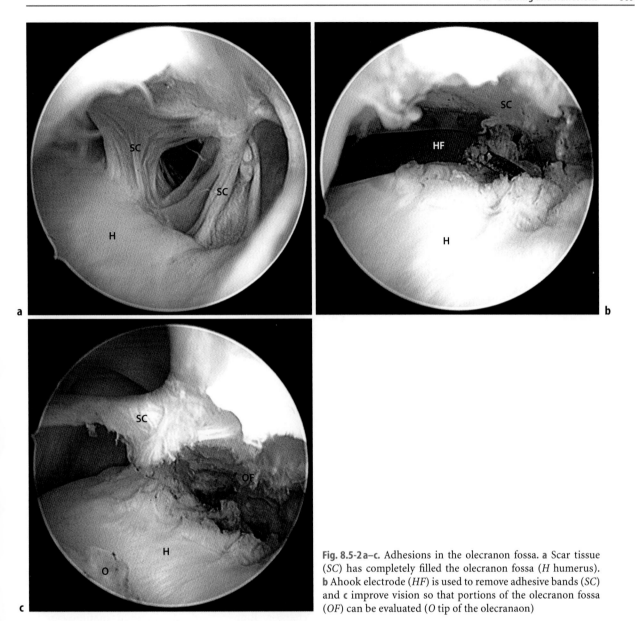

a

b

c

Fig. 8.5-2a–c. Adhesions in the olecranon fossa. a Scar tissue (*SC*) has completely filled the olecranon fossa (*H* humerus). b Ahook electrode (*HF*) is used to remove adhesive bands (*SC*) and c improve vision so that portions of the olecranon fossa (*OF*) can be evaluated (*O* tip of the olecranaon)

4. **Releasing the anterior capsule.** With a severe extension deficit, the anterior capsule can be very carefully released from the humeral shaft. If the other portions of the joint are free of adhesions, this measure alone has a good chance of improving the extension deficit.

5. **Testing range of motion.** Forcible manipulation under anesthesia is not advised. It is much better to divide the major adhesive bands and rely on gentle physical therapy to improve elbow motion. Forcible mobilization will invariably causing tearing of capsular structures, leading to a recurrence of scarring and elbow stiffness. In addition, capsular and muscular tears can cause severe postoperative pain that seriously hampers rehabilitation.

Scar Tissue in the Olecranon Fossa
(Fig. 8.5-2)

1. **Inspection.** The normal boundaries of the olecranon fossa are obscured by scar tissue (arthroscope in high posterolateral portal).

2. **Removal of scar tissue.** The scar tissue is removed with a synovial resector passed through the posterocentral portal. Scar tissue may completely fill the olecranon fossa, obliterating its normal concavity. This plaquelike tissue can be shelled out of the fossa with an electrocautery probe (hook electrode) and then extracted. Another option is to excise the scar tissue with a small meniscus cutter or synovial resector.

Postoperative Care

Physical therapy following arthrolysis for ligament-related motion loss is one of the most challenging tasks in rehabilitative therapy. Aggressive exercises can lead to pain and incite a capsular reaction or even capsular fibrosis, making it difficult or impossible to restore joint motion. The following errors are typical and all too common:

- **Exercising past the pain threshold**
- **Forcible flexion and extension exercises**
- **Long exercise sessions (lasting several hours)**

> ▶ **Caution:** Aggressive rehabilitation can actually decrease the range of elbow motion compared with the preoperative baseline.

Because of these problems, the surgeon and physical therapist must properly coordinate their efforts in order to achieve a successful outcome. We recommend inpatient treatment at a rehabilitation center that is equipped to deal with these problem cases.

It is normal for a decrease in motion to occur about 2–3 weeks into rehabilitation as a result of scar formation. This temporary deficit will usually resolve by about the 4th week.

In the absence of contraindications, an oral nonsteroidal antirheumatic agent (NSAR) such as indomethacin should be administered for 2–3 weeks.

8.6 Osteoarthritis

Cause

Degenerative changes in the elbow joint may be a result of trauma or repetitive overuse.

Symptoms

Symptoms include pain (warm-up pain), progressive limitation of motion (extension deficit), recurrent effusions, occasional warm sensation, and intraarticular crepitus.

Radiographs

Radiographs show typical degenerative changes such as joint space narrowing, marginal spurring and osteophytes. These changes are frequently accompanied by intraarticular loose bodies.

Arthroscopic Findings

In addition to varying grades of cartilage damage (see Sect. 8.2, Fig. 8.6-1), arthroscopy may reveal intraarticular loose bodies (see Sect. 8.3). Synovitis is invariably present (see Sect. 8.1). A partial synovectomy must be performed before the extent of osteophyte formation (see Sect. 8.4) can be assessed.

Therapeutic Management

The primary goal is to relieve pain by reducing joint irritation. In most patients with advanced degenerative changes, little or no gain in joint motion can be achieved.

Arthroscopic treatment consists of treating the cartilage lesions (see Sect. 8.2), loose body removal (see Sect. 8.3), partial synovectomy (see Sect. 8.1), and osteophyte removal as required (see Sect. 8.4).

Postoperative Care

Postoperative care consists of gentle exercises, especially traction techniques, and careful passive mobilization. Nonsteroidal antirheumatic agents (if not contraindicated) will support the remission of joint irritation. Activity modification (change of job or sports activities) is strongly advised in young patients and patients with advanced degenerative changes.

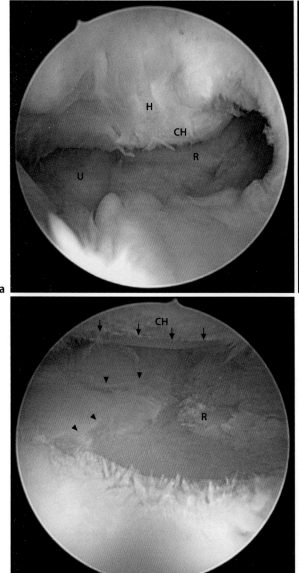

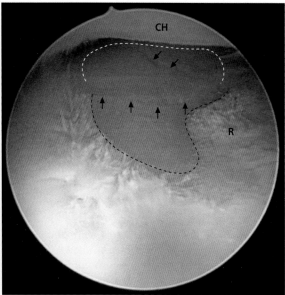

Fig. 8.6-1 a–c. Osteoarthritis following a radial head fracture. **a** Inspection from the posterior side reveals cartilage lesions on the humeral posterior surface (*H*) and capitellum (*CH*) (*R* radial head, *U* ulna) (arthroscope in high posterolateral portal). **b** The radial head features exposed bone areas (*dashed lines*) and fibrocartilage-filled gaps (*arrows*) representing old fracture lines. **c** Exposed bone (*arrows*) is also visible on the capitellum (*CH*). Note the fibrocartilage-filled fracture lines on the radial head (*arrowheads*)

8.7 Osteochondritis Dissecans (Panner Disease)

Cause

Caused by aseptic necrosis of the capitellum, Panner disease occurs predominantly in athletically active adolescents due to repetitive overloading of the radioulnar joint (gymnastics, power sports, basketball, volleyball, handball).

Symptoms

Complaints range from nonspecific pain (often misinterpreted initially as "growing pains") and intermittent snapping to intermittent or permanent locking of the joint. Effusion and intraarticular crepitus may also occur.

Diagnosis

Sites of pain and tenderness are assessed by palpation. In the initial stages, pain can be elicited by pressure over the capitellum. No specific tests are known. Osteochondritis dissecans should always be suspected in young patients with a specific history of humeroulnar joint overuse.

Radiographs

Early Panner disease is often undetected on AP radiographs, which show only a faint lucent area in the capitellum. Radiographs in advanced cases show subchondral sclerosis, contour irregularities, or an intraarticular loose body.

MRI

MRI can define the location, extent, and stage of the osteochondral process. Images may show partial or complete separation of the osteochondral fragment from its bed, possibly accompanied by intraarticular effusion (Fig. 8.7-1).

Arthroscopic Findings

The arthroscopic staging system for osteochondritis dissecans (see Sect. 2.7, p. 297) can also be used to describe osteochondritis dissecans of the capitellum.

Therapeutic Management

The goal of treatment is to preserve the cartilaginous and articular contours of the humeroradial joint. Treatment therefore includes the removal of unstable fibrillations. A sclerotic area is perforated by antegrade or retrograde drilling to prevent further separation.

If only chondral involvement is seen, the unstable cartilage areas are removed, and the remaining defect is treated by subchondral abrasion or microfracture to induce reparative fibrocartilage formation.

Partially separated fragments should be reattached if possible. If the fragment is completely separated and is associated with multiple cartilage fissures or has only a small bony component, the fragment can be removed and the crater treated by subchondral abrasion or microfracturing. In the case of a large fragment with a large bony component, reattachment should be attempted (e.g., using Ethipins or cannulated small-fragment screws).

The younger the patient and the more open the epiphyseal growth plates, the better the prognosis. Closed growth plates imply a less favorable prognosis.

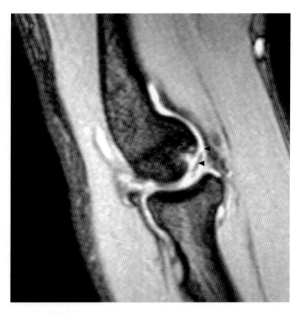

Fig. 8.7-1. MRI in Panner disease. An osteochondral fragment (*arrowheads*) has separated from the capitellum

Operative Technique

The operative technique is basically the same as for osteochondritis dissecans in the knee (see Sect. 2.7) (Figs. 8.7-2 and 8.7-3).

Postoperative Care

Patients who have undergone retrograde drilling or subchondral abrasion should avoid elbow loads and athletics for at least 8–10 weeks. Range of motion exercises are allowed starting in the second postoperative week.

Fig. 8.7-2 a–e. Osteochondritis dissecans of the capitellum (Panner disease), stage IV. **a** Inspection of the humeroulnar joint through a high posterolateral portal initially shows a large loose body (*LB*) (*H* humerus, *U* ulna). **b** The loose body and surrounding synovitis (*SY*) obscure the radial head (*R*) and capitellum. **c** A low posterolateral portal is placed using a trial needle (*N*), and **d** the loose body is removed with a grasping forceps (*G*). **e** The loose body is extracted under arthroscopic control to avoid (or promptly detect) losing the loose body within the joint or subcutaneous tissue

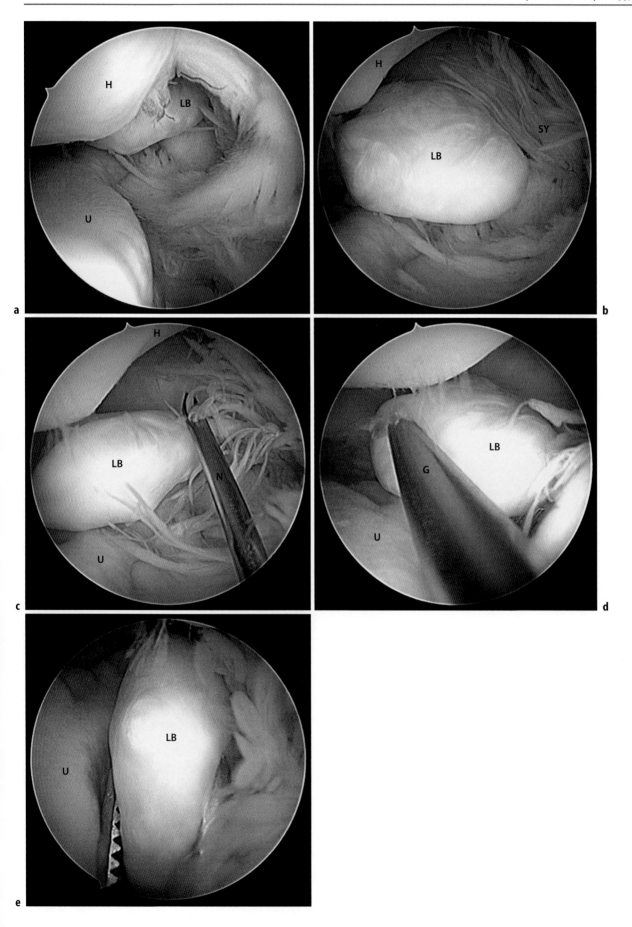

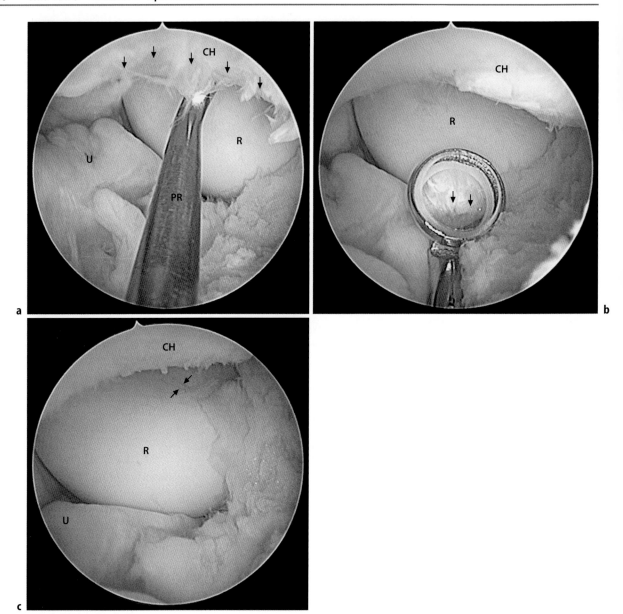

Fig. 8.7-3 a–c. Osteochondritis dissecans of the capitellum (stage IV) (continued from Fig. 8.7-2). **a** The capitellum (*CH*) probed to identify unstable areas and locate the origin of the osteochondral fragment (*arrows*) (*PR* probe). Note the fibrillated cartilage lesions (*arrows*) along the margin of the defect (*R* radial head, *U* ulna). **b** Inspection of the cartilage surface with a mirror reveals fine cartilage fibrillations (*arrows*). **c** After the fibrillations have been debrided from the capitellum, the radial head is inspected. The cartilage fissures (*arrows*) on the radial head were caused by intermittent catching of the osteochondral fragment between the articular surfaces

8.8 Radial Head Fracture

Cause

A fall onto the arm.

Symptoms

Pain, swelling, and limitation of motion.

Clinical Examination

Physical examination reveals tenderness and swelling over the radial head. With a fresh injury, radiographs should be obtained before a detailed clinical examination is performed.

Radiographs

Radiographs confirm the occurrence of a fracture and define its pattern and displacement.

Arthroscopic Findings

Arthroscopy can demonstrate the fracture line and fragment angulation after blood clots are removed. The scope is placed in the anteromedial or high posterolateral portal.

Therapeutic Management

Treatment may be open or arthroscopic. Arthroscopically assisted internal fixation is an option for wedge fractures and minimally displaced fractures but is still in its clinical "infancy." A routine technique has not yet been established.

Arthroscopic treatment includes clearing the joint of old blood clots, removing small loose chondral fragments, and arthroscopically assisted internal fixation.

Attention should be given to the capsular tears that may accompany a radial head fracture. These can allow considerable fluid extravasation into the periarticular tissues, causing massive soft-tissue swelling or even a compartment syndrome in the forearm. These complications are detected by intermittently palpating the proximal forearm during arthroscopically controlled stabilization of the fracture.

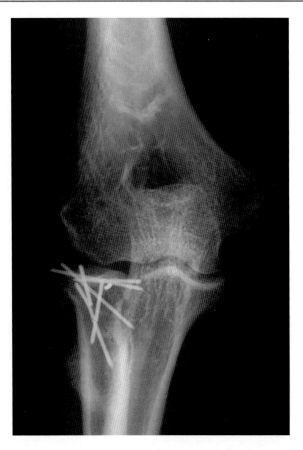

Fig. 8.8-1. Limitation of motion following the internal fixation of a comminuted radial head fracture with multiple Kirschner wires

Operative Technique

Internal Fixation

The displaced fragment is reduced with the arthroscopic probe or a Kirschner wire "joy stick" under arthroscopic control. The reduced fracture is then temporarily fixed with a Kirschner wire. A cannulated small-fragment screw is inserted over the wire (or over a second K-wire) into a predrilled and tapped hole, and the Kirschner guidewire is removed. Two screws are recommended for secure fixation. Reduction and screw insertion are performed under fluoroscopic control.

We cannot yet offer a standard operative technique, because the procedure is not (yet) routine.

Hardware Removal
(Figs. 8.8-1 to 8.8-3)

Arthroscopy can be used to evaluate the condition of the stabilized fracture and also remove the internal fixation hardware. This can be difficult in the presence of intra-articular adhesions or anterior capsular fibrosis with elbow stiffness (Fig. 8.8-1).

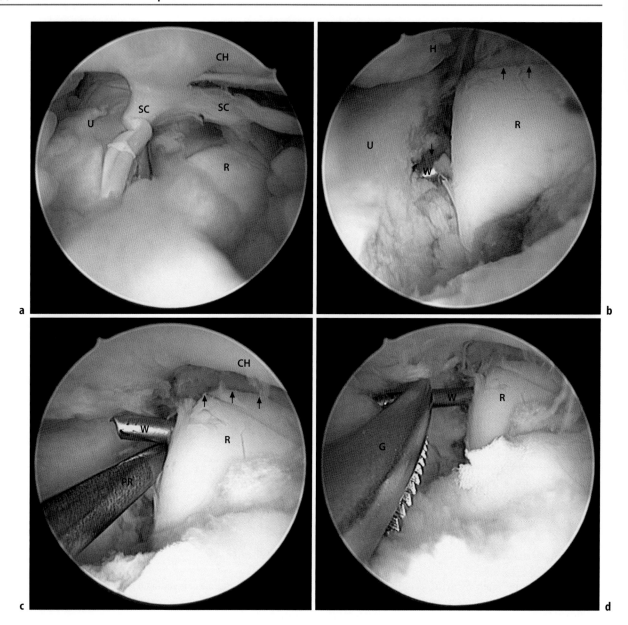

1. **Inspection and probing.** The internal fixation hardware is often covered by scar tissue and fibrocartilage, making it difficult to locate (Fig. 8.8-2).

2. **Identifying the hardware.** The internal fixation hardware can be exposed by performing a partial synovectomy and removing the scar tissue. The intraarticular findings should be correlated with the radiographic findings at this stage to ensure that the correct portion of the radial head is being searched. The surgeon should proceed very carefully if radiographs show hardware projecting from the radial head that may impinge on adjacent bones (ulna, humerus). If a shaver is used to expose the internal fixation material, the inner blade of the instrument may break if it

Fig. 8.8-2 a–d. Limitation of motion 6 months after the internal fixation of a comminuted radial head fracture with multiple Kirschner wires (see Fig. 8.8-1). **a** Inspection from the posterior side shows multiple adhesive bands (*SC*) that obscure the radial head (*R*) (*CH* capitellum, *U* ulna). **b** Removal of the adhesions reveals unhealed fracture lines (*arrows*) on the ulnar portion of the radial head (*R*). A Kirschner wire (*W, arrow*) extends from the radial head into the ulna (*U*) and thus contributes to the loss of pronation and supination (*H* humerus). **c** The wire is palpated with the probe (*PR*). The ulnar fragment of the radial head is still unstable. **d** The wire (*W*) is extracted with a grasping forceps (*G*)

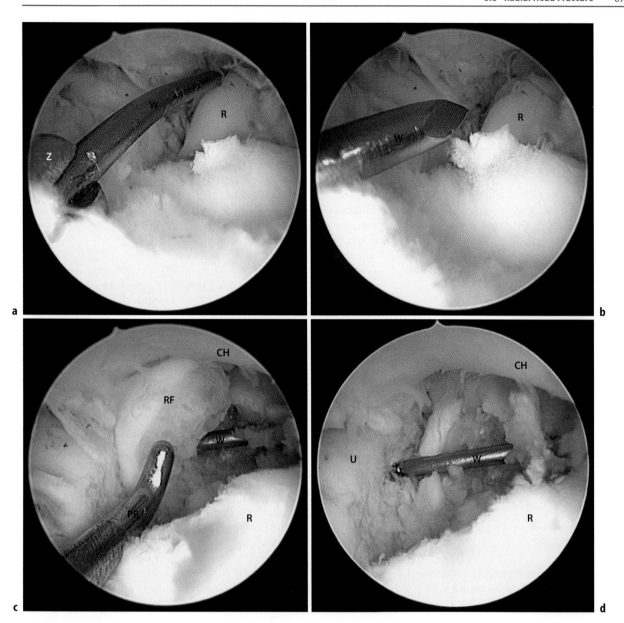

strikes the projecting hardware (see Fig. 7.15-1). The surgery can be facilitated by using probes to retract adhesive bands or using electrocautery to transect obstructive adhesions.

3. **Removing the hardware.** The removal technique depends on the type of hardware used (Kirschner wires, screws). Screws are partially removed with a screwdriver and then grasped and twisted the rest of the way out with a grasping forceps (see Sect. 2.7, p. 297, for technique). Kirschner wires can be removed from the bone with a fine grasping forceps or mosquito clamp (Fig. 8.8-2) and extracted from the joint with a small grasper or needle holder (Fig. 8.8-3). If the fixation hardware is difficult to locate, it may be better

Fig. 8.8-2a–d. Limitation of motion following a comminuted radial head fracture (continued from Fig. 8.8-2). **a, b** The Kirschner wire (*W*) is removed with a grasping forceps (*G*) (*R* radial head). **c** Probing of the unstable radial head fragment (*RF*) reveals another Kirschner wire (*W*). The stable portion of the radial head (*R*) is at the bottom of the field. **d** Removal of the unstable radial head fragment shows that the second wire also fixes the radial head to the ulna, creating an "arthrodesis" of the proximal radioulnar joint. The second wire is also removed

to leave the material in situ if it does not project past the circumference of the radial head. Otherwise it should be removed under fluoroscopic control to shorten the operating time and avoid a traumatizing and perhaps fruitless search for the internal fixation material.

8.9 Infection

Cause

An elbow infection may result from an intraarticular injection, percutaneous aspiration, arthroscopy, or hematogenous spread from an extraarticular focus. The main causative organism is Staphylococcus aureus.

Symptoms

Patients manifest typical signs of inflammation. If the infection develops after an intraarticular cortisone injection, the symptoms may be masked, causing considerable delay in diagnosis and treatment.

Clinical Diagnosis

If infection is suspected from the history and clinical signs, the joint should be aspirated for white blood count and sensitivity report. A WBC higher than 35,000 confirms intraarticular infection (see also Sect. 2.18, p. 663).

Radiographs

Radiographic changes (joint space narrowing, articular surface destruction) are seen only in more advanced stages.

MRI

MRI can demonstrate the intraarticular effusion and reactive synovitis that are associated with intraarticular infection. Gadolinium-enhanced images are more accurate in defining the extent of the infection.

Arthroscopic Findings

As in any infected joint, elbow arthroscopy will reveal the variable morphologic changes that are characteristic of intraarticular infection (see Sect. 2.18, p. 663).

Therapeutic Management

Infection constitutes an emergency indication for elbow arthroscopy. There is no time to wait for culture results, but the WBC of the aspirate can be determined quickly and easily (see Sect. 2.18).

Arthroscopic treatment is basically the same as in other joints (see Sect. 2.18).

If the infection has already caused advanced destructive joint changes, the patient should understand that a complete functional recovery cannot be achieved and that additional surgical procedures may be necessary.

Postoperative Care

Early, gentle postoperative mobilization of the elbow is desired. Exercises should be below the pain threshold and should be planned in close cooperation with the physical therapist. The therapist should contact the surgeon at once if there is any recurrence of pain, swelling, or redness during rehabilitation in an ambulatory setting.

8.10 Outlook and Personal Experience

The elbow is probably one of the most sensitive of the human joints in its response to trauma. Thus one can appreciate the special importance of arthroscopy and arthroscopically assisted internal fixation and implant removal in the elbow. At the same time, the tight confines of the elbow joint place limits on what can be accomplished using arthroscopic techniques. It is reasonable to expect that the arthroscopically assisted treatment of radial head fractures in particular will become increasingly popular during the next few years. Our experience to date in based on 394 elbow arthroscopies performed at our center from 1992 to 2000. We have had very encouraging results with arthroscopic arthrolysis, finding the cause of the motion loss to be a significant factor. Posttraumatic joint stiffness with anterior capsular fibrosis or periarticular calcifications have proven to be problem cases that cannot be satisfactorily treated with arthroscopy. Nevertheless, when we consider the variety of pathologic changes that can be addressed and the range of technical options that are available, we must conclude that the future outlook of elbow arthroscopy holds great promise.

PART V

Shoulder Joint

Shoulder – General Part

The shoulder ranks second only to the knee in terms of the frequency of arthroscopic procedures. The shoulder consists of the glenohumeral joint, whose capacious size makes it excellent for arthroscopy, and the subacromial space. Strictly speaking, the term "arthroscopy" can be applied only to the glenohumeral joint, and "bursoscopy" is more appropriate for the bursa-occupied subacromial space. The acromioclavicular (AC) joint is also part of the shoulder and is accessible to arthroscopic procedures, if only to a limited degree.

9.1 Historical Development

As early as 1931, the American surgeon Michael Burman examined 25 shoulder joints in cadavers with an arthroscope. Almost 50 years passed before shoulder arthroscopy began to develop as a clinical tool. Older reported his initial experience with shoulder arthroscopy in 1976, and similar reports were published by Johnson in 1980 and 1981 and by Caspari in 1982. Andrews published a 1983 report on shoulder arthroscopies in 120 patients.

While shoulder arthroscopy was initially done solely as a diagnostic procedure (as in other joints), today arthroscopy of the glenohumeral joint and subacromial space has gained an established role in both diagnosis and treatment.

9.2 Instrumentation (Arthroscopy System)

The same instruments are required as in the knee joint (see Sect. 1.2). A large-bore sheath (at least 6 mm) should be used to deliver adequate fluid pressure for distention. A smaller sheath diameter may require establishing a separate inflow portal in some procedures.

9.3 Video System

The video system components are the same as those used in knee arthroscopy (see Sect. 1.3). The surgeon performs shoulder arthroscopy in a standing position, and this should be considered when positioning the monitor (just below eye level).

9.4 Probe

The probing hook is an essential tool. It is used both to palpate intraarticular structures and to assess the result of the surgery (e. g., checking the extent of bone removal for subacromial decompression; see Fig. 10.10-9).

9.5 Operating Instruments

Shoulder arthroscopy utilizes the same mechanical, motorized, and electrosurgical instruments that are used in the knee (see Sect. 1.6).

Laser use has been described in the arthroscopic treatment of shoulder instability, but its efficacy has not yet been established. Detailed studies are still needed on arthroscopic laser-assisted capsular shift procedures based on thermal shrinkage of the capsule.

Specialized instruments for repairing the anterior glenoid labrum and other applications are described under the appropriate headings.

9.6 Anesthesia

General or regional anesthesia can be used. Given the potential for circulatory compromise in the beach chair position (see Sect. 9.7.2), general anesthesia is preferred. This also provides effective muscular relaxation and the

option for controlled hypotension if vision is obscured by intraoperative bleeding.

The best of the regional techniques (supraclavicular and interscalene blocks) for postoperative plain relief is the interscalene plexus block described by Winnie.

9.7 Positioning

Two positioning methods are commonly used for shoulder arthroscopy: the lateral decubitus position and the beach chair position. Each has its own advantages and disadvantages.

9.7.1 Lateral Decubitus Position

The patient is placed in a lateral position with the back even with the edge of the table (Fig. 9.7-1). The torso is supported by side rests mounted anteriorly at the level of the thoracic outlet and posteriorly at the level of the pelvis. Bony prominences (elbow and fibular head on the downside) are carefully padded.

It should be considered that the glenoid cavity of the scapula serves as the reference plane for the glenohumeral joint. If the patient is positioned in strict lateral decubitus, the articular surface of the glenohumeral joint will be tilted anteriorly. This joint is directed laterally either by rolling back the patient's torso about 30° onto a beanbag or by tilting the operating table.

This position requires a special shoulder traction system that permits adjustments in abduction, anteversion, and distraction. A forearm wrap connects the arm

Fig. 9.7-1. Shoulder arthroscopy in the lateral decubitus position with an overhead traction system

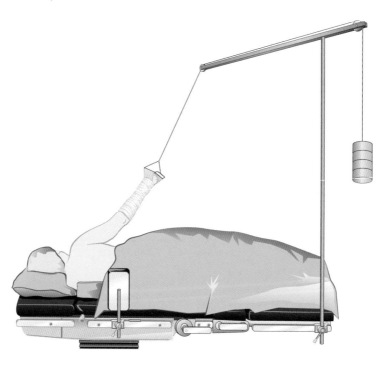

securely to an overhead traction device without risk of localized compression injury to the soft tissues. The arm is positioned in approximately 45° of abduction and 15° of anteversion with a traction weight of 4–8 kg. More than 45° of abduction or heavier traction could lead to brachial plexus injury.

▶ **Advantages**
- Free access to the scapula
- Controlled amount of arm traction
- Facilitates glenohumeral surgery

▶ **Disadvantages**
- Need for traction device (arm holder)
- Time consuming
- Greater risk of position-related injuries (localized pressure injury to the down arm, plexus stretch injury)
- Complex padding
- Complex draping
- Difficult conversion to an open procedure

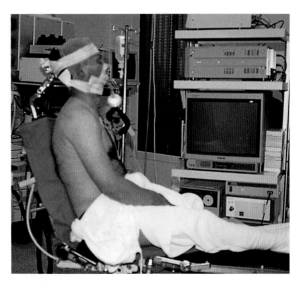

Fig. 9.7-2. Beach chair position

9.7.2 Beach Chair Position

When this position is used, it is important to keep the full circumference of the shoulder accessible during the operation. An extended head rest is used that supports the head and places the shoulder past the edge of the operating table so that it is accessible from both the anterior and posterior sides (Fig. 9.7-2).

▶ **Advantages**
- Allows for rapid conversion to an open procedure
- Normal vertical orientation of shoulder anatomy
- Well suited for subacromial procedures
- Lower cost
- Saves time
- Facilitates draping

▶ **Disadvantages**
- Difficult or poor visualization of the medial scapular margin
- Risk of hypotension

The position that is chosen depends on the experience of the surgeon and the type of surgery that is planned. With its relative simplicity and conversion options, the beach chair position has become our standard position for shoulder arthroscopy.

9.8 Draping

Draping technique depends on the position.

Lateral Decubitus Position
For arthroscopy in the lateral decubitus position, the patient should be covered with a drape prior to skin preparation to protect the patient from antiseptic solution running off the skin. The arm is sterilely wrapped and secured in the traction device, and the shoulder area is covered with two sterile aperture drapes, one placed from the axillary side and the other from the cranial side.

Beach-Chair-Position
For beach-chair arthroscopy, the arm is abducted at the shoulder during the skin preparation; a towel protects the patient's body from solution running off the skin. Next the patient is covered to the chest with sterile fabric drapes. A waterproof adhesive aperture sheet is placed over the shoulder from the cranial side, and a smaller adhesive drape is placed from the axillary side. The arm is wrapped in a waterproof towel drape secured with adhesive tape (Fig. 9.8-1). The cranial sheet is stretched over the patient's head to form a screen for the anesthesiologist, who sits next to the contralateral shoulder.

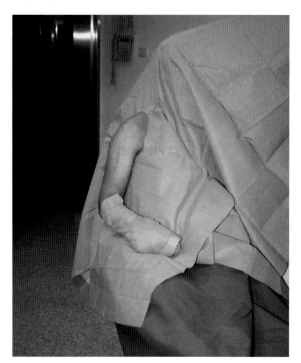

Fig. 9.8-1. Draping for shoulder arthroscopy in the beach chair position

9.9 Distention Medium

Because shavers and electrocautery will be used, the joint is distended with a nonelectrolytic solution (e.g., Purisole).

Intraoperative bleeding is a greater threat to arthroscopic vision than in any other joint. Thus, a gas medium may be considered for the diagnostic survey. When a fluid medium is used, a high intraarticular pressure must be maintained to improve vision. This can be done by suspending the reservoir bag from a ceiling lift or a special motor-driven stand (see Fig. 1.11-4). But since most modern operating rooms have lower ceilings than "old" suites built more than 40 years ago, it can be difficult to increase the distention pressure by raising the fluid reservoir. This problem can be solved by using a pressure-controlled roller pump (see Fig. 1.11-2).

9.10 Setup and Preparations for Arthroscopy

When the beach chair position is used, the surgeon stands posterolateral to the operative shoulder. This area is not accessible to the anesthesiologist, who sits cranial to the contralateral shoulder. The first assistant stands lateral to the patient's upper arm, and the scrub nurse stands next to the instrument table at the level of the patient's pelvis. The arthroscopy cart is on the opposite side of the operating table.

9.11 Portal Placement

Portals are available for accessing the glenohumeral joint, subacromial space, and AC joint.

9.11.1 Gross Anatomy

Before the portals are created, it is necessary to palpate the bony structures about the shoulder. The principal landmarks are the clavicle, AC joint, acromion, coracoid process, and scapular spine. Surgeons with little experience in shoulder arthroscopy should outline these structures with a marking pen.

The entire shoulder is covered by the deltoid muscle. The anterior portion of the muscle arises from the lateral half of the clavicle, its middle portion from the acromion, and its posterior portion from the scapular spine. It inserts on the deltoid tuberosity of the humerus. The anterior, lateral, and posterior portals penetrate the deltoid muscle, and its fibers can be seen as the arthroscope is withdrawn at the end of the procedure.

The axillary nerve supplies the deltoid muscle and passes with the posterior circumflex humeral artery through the axillary quadrangular space, which is bounded above by the inferior border of the teres minor muscle. Thus, the axillary nerve relates closely to the "classic" posterior portal for glenohumeral arthroscopy (Fig. 9.11-1).

9.11.2 Glenohumeral Portals

Posterior Portal

This portal serves as the primary arthroscope portal. It is placed approximately 2–3 cm inferior and 1–2 cm medial to the posterolateral corner of the acromion. This position corresponds to the palpable "soft spot" of the posterior shoulder (Fig. 9.11-1).

▶ **Tip:** Because this portal is also used for subacromial arthroscopy, we recommend placing it approximately 1–2 cm inferior to the posterolateral corner of the acromion, or slightly higher than the standard posterior portal site.

Anterior Portals

The two anterior portals – anterior superior and anterior inferior – are used for instrumentation or inflow. They can also be used to inspect the posterior portion of the glenohumeral joint after the arthroscope and instrument portals have been switched.

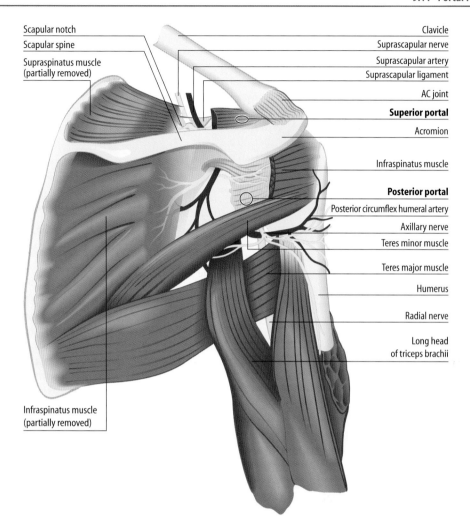

Scapular notch
Scapular spine
Supraspinatus muscle
(partially removed)

Clavicle
Suprascapular nerve
Suprascapular artery
Suprascapular ligament
AC joint
Superior portal
Acromion

Infraspinatus muscle

Posterior portal
Posterior circumflex humeral artery
Axillary nerve
Teres minor muscle

Teres major muscle

Humerus

Radial nerve

Long head
of triceps brachii

Infraspinatus muscle
(partially removed)

Fig. 9.11-1. Location of the posterior glenohumeral portal and the superior subacromial portal. The deltoid muscle and portions of the supraspinatus and infraspinatus muscles have been removed (posterior aspect, see text for details). (After Esch 1993)

▶ **Caution:** To avoid neurovascular injury when creating the anterior portals, keep the following rules in mind:
- **Do not abduct the arm more than 45°.**
- **Always place the portals above the subscapularis tendon.**
- **Never place portals medial to the coracoid process.**

Superior Portal

- **Anterior superior portal.** This portal is established just anterior to the biceps tendon.

- **Anterior inferior portal.** This portal is placed just proximal to the subscapularis tendon. Structures most at risk from the anterior portals are the cephalic vein in the deltopectoral interval and the musculocutaneous nerve. The latter runs about 4–5 cm inferior to the coracoid process but may be as close as 1 cm to the coracoid process if it perforates the coracobrachialis muscle at that level.

The superior portal (Neviaser portal, supraspinatus portal) is placed approximately 1 cm medial to the acromion between the clavicle and scapular spine and is used for instrumentation or inflow. Structures at risk are the suprascapular nerve and suprascapular artery, which run in the scapular notch. The scapular notch is located about 2 cm medial to this portal.

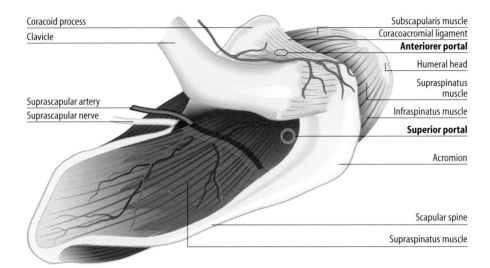

Coracoid process
Clavicle

Suprascapular artery
Suprascapular nerve

Subscapularis muscle
Coracoacromial ligament
Anteriorer portal
Humeral head
Supraspinatus muscle
Infraspinatus muscle
Superior portal
Acromion

Scapular spine
Supraspinatus muscle

Fig. 9.11-2. Location of the anterior and superior portals for subacromial arthroscopy (superior aspect, see text for details)

9.11.3 Subacromial Portals

Subacromial arthroscopy is possible through posterior, anterior, lateral, and superior portals (Fig. 9.11-2).

1. **Posterior subacromial portal.** The same skin incision is used as for the posterior glenohumeral portal (see above). Creation of the portal is facilitated by placing it just 1–1.5 cm inferior to the posterolateral corner of the acromion (see above).

2. **Anterior subacromial portal.** This portal is placed lateral to the coracoacromial ligament.

3. **Lateral subacromial portal.** This portal is placed distal to the lateral acromial border under arthroscopic vision. It is located approximately 2 cm posterior to the anterolateral acromion and just below the subacromial sulcus, which is usually palpable. The portal should take the shortest path through the soft tissues into the subacromial space to facilitate outflow and avoid excessive fluid collection in the subcutaneous tissue.

4. **Superior subacromial portal.** The subacromial space can also be reached from the superior glenohumeral portal.

9.11.4 Acromioclavicular Portals

An anterior and a posterosuperior portal are known. Both give direct access to the AC joint. Alternatively, the AC joint can be reached through the subacromial space.

9.11.5 Creating the Glenohumeral Arthroscope Portal: Technique

The posterior portal is the standard primary arthroscope portal. In creating this portal, it is helpful to mark the anatomic landmarks on the skin (clavicle, acromion, scapular spine) along with the coracoid process and coracoacromial ligament. The portal is created in the following sequence of steps:

1. **Palpation.** The soft spot between the infraspinatus and teres minor muscles is palpated approximately 1–2 inferior and 1 cm medial to the posterolateral corner of the acromion.

2. **Skin incision.** A 3–4 mm incision is made through the skin only. A deeper incision is avoided, as it could needlessly transect deltoid muscle fibers and cause bleeding.
   ▶ **Tip:** Preliminary joint distention, though recommended in other joints like the ankle and elbow, is not advised in the shoulder, because failure to place the needle precisely in the glenohumeral joint will result in troublesome fluid extravasation.

3. **Sheath insertion.** The sheath with blunt obturator is advanced toward the glenohumeral joint and coracoid process with a careful twisting motion.
   ▶ **Tip:** Placing the thumb of the free hand just proximal to the palpable posterior soft spot and the index finger on the coracoid process will help the surgeon aim for the glenohumeral joint (Fig. 9.11-3).

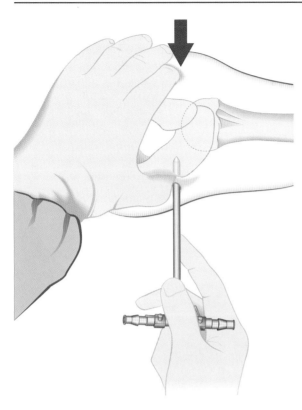

Fig. 9.11-3. Insertion of the sheath and blunt obturator. The tip of the coracoid process (*arrow*) is palpated with the index finger during sheath insertion

As the sheath is twisted during insertion, the obturator will penetrate the deltoid bluntly by pushing its fibers aside. The tip of the blunt obturator is used to palpate the posterior glenoid rim and humeral head and locate the intervening joint space. The capsule is penetrated on the joint line. A marked decrease in resistance confirms that the sheath has entered the glenohumeral joint.

4. Distention. The joint is distended with fluid. To make certain that the fluid is distending the glenohumeral joint rather than extraarticular soft tissues, the blunt obturator is removed and the scope inserted. If intraarticular structures can be seen after several milliliters of fluid has been instilled, the distention is continued. If articular structures (humeral head or biceps tendon) cannot be seen, the sheath may be outside the joint.

9.11.6 Creating the Glenohumeral Instrument Portal: Technique

Either of two techniques can be used to create the anterior instrument portals:

- Inside-out technique using a switching stick (Wissinger rod).
- Outside-in technique using a percutaneous needle.

Switching Rod (Wissinger Rod) Technique of Portal Placement
(Fig. 9.11-4)

1. Visualizing the portal site. The anterior superior portal is placed just anterior to the biceps tendon, and the anterior inferior portal just proximal to the subscapularis tendon. The arthroscope is advanced to the desired portal area, which is within a triangle formed by the biceps tendon, glenoid, and subscapularis tendon.

2. Advancing the Wissinger rod. The arthroscope is fixed in this position and pressed lightly against the anterior capsule. Then the scope is removed, and the Wissinger rod or switching stick is inserted through the sheath from the posterior side and advanced

Fig. 9.11-4. Inside-out placement of the anterior glenohumeral portal using a switching rod (*SR*) (Wissinger rod). The skin is incised at the point where the rod tents the skin over the anterior shoulder (*arrow*)

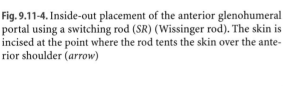
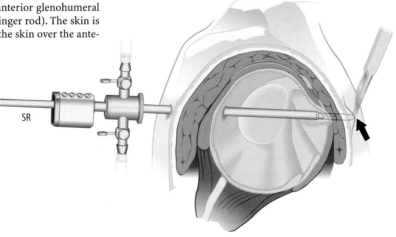

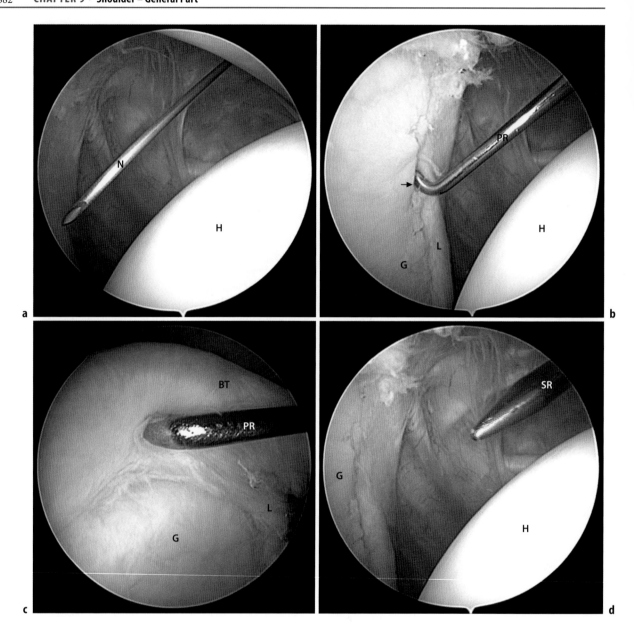

through the anterior capsule above the subscapularis tendon. The surgeon palpates the tip of the rod subcutaneously on the anterior side of the shoulder.

3. **Skin incision.** A 2–3 cm skin incision is made over the palpable tip of the rod, and the rod is advanced through the anterior skin.

4. **Inserting a working cannula.** A working cannula is passed over the rod and into the joint from the anterior side. Then the Wissinger rod is withdrawn, and the scope is reinserted into the sheath. When the joint has been redistended, the working cannula can be seen in the anterior inferior portal. It is used to introduce the probe and operating instruments (shaver, electrocautery, etc.).

Fig. 9.11-5 a–d. Placement of the anterior glenohumeral portal. **a** The optimum portal site is located with a percutaneous needle (*N*) (*H* humeral head). **b** The probe (*PR*) is introduced. An irregularity (*arrow*) in the labrum (*L*) is palpated with the probe (*G* glenoid). **c** The origin of the long biceps tendon (*BT*) is probed. **d** A switching rod (*SR*) is inserted to interchange the arthroscope and instrument portals

Needle Technique of Portal Placement
(Fig. 9.11-5)

1. **Positioning.** The arthroscope is advanced to the area in which the anterior inferior portal will be placed (see above). In thin patients, the light spot from the arthroscope can be seen through the anterior skin.

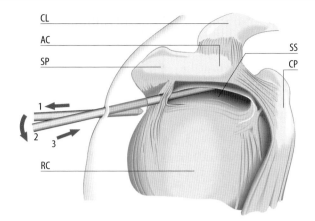

CL
AC
SP
SS
CP
1
2
3
RC

9.11-6

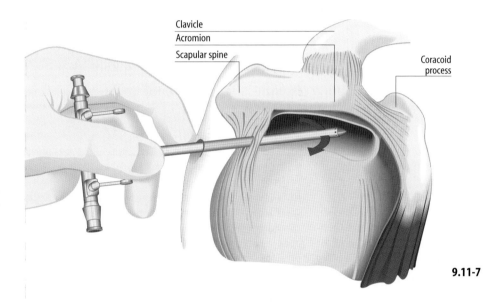

Clavicle
Acromion
Scapular spine
Coracoid process

9.11-7

2. **Locating the portal site with the needle.** A percutaneous needle is inserted from the anterior side. It should penetrate the anterior capsule just above the subscapularis tendon. If the needle is incorrectly placed, it is reinserted at a different site.

3. **Skin incision.** When the needle is properly positioned, a 3–4 cm skin incision is made at the insertion site, the needle is removed, and the subcutaneous tissue is spread open.

4. **Inserting a working cannula.** A working cannula with blunt obturator is carefully inserted with a twisting motion until it enters the glenohumeral joint. Arthroscopic vision confirms intraarticular placement of the cannula at the intended portal site. Another technique is to develop the portal with a blunt clamp, which is opened after perforating the capsule. Then a probe, operating instrument, or switching stick can be introduced (Fig. 9.11-5 b, c).

Fig. 9.11-6. Establishing access to the subacromial space. After insertion of the blunt obturator, the sheath and obturator are first pulled back (*1*) and then angled superiorly (*2*) and advanced into the subacromial space (*3*) (*SP* scapular spine, *AC* acromion, *CL* clavicle, *CP* coracoid process, *RC* rotator cuff, *SS* subacromial space)

Fig. 9.11-7. The sheath with blunt obturator is swept medially and laterally to lyse adhesions in the subacromial bursa

9.11.7 Creating the Subacromial Arthroscope Portal: Technique

This portal is created following arthroscopic inspection of the glenohumeral joint (Figs. 9.11-6 and 9.11-7)

1. **Positioning the patient.** When arthroscopy is performed in the lateral decubitus position, it may be

necessary to decrease arm abduction to 15° and rotate the arm slightly forward while keeping it extended. Initially the arthroscope remains in the glenohumeral joint. The scope is then withdrawn, and a blunt obturator is inserted into the sheath.

2. **Entering the subacromial space.** The sheath with obturator inserted is backed out of the glenohumeral joint (Fig. 9.11-6). The sheath can be felt exiting the joint space. The obturator-armed sheath is then angled superiorly and advanced toward the acromion (Fig. 9.11-7). It is first swept medially and laterally to lyse bursal adhesions that would obstruct vision.

▶ **Caution:** Avoid injuring the subdeltoid fascia during this maneuver. Lesions of the fascia can increase fluid extravasation into the soft tissues, hampering the rest of the procedure.

3. **Improving orientation.** Percutaneous needles can be inserted at the lateral border and anterolateral corner of the acromion and at the AC joint to improve orientation in the subacromial space after insertion of the scope.

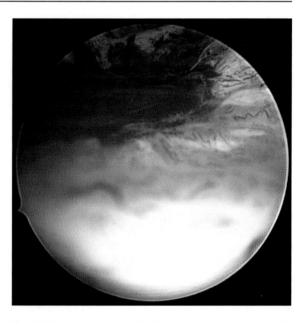

Fig. 9.12-1. Intraoperative bleeding can obscure vision in the subacromial space

9.11.8 Creating the Subacromial Instrument Portal: Technique

An anterior instrument portal is created next. This can be done from inside out using a Wissinger rod or switching stick, as described for the glenohumeral joint, or from outside in using a percutaneous needle (see above).

9.11.9 Acromioclavicular Portals

This superficial joint can be entered with a percutaneous needle from the anterior side and distended with fluid. The arthroscope portal is created by inserting a second needle from the posterosuperior side. Fluid backflow confirms that the needle is intraarticular. A 1–2 mm skin incision is made at the insertion site, the subcutaneous tissue is carefully spread open, and a sheath with blunt obturator is inserted. Because the AC joint is very small, we recommend using the "wrist scope" from the small-joint instrument set (see p. 748, Fig. 5.2-1). The anterior needle remains in the AC joint and if necessary can be used to redistend the joint.

When the sheath is within the joint and the scope has been inserted, the inflow line is connected to the sheath. The needle technique is used to establish the anterior portal, which is used for instrumentation (e.g., motorized instruments for resecting the articular disk or the lateral end of the clavicle).

9.12 Obscured Vision

Intraoperative bleeding can be a serious impediment to arthroscopy and arthroscopic surgical procedures in the shoulder (Fig. 9.12-1). Bleeding may result from the opening of cancellous bone spaces (subacromial decompression, freshening the bone for an anterior capsule repair) or from the plication, suturing, or division of ligaments when arthroscopy is performed without a tourniquet or exsanguination.

The difficulties are compounded when irrigating fluid extravasates through the various portals into the periarticular tissues, leading to pronounced "shoulder swelling" that increases with the duration of the procedure. This soft-tissue swelling makes it difficult to insert operating instruments and prolongs the operating time.

▶ **Note:** Inadequate visualization due to bleeding is the main problem in arthroscopic procedures.

Various techniques can be used to prevent bleeding and improve vision:

1. **Increasing the distention pressure.** Increasing the distention pressure by raising the reservoir bag or using a roller pump is a simple way to improve arthroscopic vision. However, if multiple instrument portals have been placed, a higher distention pressure will cause increased fluid collection in extraarticular tissues, making it difficult to insert operating instruments and hampering the rest of the procedure.

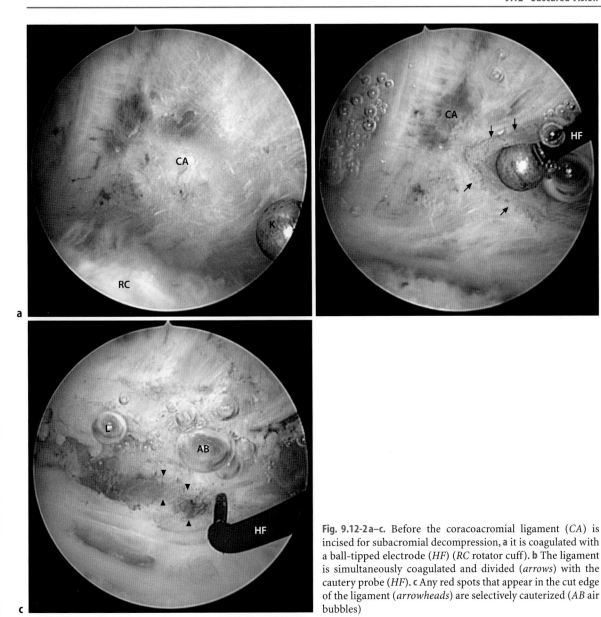

Fig. 9.12-2a–c. Before the coracoacromial ligament (*CA*) is incised for subacromial decompression, **a** it is coagulated with a ball-tipped electrode (*HF*) (*RC* rotator cuff). **b** The ligament is simultaneously coagulated and divided (*arrows*) with the cautery probe (*HF*). **c** Any red spots that appear in the cut edge of the ligament (*arrowheads*) are selectively cauterized (*AB* air bubbles)

2. **Electrocautery.** Actively bleeding vessels or areas of bloody imbibition that are a presumed bleeding source can be coagulated with a ball-tipped cautery probe. We recommend the prophylactic coagulation of tissues that are to be resected or divided (Fig. 9.12-2). This is particularly advised prior to subacromial decompression (see Sect. 10.10).

3. **Epinephrine.** Epinephrine can be added to the irrigating solution to induce vasoconstriction and reduce bleeding. This should be done only after consulting with the anesthesiologist to determine whether the patient's cardiovascular status would contraindicate epinephrine use.

4. **Laser use.** The use of a laser for synovectomy or bone removal (e.g., in subacromial decompression) reduces bleeding owing to the hemostatic effect of laser ablation. Laser use significantly prolongs the operating time, however, and can cause deep osseous lesions that predispose to unpredictable late sequelae (osteonecrosis).

5. **Controlled hypotension.** Hypotensive anesthesia is a proven method of reducing intraoperative bleeding but can be used only in patients without cardiovascular problems.

6. Local infiltration of the portals. The portal sites can be infiltrated with a local anesthetic solution containing epinephrine (1:200,000).

The best way to maintain a clear field is to prevent bleeding through precautionary measures:

- **Practice atraumatic technique.** Never advance the arthroscope or operating instruments "boldly or blindly."
- **Selectively coagulate bleeding sites with the cautery tip.**
- **Coagulate ligamentous structures before cutting them** (Fig. 9.12-2).
- **Coagulate opened cancellous bone areas** (e.g., after subacromial decompression).
- **Coagulate the cut edges of ligaments** (Fig. 9.12-2 c).
- **Keep the operating time as short as possible.**
- **Using sparing, atraumatic technique when establishing portals.**

If bleeding still obscures vision despite these measures, we recommend a slightly increased fluid inflow combined with hypotensive anesthesia.

9.13 Anatomy and Examination Sequence

9.13.1 Anatomy

Humeral Head

The humeral head articulates with the glenoid cavity. It is covered with hyaline cartilage. At the junction of the rotator cuff with the articular cartilage of the posterior humeral head is a cartilage-free area called the "bare spot." This area may present foramen-like irregularities, and blood vessels are occasionally seen (Fig. 9.13-1). The bare spot should not be confused with the Hill-Sachs lesion that results from shoulder dislocation.

Glenoid Cavity

The glenoid cavity of the scapula (hereafter called the glenoid) articulates with the humeral head and is also covered with hyaline cartilage. The glenoid cartilage is usually thinned in its central portion, and this should not be mistaken for chondromalacia.

Glenoid Labrum

The glenoid labrum (hereafter called the labrum) encircles the glenoid, enlarging and deepening its articular surface. The long biceps tendon inserts in the superior portion of the labrum, and the capsule-reinforcing glenohumeral ligaments insert anteriorly.

Two variants in the attachment of the labrum to the glenoid are known. In 60% of cases the central and superior labrum is partially detached from the glenoid

surface. In these cases the labrum can be elevated from the glenoid with an arthroscopic probe. The remaining portions of the labrum (anterior, inferior, and posterior) are firmly attached to the glenoid rim. In the second variant, seen in about 40% of cases, the entire central portion of the labrum is attached to the glenoid. In this case the labrum cannot be separated from the glenoid with a probe.

In 10% to 19% of patients, the anterior superior portion of the labrum contains an opening called the "sublabral hole." This normal variant should not be confused with a Bankart lesion.

Biceps Brachii Muscle

The long head of the biceps brachii arises from the supraglenoid tubercle and partly from the superior labrum (Fig. 9.13-1). The tendon passes anteriorly over the humeral head and enters a funnel-shaped, synovium-lined groove between the greater and lesser tuberosities (the bicipital groove) before descending toward the forearm.

The passage of the long biceps tendon over the top of the humerus accounts for its function as a depressor of the humeral head. As a result, this tendon plays a significant role in rotator cuff tears. Because the long biceps tendon is easy to locate arthroscopically, it provides a key landmark for initiating the arthroscopic survey.

Rotator Cuff

The tendons of the subscapularis, supraspinatus, infraspinatus, and teres minor muscles form the functionally important complex of the rotator cuff. The infraspinatus muscle arises in the infraspinous fossa and inserts on the posterior facet of the greater tuberosity of the humerus. The teres minor muscle runs just inferior to the infraspinatus.

The supraspinatus muscle arises in the supraspinous fossa and inserts on the middle facet of the greater tuberosity. The subscapularis muscle, which arises in the subscapular fossa and inserts on the lesser tuberosity, completes the rotator cuff. The subscapularis tendon is always visible arthroscopically and is an important landmark for placing the anterior glenohumeral portals. The rotator cuff forms the roof of the glenohumeral joint and the floor of the subacromial space. Thus, an intact rotator cuff prevents entry into the subacromial space from the glenohumeral joint.

The most important part of the rotator cuff is formed by the supraspinatus muscle, which is supplied by the suprascapular nerve. This nerve runs through the suprascapular notch in company with the suprascapular artery. The nerve also supplies the infraspinatus and teres minor muscles. The branch to the infraspinatus is at risk during arthroscopic repairs of the anterior capsule and ligaments in shoulder instabilities (transglenoid techniques).

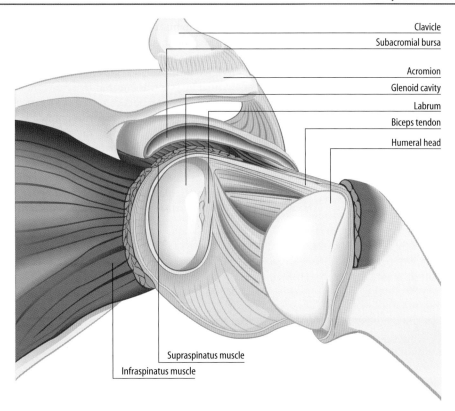

Clavicle
Subacromial bursa
Acromion
Glenoid cavity
Labrum
Biceps tendon
Humeral head
Supraspinatus muscle
Infraspinatus muscle

Fig. 9.13-1. Anterior capsule of the glenohumeral joint under extreme distraction. (Posterior view after removal of the posterior capsule, see text for details) (After Esch 1993)

Joint Capsule

The glenohumeral joint capsule is very capacious and has a large inferior recess called the axillary recess or axillary pouch (Fig. 9.13-1). The large size of the capsule is necessary for adequate shoulder mobility. The anterior and inferior portions of the capsule are reinforced by ligamentous structures. The posterior portion of the capsule is thinner and is devoid of known reinforcing ligaments.

The capsule is attached to the glenoid labrum and inserts into the scapular neck at the base of the labrum. At the origin of the long biceps tendon, the capsule extends past the labrum to the base of the coracoid process. On the humeral side, the capsule arises from the anatomic neck of the humerus, leaving a gap for the long biceps tendon.

The ligaments that reinforce the anterior and inferior capsule are called the glenohumeral ligaments. Three in number, they consist of the superior, middle, and inferior glenohumeral ligaments (Fig. 9.13-1).

1. **Superior glenohumeral ligament.** This ligament is narrow and usually is not visible arthroscopically because it is covered by synovium. Sometimes it winds around the long biceps tendon just before that tendon descends into the bicipital groove.

2. **Middle glenohumeral ligament.** This ligament originates on the anterior superior neck of the humerus medial to the lesser tuberosity and runs to the subscapularis tendon at about a 60° angle before inserting on the anterior and midsuperior glenoid rim. Ranging from a thick band to a thin cord, this ligament is visible arthroscopically between the subscapularis tendon and inferior glenohumeral ligament. Sometimes it relates very closely to the inferior glenohumeral ligament.

3. **Inferior glenohumeral ligament.** This ligament is the most important anterior stabilizing structure. It is actually a ligament complex consisting of an anterior superior band, an inferior axillary band, and a posterior superior band. The anterior superior band arises from the lower humeral neck and inserts on the anterior inferior half of the labrum and glenoid. The axillary band inserts on the inferior circumference at the margin of the labrum and glenoid.

   The posterior superior band inserts on the posteroinferior portion of the labrum. The anterior superior and posterior superior bands form the medial wall of the axillary recess. All the bands show considerable variation in their size, thickness, and location.

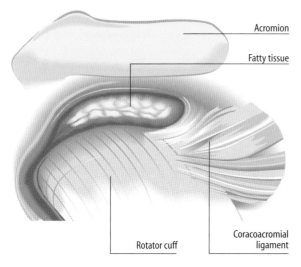

Acromion

Fatty tissue

Coracoacromial
ligament

Rotator cuff

Subacromial Bursa (Fig. 9.13-2)

The rotator cuff and the top of the coracoacromial ligament form the floor of the subacromial space, which is
lined by the subacromial bursa. Because the coracoacromial ligament is covered by synovium and fatty tissue,
often it cannot be recognized as a ligamentous structure
unless exposed. The superior boundary of the subacromial space is formed by the undersurface of the acromion, which is also covered by synovial tissue. The subacromial space is bounded laterally and posteriorly by
the deltoid muscle. The bursa is bounded medially by
very vascular fatty tissue located between the acromial
undersurface and the supraspinatus muscle.

Fig. 9.13-2. Anatomic boundaries of the subacromial space
(after Esch 1993)

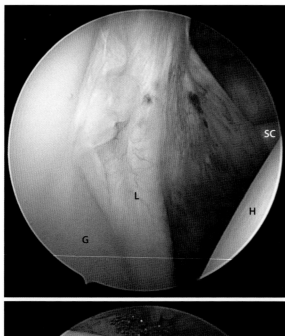

a

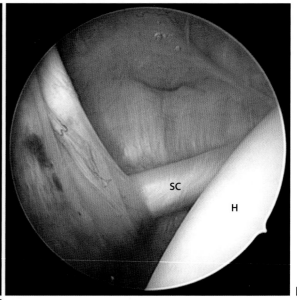

b

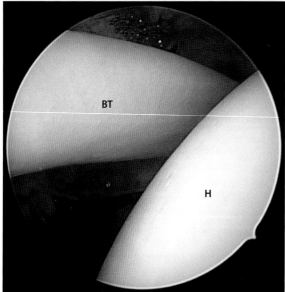

c

Fig. 9.13-3 a–c. Intraarticular orientation. **a** After the arthroscope is inserted into the sheath and the joint is distended, the
labrum (*L*) and part of the glenoid (*G*) can be identified (*H*
humeral head, *SC* subscapularis tendon). **b** The subscapularis
tendon should not be confused with the biceps tendon. **c** The
biceps tendon (*BT*) runs anteriorly over the humeral head

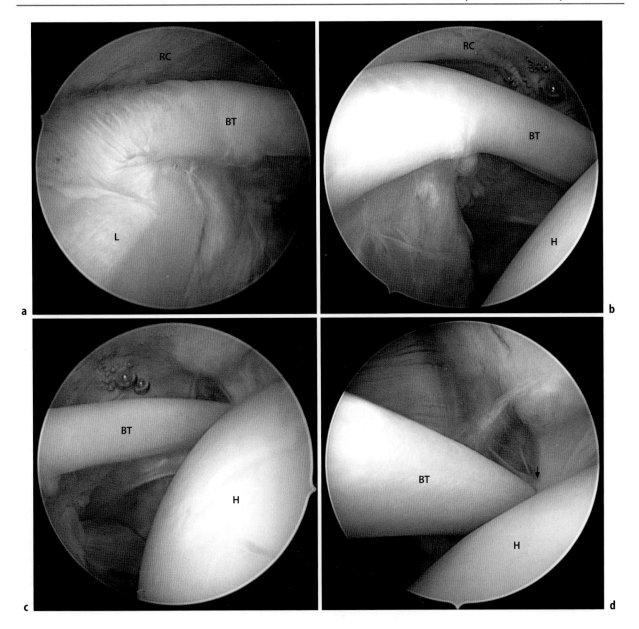

9.13.2 Examination of the Glenohumeral Joint

After the arthroscope has been inserted into the joint and carefully retracted, the first structures to be identified are usually the glenoid and the anterior part of the labrum (Fig. 9.13-3). Angling the arthroscope upward brings the long biceps tendon into view. This tendon is the most important primary landmark for intraarticular orientation. Its entire course can be seen, including its origin on the supraglenoid tubercle and labrum. The biceps tendon runs forward over the humeral head and enters the bicipital groove (Fig. 9.13-4).

Next the anterior capsule and the anterior part of the glenoid and labrum are evaluated. An important land-

Fig. 9.13-4a–d. Inspection of the long biceps tendon. **a** The long biceps tendon (*BT*) arises from the supraglenoid tubercle and partly from the labrum (*L*). It is directly adjacent to the rotator cuff (*RC*). **b** The biceps tendon runs forward and downward over the humeral head (*H*). **c, d** Anterior to the humeral head, the tendon runs distally in a synovial pouch (*arrow*) and enters the bicipital groove

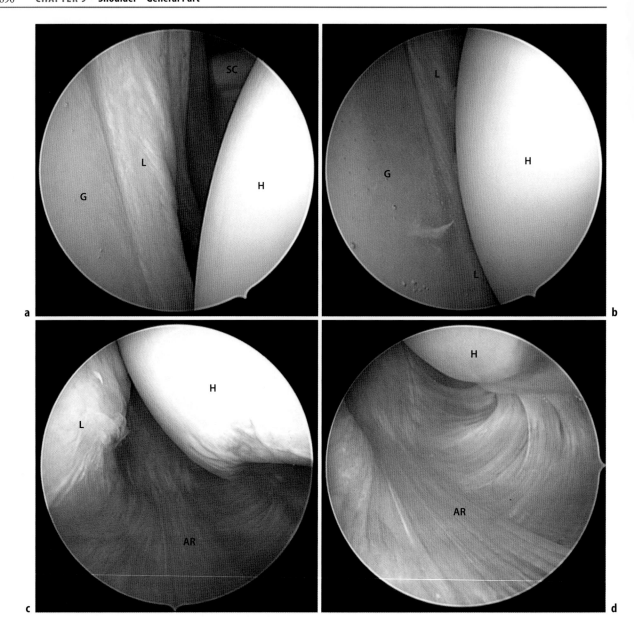

mark on the anterior capsule is the triangle between the subscapularis tendon, superior glenohumeral ligament, and middle glenohumeral ligament (foramen of Weitbrecht). The free edge of the subscapularis tendon is easily identified in most cases (Fig. 9.13-3 b). It is an important landmark for placing the anterior inferior portal.

The anterior portion of the labrum is inspected. It can display many possible anatomic variants in addition to pathologic separations (SLAP lesions, Andrews lesion).

Distal to the middle glenohumeral ligament, the inferior glenohumeral ligament runs almost parallel to the glenoid. It usually appears as a bandlike thickening of the capsule that opens distally toward the inferior recess.

The arthroscope can be retracted to evaluate the glenoid and the posterior glenoid rim as far as the inferior

Fig. 9.13-5 a–d. Inspection of the anterior glenohumeral joint space. The anterior part of the labrum (*L*), the glenoid (*G*), and the humeral head (*H*) can be identified. **a** The subscapularis tendon (*SC*) is visible in the deep portion of the field. **b** Angling the scope downward demonstrates the inferior portions of the labrum (*L*) and glenoid. **c, d** Additional downward angulation of the scope brings the axillary recess (*AR*) into view

recess (Fig. 9.13-5). Angling the scope downward demonstrates the inferior part of the labrum and, below it, the axillary recess (Fig. 9.13-5 c, d).

From there the arthroscope is swung back upward along the humeral head. The posterior aspect of the humeral head features the "bare spot," which should not be mistaken for a Hill-Sachs lesion. The insertion of the rotator tendons on the greater tuberosity (supra- and infraspinatus tendons) can be identified and inspected for partial or complete tears. The arm should be abducted at this time to better visualize the area of insertion.

The posterior joint capsule can be inspected by moving the arthroscope to an anterior portal. The capsule is considerably thinner posteriorly than anteriorly. Sometimes it is reinforced by a cordlike structure representing the posterior inferior band of the inferior glenohumeral ligament.

9.13.3 Examination of the Subacromial Space

First the sheath with blunt obturator is been swept back and forth to lyse fibrous bands and adhesions, and then the subacromial space is distended. At this point the extent of the space can be appreciated. Some anatomic structures are usually difficult or impossible to identify because they are covered by synovium. When a partial synovectomy is performed, the rotator cuff on the floor of the subacromial space can be identified and evaluated for pathology. The acromion and coracoacromial ligament can be identified in the superior portion of the space.

9.14 Complications

Complication rates of 0.8% to 3% have been reported for shoulder arthroscopy. As in other joints, there is probably a high unreported incidence of iatrogenic cartilage lesions. It should be stressed, however, that fluid extravasation occurs in almost every arthroscopic shoulder operation and is not considered a complication (Fig. 9.14-1). Even pronounced extravasation will generally resolve in 1–2 hours without sequelae. It may interfere with the surgical procedure, however, by making it difficult to insert operating instruments. Obscured vision due to bleeding is another very frequent problem in arthroscopic operations.

The following types of complication are discussed below:
- Position-related complications
- Distraction-related complications
- Portal-related complications
- Technique-related complications

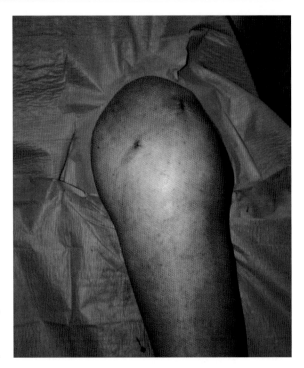

Fig. 9.14-1. "Normal" swelling of the shoulder following arthroscopic subacromial decompression

9.14.1 Position-Related Complications

The beach chair position is associated with postural hypotension, and the anesthesiologist must be prepared for this. Hypoglossal nerve injury has also been reported with this position; it can be prevented by adequate padding.

The lateral decubitus position may be associated with pressure injury to the ulnar nerve in the arm and peroneal nerve in the leg on the downside. Careful padding is necessary.

9.14.2 Distraction-Related Complications

More than 8 kg of traction places strain on the brachial plexus and may even cause traction injury. The traction weight should not exceed 8 kg, therefore. Also, the arm should not be abducted by more than 45°. Traction injuries to the musculocutaneous nerve have been described. The hand and forearm should be carefully padded and adequately secured to the traction device to avoid local pressure injuries and skin lesions.

9.14.3 Portal-Related Complications

A faulty insertion angle can cause undesired entry of the sheath into the subdeltoid bursa or axilla.

Cartilage Lesions

Forcible or aggressive sheath insertion can cause scuffing or scraping injuries to the articular cartilage on the humeral head or glenoid. Labral lesions can also occur.

▶ **Tip:** As in other joints, avoid using a sharp trocar in shoulder arthroscopy.

Nerve Lesions

- **Axillary nerve.** Placing the posterior glenohumeral portal 3–5 cm inferior to the acromion poses a risk to the axillary nerve. Since the nerve is also very close to the axillary recess, it may be injured by an aggressive synovectomy or capsular incisions in the lower part of the joint.

- **Suprascapular nerve.** This nerve runs an average of 1.8 cm medial to the glenohumeral joint. It runs about 3 cm medial to the superior glenohumeral portal.

- **Infraspinous branch of the suprascapular nerve.** This nerve branch is at risk during repairs of the anterior capsule and ligaments and transglenoidal fixation (see Sect. 10.6).

- **Brachial plexus.** The brachial plexus or its branches (median nerve, ulnar nerve, musculocutaneous nerve) are at risk during placement of the anterior portals. As a result, the inside-out Wissinger rod technique is often used in establishing the anterior inferior glenohumeral portal (see p. 881).

- **Musculocutaneous nerve.** This nerve arises from the lateral part of the brachial plexus and runs 2.5–4 cm distal to the tip of the coracoid process. It can penetrate the coracobrachialis muscle at varying levels, and sometimes it runs just 1 cm inferior to the coracoid process. Consequently, the anterior portals should not be placed distal and medial to the tip of the coracoid process.

9.14.4 Technique-Related Complications

Instrument breakage. Instrument breakage is a danger in shoulder arthroscopy as in any other arthroscopic procedure. It can be very difficult to locate instrument fragments that have slipped into the variable recesses of the glenohumeral joint. Retrieval techniques are described in Sect. 1.15.1.

- **Nerve lesions.** Nerves that run anterior or posterior to the glenoid (e.g., the suprascapular nerve and infrascapular branch) are at risk during repairs of the anterior capsule and ligaments (see above).

- **Loosening or breakage of fixation hardware.** Staple fixation was commonly used in the early days of arthroscopic shoulder stabilization. It was not unusual for the staples to loosen or break out of the bone. As a result, staple fixation is no longer practiced today.

- **Bony lesions.** A bone fragment may be broken from the glenoid during the fixation of anterior labral structures.

- **Rotator cuff tears.** Aggressive debridement can convert a partial rotator cuff tear to a full-thickness tear. Partial cuff tears should be debrided with extreme care, therefore.

- **Acromial fracture.** Excessive resection during subacromial decompression can greatly thin the acromion, predisposing it to fracture by even minor trauma. Thus, before performing subacromial decompression the surgeon should evaluate the thickness of the acromion, which is highly variable.

- **Clavicular fracture.** Part of the inferior clavicle is often removed during subacromial decompression. Excessive resection in this area can predispose to clavicular fracture.

- **Infection.** Without doubt, infection is the most feared complication of shoulder arthroscopy. Its management is discussed in Sect. 10.9.

- **Postoperative hemarthrosis.** This complication may follow an extensive synovectomy.

In summary, many unsatisfactory results of arthroscopic shoulder surgery are not the result of complications but of inadequate preoperative evaluation and an undiscriminating approach to patient selection. Arthroscopic stabilizing procedures are particularly demanding and require the use of sound criteria in selecting arthroscopic surgery over open techniques.

9.15 Documentation

Documentation in shoulder arthroscopy should meet the same requirements as in other joints, including a standard report sheet and visual documentation (e.g., video prints; see Sect. 1.16).

9.16 Outpatient Arthroscopy

Most arthroscopic procedures on the shoulder can be performed on an ambulatory basis. This includes numerous arthroscopic stabilization techniques that are used in treating anterior shoulder dislocations. At the same time, it should be possible to convert to an open procedure if technical difficulties arise or unfavorable anatomic conditions are encountered. Often this can be accomplished only in an inpatient setting.

Because subacromial syndromes commonly affect older patients (see Sect. 10.10), facilities must be available to provide appropriate postoperative care following outpatient surgery.

Intraarticular infections should always be treated in a hospital setting.

9.17 Indications

Increasing experience in shoulder surgery and new discoveries in pathomechanics have significantly broadened the range of diagnostic and therapeutic options for shoulder disorders. In almost every case, an accurate preoperative diagnosis can be established by a detailed clinical examination and by ultrasound imaging, which is useful in detecting structural changes. Purely diagnostic arthroscopy should be reserved for highly selected cases.

Whenever a diagnosis is made or confirmed arthroscopically, the surgeon must be able to provide the necessary surgical treatment (arthroscopic or open) in the same sitting.

As in other joints, the indication for arthroscopy is based not on symptoms but on objective findings.

9.17.1 Chronic Pain

If a definitive diagnosis cannot be made despite a detailed clinical examination and noninvasive imaging studies, it is appropriate to proceed with arthroscopy to exclude or confirm intraarticular pathology. Local synovitis, irritation of the long biceps tendon (tendinitis), or generalized synovitis (e.g., due to rheumatoid disease) can lead to chronic shoulder pain.

9.17.2 Locking

Joint locking may be caused by loose bodies, labral tears, or subluxation. Arthroscopy can be used both to establish the diagnosis and, in most cases, to provide definitive treatment.

9.17.3 Loose Bodies

If loose bodies are confirmed radiologically or presumed from clinical findings, it is appropriate to proceed with arthroscopic examination and removal.

9.17.4 Labral Lesions

Labral lesions can lead to pain, limited motion, and intermittent locking. Anatomic variants can be differentiated arthroscopically from labral pathology. In particular, the various types of lesion (e.g., SLAP lesions) can be classified and treated as required.

9.17.5 Rotator Cuff Tears

If a rotator cuff tear is detected by clinical examination and ultrasound imaging, a partial tear can be managed by arthroscopic subacromial decompression, debridement, or a combination of both, depending on the findings. In the case of larger rotator cuff defects (rotator cuff defect arthropathy), the overall condition of the joint should be evaluated.

9.17.6 Subacromial Syndrome

Nonoperatively treated subacromial syndrome, whether caused by impingement, calcium deposits in the rotator cuff, subacromial adhesions, or partial- or full-thickness rotator cuff tears, is an indication for arthroscopy of the subacromial space and is usually an indication for endoscopic subacromial decompression (ESD).

9.17.7 Limitation of Motion

Limitation of shoulder motion requires an accurate differential diagnosis. Adhesive capsulitis ("frozen shoulder") is not based on subacromial pathology but is classified as a separate entity. Limited motion may also be caused by subluxation, loose bodies, labral tears, or a very painful subacromial syndrome.

9.17.8 Biceps Tendon

Besides tendinitis of the long biceps tendon, partial ruptures can be confirmed arthroscopically. Partial and complete tendon ruptures can be managed by debridement of the rupture site.

9.17.9 Shoulder Instabilities

Arthroscopy in shoulder instabilities can exclude or confirm a Bankart lesion, SLAP lesion, local synovitis, a Hill-Sachs lesion, cartilage lesions, glenoid fractures, and loose bodies. In properly selected cases, the anterior capsule and ligaments can be stabilized using arthroscopic techniques.

9.17.10 Infection

Infection of the glenohumeral joint, whether it results from arthroscopy, intraarticular injection, or percutaneous joint aspiration, is a suitable indication for arthroscopic treatment.

9.17.11 Acromioclavicular Joint

Osteoarthritis of the AC joint can be managed in selected cases by arthroscopic resection of the lateral clavicle.

This chapter is divided into sections based on lesions of the glenohumeral joint (Sections 10.1–10.9), the subacromial space (Sect. 10.10), and finally the AC joint (Sect. 10.11).

10.1 Synovitis

Cause

The causes of synovitis in the shoulder are similar to those in other joints (see Sect. 2.3). Local synovitis is commonly found in association with labral lesions and rotator cuff tears. With degenerative changes in the AC joint, osteophytes projecting into the subacromial space can incite a local synovitis (see Sect. 10.11).

Systemic synovial diseases such as rheumatoid arthritis, ankylosing spondylitis, and lupus erythematosus can also be manifested in the shoulder. This is particularly common in rheumatoid arthritis patients.

Symptoms

In addition to pain at rest and during movement, patients complain of swelling and limited motion, particularly when the subacromial space is affected.

Clinical Diagnosis

The clinical examination covers the full battery of diagnostic tests for lesions of the subacromial space (see Sect. 10.10), biceps tendon (see Sect. 10.5), and rotator cuff (see Sect. 10.7).

Radiographs

If destructive cartilage lesions have occurred, secondary degenerative bony changes will usually be apparent on radiographs. Indirect signs such as elevation of the humeral head may indicate concomitant rotator cuff lesions. The AC joint should be evaluated for degenerative changes.

Ultrasound

Ultrasound imaging can demonstrate synovial fronds and effusion in the glenohumeral joint and subacromial space. Associated pathology (rotator cuff tears, biceps tendon lesions, erosive lesions of the humeral head) should also be excluded.

Arthroscopic Findings

The arthroscopic features of synovitis are basically the same as in other joints (see Sect. 2.3) (Fig. 10.1-1). Synovitis in the glenohumeral joint is very often accompanied by subacromial bursitis.

Therapeutic Management

Treatment is geared mainly toward the cause of the synovial changes. In cases of reactive synovitis, it is necessary to treat the inciting cause such as shoulder instability, a labral lesion, or a rotator cuff tear. The same applies to associated pathology such as cartilage lesions and loose bodies.

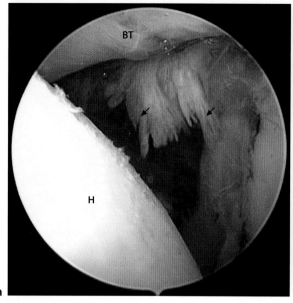
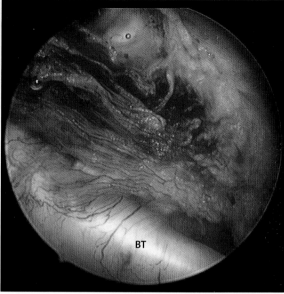

The prognosis depends on the cause. Partial, subtotal, or complete synovectomy can be performed arthroscopically in patients with systemic disease (pigmented villonodular synovitis, synovial chondromatosis, rheumatoid arthritis).

No comprehensive studies have yet been published on arthroscopic complete synovectomy in the shoulder. In theory, however, arthroscopic synovectomy should offer definite advantages in terms of earlier mobilization and less postoperative pain. Arthroscopic synovectomy should be considered, therefore, in settings where the necessary personnel and equipment are available.

Operative Technique

Partial Synovectomy, Synovial Biopsy

Affected areas are removed with a shaver (synovial resector) introduced through an anterior portal.

▶ **Tip:** Proceed very carefully when resecting localized synovitis in the axillary recess due to the close proximity of the axillary nerve.

Complete Synovectomy

It is important to obtain adequate joint distention when performing a complete synovectomy. We recommend using a roller pump to maintain a sufficiently high distention pressure (see Fig. 1.11-2).

1. **Orientation.** If synovial tissue completely fills the joint cavity, the first priority is to establish orientation. Even the anterior inferior portal can be difficult to establish when vision is poor (Fig. 10.1-2 a, b).

Fig. 10.1-1 a, b. Synovitis in the glenohumeral joint. **a** Coarse synovial villi (*arrows*) project into the joint space (*BT* biceps tendon, *H* humeral head). **b** Synovium (*SY*) has partially overgrown the biceps tendon

2. **Anterior synovectomy.** After an anterior portal has been created, it is unnecessary to establish a separate portal for inflow when a roller pump is used. The anterior capsule is synovectomized first. The entire anterior capsule, the anterior part of the axillary recess, and the floor of that recess are accessible through the anterior portal.

▶ **Tip:** Avoid placing additional instrument portals right away in order to minimize fluid extravasation into the periarticular soft tissues.

3. **Superior synovectomy.** An attempt is made to reach the superior joint region, including the long biceps tendon and rotator cuff undersurface, through the anterior portal (Fig. 10.1-2 c). The synovectomy should proceed carefully to avoid the partial or complete resection of a damaged biceps tendon or rotator cuff.

4. **Switching portals.** The arthroscope and instrument portals are interchanged using a switching stick (see p. 881). If it is feared that this will cause excessive fluid extravasation, a working cannula should first be inserted into the posterior portal to seal off the capsular incision.

5. **Posterior synovectomy.** The posterior glenohumeral joint and the posterior wall of the axillary recess can

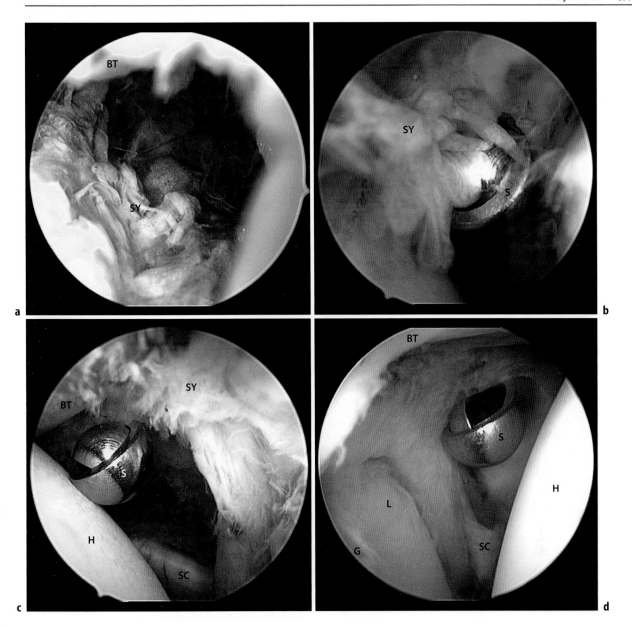

Fig. 10.1-2 a–d. Synovectomy in the glenohumeral joint. **a** Initial inspection shows generalized synovitis (*SY*) with coarse synovial villi obscuring much of the joint interior (*BT* biceps tendon). **b** First, synovectomy is performed with a shaver (*S*) to improve visualization. **c** Then the anatomic structures can be more clearly identified (*H* humeral head, *BT* biceps tendon, *SC* subscapularis tendon). **d** The arthroscope is moved to the anterior portal, and the shaver is inserted through the posterior portal to synovectomize the posterior capsule (*G* glenoid, *L* labrum)

be synovectomized through the posterior portal. The areas of the capsule directly bordering the posterior portal (Fig. 10.1-2 d) may be difficult to reach, and it may be necessary to establish an accessory portal (e.g., anterior superior or Neviaser) (see p. 878).

6. **Synovectomy in the subacromial space.** When the synovectomy in the glenohumeral joint has been completed, the arthroscope is advanced through the posterior skin incision toward the subacromial space, and a lateral instrument portal is created (see p. 880). First the space should be cleared of coarse synovial villi to facilitate orientation. Altered areas of synovium are removed. This may require switching the arthroscope and instrument portals.

7. Drainage. After an extensive synovectomy, an intraarticular suction drain is left in the glenohumeral joint.

Postoperative Care

Gentle mobilization of the shoulder is desired after a complete synovectomy to prevent adhesion formation in the axillary recess. A continuous passive motion splint may be used. Full range of motion should be achieved as quickly as possible.

10.2 Cartilage Lesions

Cause

Cartilage lesions are most commonly the result of shoulder dislocations (e. g., Hill-Sachs deformity). Degenerative changes are rare compared with the knee joint. Cartilage lesions are frequently encountered in joints with chronic synovitis (e. g., due to rheumatoid arthritis).

Symptoms

Complaints are usually based on the inciting cause, such as shoulder instability. When degenerative changes are present, the predominant features are limited motion, rest pain, and/or intraarticular crepitus.

Clinical Diagnosis

Besides a detailed examination of the capsule and ligaments (see Sect. 10.6) and rotator cuff (see Sect. 10.7), the range of motion is determined. The shoulder is also checked for intraarticular crepitus.

Radiographs

Pronounced chondral changes lead to typical degenerative changes that are visible on radiographs (joint space narrowing, marginal osteophytes). With localized cartilage lesions, radiographs may be unrevealing.

Ultrasound

Localized cartilage lesions usually cannot be detected with ultrasound. Other changes such as reactive effusion or a Hill-Sachs lesion can be visualized, but a Bankart lesion cannot.

Arthroscopic Findings

The humeral head and glenoid may display various traumatic and degenerative cartilage lesions that are identical in appearance to cartilage lesions in other joints (see Sect. 2.2). Hill-Sachs cartilage lesions are usually localized to the posterior aspect of the humerus (see Fig. 10.6-4). With advanced osteoarthritic changes (omarthrosis) or rotator cuff defect arthropathy, it is common to find areas of exposed subchondral bone. This may be accompanied by intraarticular loose bodies and variable degrees of reactive synovitis.

Therapeutic Management

Treatment is determined by the underlying disorder, such as shoulder instability. In joints with advanced degenerative changes, treatment consists of intraarticular lavage to remove loose bodies and cellular debris. A partial synovectomy may be necessary for reactive synovitis.

When advanced osteoarthritis is present, the prospects for a successful outcome are diminished, especially in patients with a concomitant severe rotator cuff defect.

The treatment of localized cartilage damage consists of removing unstable cartilage fragments and stabilizing the edges of the defect. This may be supplemented by subchondral abrasion or microfracturing to induce fibrocartilage formation. Because these cartilage lesions are rare in the glenohumeral joint, there is still no experience to report with these techniques in large clinical series.

Operative Technique

The operative technique is basically the same as described in the knee joint (see p. 201). Fibrocartilage induction is described on p. 217.

Postoperative Care

The shoulder joint should be mobilized as early as possible to prevent adhesions. Pushups and other shoulder-loading activities should be avoided for at least four months.

10.3 Loose Bodies

Cause

Chondral or osteochondral fragments may be sheared off by trauma or shoulder dislocation. Synovial chondromatosis is a relatively frequent cause compared with other joints. Avascular necrosis of the humeral head is less common.

Symptoms

Besides the underlying disorder (dislocation, chondromatosis), intraarticular loose bodies can cause sudden shooting pain and locking. Usually, however, typical complaints such as catching, locking, and effusion take some time to develop due to the large capacity of the glenohumeral joint capsule. This also explains why chondromatosis frequently goes undiagnosed until secondary degenerative changes appear.

Clinical Diagnosis

No specific tests are known for diagnosing intraarticular loose bodies. Intraarticular crepitus may be noted in some cases. Clinical diagnosis is geared toward the underlying disorder, such as a shoulder dislocation (see Sect. 10.6).

Radiographs

Calcified loose bodies are visible on X-ray films, and therefore radiography is considered the most important diagnostic modality.

Ultrasound

Ultrasound can demonstrate changes such as Hill-Sachs deformities and intraarticular effusion.

MRI

MRI is unnecessary in cases where a loose body has been detected radiographically and the shoulder has been examined with ultrasound. MRI is recommended, however, to investigate recurrent locking of unknown cause.

Arthroscopic Findings

One or more loose bodies of varying size may be found, depending on the cause. Often they are accompanied by a reactive synovitis that hampers evaluation of the loose bodies. Meanwhile, loose bodies may hide in various joint recesses where they are inaccessible to arthroscopic inspection.

Therapeutic Management

The treatment of choice for loose bodies is removal. When loose bodies are accompanied by other pathology, as in the setting of shoulder instability, it should be determined whether arthroscopic or open repair is necessary or feasible (see Sect. 10.6).

When multiple loose bodies are present, it may not be possible to find all the loose bodies since smaller fragments may "hide" in the various joint recesses. With synovial chondromatosis, a complete synovectomy should be performed and the patient should be informed about the potential for recurrence.

The tactical approach to loose body removal in the shoulder is basically the same as in the knee (see p. 319). To prevent loose bodies from entering the subcutaneous tissue and avoid excessive subcutaneous extravasation, smaller loose bodies are removed first, followed by medium-size and larger bodies. Smaller loose bodies are most easily removed with an irrigation cannula (see Fig. 1.6-23). It is helpful to have a separate instrument portal for inflow if a roller pump is not available. Medium-size loose bodies are extracted with a grasping forceps. With large loose bodies, it may be necessary to fragment the object within the joint and remove it piecemeal.

▶ **Tip:** Because the distance between the skin and joint capsule may be several centimeters (especially if there has been subcutaneous extravasation into the periarticular soft tissues), grip the loose body securely with the grasping forceps so that it will not get lost in the periarticular or subcutaneous tissues.

Postoperative Care

If surgery did not go beyond loose body removal, it is unnecessary to immobilize the shoulder, and normal motion may be resumed on the first postoperative day. Otherwise the postoperative protocol is geared toward the associated pathology.

10.4 Labral Lesions

Cause

Tearing and degenerative changes in the labrum become increasingly common with aging. Hence, the normal aging process should be taken into consideration when evaluating labral pathology. Trauma to the shoulder, such as a fall onto the outstretched arm, can cause traumatic labral tears. Fraying and tearing of the anterior labrum also result from subluxations of the humeral head and are not uncommon in throwing athletes.

Symptoms

Degenerative changes may remain asymptomatic. Larger tears can cause intermittent catching and locking. Often, however, the symptoms are determined by the causal mechanism such as a shoulder dislocation or a direct fall onto the shoulder.

Clinical Diagnosis

No specific tests are known for diagnosing a labral lesion. Pressing the humeral head against the glenoid may elicit a click or snap caused by the torn labral fragment catching between the humerus and glenoid.

Radiographs, MRI

Specific signs of a labral lesion cannot be seen on radiographs. Most larger labral lesions are clearly defined with MRI, however.

Arthroscopic Findings

Numerous anatomic variants of the glenoid labrum have been described. It may extend over the articular surface of the glenoid in a meniscus-like fashion, or its undersurface may be attached to the glenoid. In approximately 10 % of the normal population, there are openings beneath the labrum that should not be confused with a Bankart lesion or labral tear. Anatomic variants are always found in the anterior superior half of the labrum, whereas the detachment that is characteristic of a Bankart lesion usually involves the anterior inferior half of the labrum.

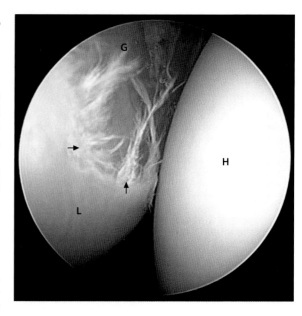

Fig. 10.4-1. Fraying of the glenoid labrum (*arrows* labral fibers, *L* labrum, *G* glenoid, *H* humeral head)

Various types of labral lesion have been identified:

- **Flap tears.** These lesions consist of variable-sized flaps, which may produce corresponding symptoms. It is not unusual for flap tears to occur in association with anterior shoulder instability.

- **Bucket-handle tear.** When a full-thickness tear develops, the central part of the labrum may act like a bucket handle and cause intermittent locking.

- **Degenerative lesions.** These lesions consist of incomplete flap tears and fraying of the free edge (Fig. 10.4-1). They are often found in association with cartilage lesions, omarthrosis, or extensive rotator cuff tears.

- **SLAP lesion** (see Sect. 10.4.1).

Therapeutic Management

Smaller unstable labral flaps or degenerative tears should be removed, as they have the potential to disrupt joint mechanics through intermittent locking. Bucket-handle tears and other large tears should be repaired whenever possible, using open technique if necessary.

▶ **Note:** In many cases, the locking symptoms that patients describe are caused not by the labral tear but by the accompanying instability or rotator cuff tear. We caution the surgeon against overinterpreting the significance of labral abnormalities.

Operative Technique

Resection

The principles are the same as in the resection of meniscal lesions. A small labral fragment is partially detached, grasped and avulsed with a grasping forceps, and extracted under arthroscopic control.

Postoperative Care

The simple resection of a small labral fragment does not require immobilization or prolonged shoulder rest. The range of shoulder motion should be restored as quickly as possible. In many cases the postoperative protocol is dictated by associated pathology such as shoulder instability.

10.4.1 SLAP Lesion

A SLAP lesion is a traumatic separation of the superior labrum involving the attachment of the long biceps tendon. The acronym SLAP describes the lesion morphology: a tear of the superior labrum extending from anterior to posterior.

Cause

Various mechanism of injury are known. Extreme tension on the long biceps tendon, as may occur in the terminal phase of throwing when the arm is decelerating and the elbow is maximally extended, can produce a labral lesion. Also, a fall onto the elbow with the arm flexed can cause a superior subluxation of the humeral head with a proximal avulsion of the superior labrum and biceps anchor. Shoulder dislocation can produce the same effect.

Symptoms

Patients describe the mechanism of the injury (fall, throwing movement). Isolated SLAP lesions can cause considerable pain.

Clinical Diagnosis

There is no specific test for diagnosing a SLAP lesion. The biceps tendon tests (see Sect. 10.5) may be positive.

Radiographs

Radiographs are unrevealing in the absence of an associated bony injury.

MRI

MRI can delineate lesions of the superior labrum.

Arthroscopic Findings

Snyder described SLAP lesions and classified them into five types (Fig. 10.4-2):

Type I: Degenerative fraying of the superior labrum, which is still firmly attached to the glenoid and long biceps tendon.
Type II: In addition to degenerative changes, the labrum and biceps anchor are detached from the glenoid, resulting in an unstable biceps-labrum complex.
Type III: Bucket-handle tear of the superior labrum with an intact biceps anchor.
Type IV: Bucket-handle tear of the superior labrum into the long biceps tendon, which is displaced with the torn labrum.
Type V: Complex tears (combinations of types I–IV).

Therapeutic Management

The treatment of SLAP lesions depends on the arthroscopic classification and on associated lesions:

Type I: Degenerative portions of the labrum are debrided with a synovial resector. This is done very carefully to avoid excessive resection of labral tissue and preserve the long biceps tendon.
▶ **Caution:** Avoid iatrogenic biceps tendon injury.
Type II: The unstable detached portion of the labrum should be repaired if possible; at least the tear site should be debrided. Various repair techniques are known:
1. Staple fixation
2. Screw fixation
3. Anchor suture repair
4. All-inside suture repair
Type III: The mobile bucket-handle tear is resected and the site freshened. The remaining labrum should be sutured if possible.
Type IV: Interposed labral fragments are resected. With an unstable long biceps tendon or impending complete rupture, biceps tenodesis is recommended. If possible, the labrum should be reduced and repaired (e. g., with an over-the-top suture).
Type V: Resection and repair are combined as needed, depending on the lesion.

Type I

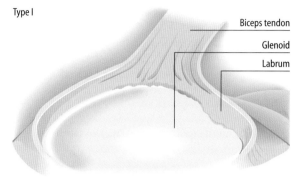

Biceps tendon

Glenoid

Labrum

Type II

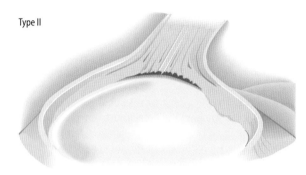

Type III

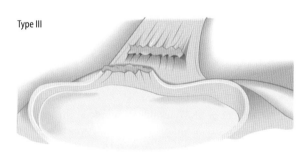

Type IV

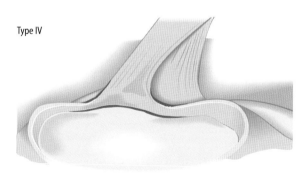

Fig. 10.4-2. Classification of SLAP lesions (see text for explanation)

Surgeons have had only limited experience with the conservative and operative treatment of SLAP lesions. There is a need for intermediate- and long-term studies in large clinical series.

Operative Technique

The repair techniques are like those used for anterior shoulder instability and are modified for use on the superior labrum. Thus, we may dispense with a detailed description of these techniques and simply cover the basics:

1. **Inspection and probing.** The lesion is probed through an anterior superior portal and its extent is determined.

2. **Freshening the glenoid.** The superior portion of the glenoid that underlies the lesion is freshened with a motorized bur or rasp to bleeding bone. This step is as important as in the arthroscopic Bankart procedure (see p. 910).

3. **Fixation of the labrum.** Various fixation techniques are available:

• **Staple or screw fixation.** The fixation is carried out through a superior portal centered over the labral lesion. As in the repair of a Bankart lesion, the labrum is reattached to the superior glenoid rim. The main drawback of this technique is the need to remove the fixation hardware (screw) at 3 months. However, absorbable fixation devices are available that do not require removal.

• **Anchor suture technique (over-the-top repair).** This technique corresponds to the transglenoid labral repair with anchor knots (see p. 912), taking note of the altered drilling direction in the posterior part of the infraspinous fossa. A second drill hole is made through the labrum at a more anterior superior level to create a three-point fixation (Fig. 10.4-3; see p. 910 for technical details).

• **Suture anchors.** Except for a different insertion direction, the technique corresponds to that in the arthroscopic Bankart procedure (see Fig. 10.6-7).

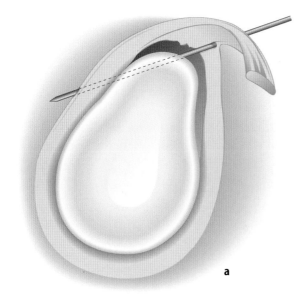

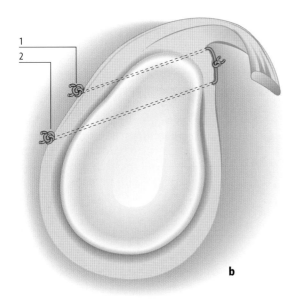

Fig. 10.4-3 a, b. Arthroscopic repair of a type II SLAP lesion with an over-the-top anchor suture. **a** A Kirschner wire is drilled through the superior glenoid rim after penetrating the detached labrum. **b** Final appearance of the repair. Two knots (*1, 2*) are placed on the anterior side of the glenoid (anchor knots), and one heavy knot (*arrow*) is tied on the opposite side. (After Habermeyer 1996)

Postoperative Care

The arm is immobilized for 4–6 weeks (Gilchrist bandage) following a labral repair. Except for biceps conditioning, muscle strengthening exercises are allowed. Free motion is allowed in week 6, and weight exercises may be started in week 12.

10.5 Biceps Tendon

Cause

Because the biceps tendon is closely related to the rotator cuff as it traverses the bicipital groove, partial- or full-thickness rotator cuff tears may be associated with inflammatory changes or partial or complete ruptures of the biceps tendon. Bony changes in the bicipital groove can also produce tendon irritation and can even cause partial or complete ruptures in long-standing cases. It should be kept in mind that the tendon itself does not move, and that the humeral head glides past it.

Symptoms

Patients with biceps tendinitis complain of anterior shoulder pain. Patients with a complete rupture give a history of trauma, but often the trauma itself is not adequate to account for the lesion. Patients suddenly notice a bulge in the distal upper arm caused by the displaced muscle belly.

Clinical Diagnosis

Physical examination in tendinitis shows tenderness of the long biceps tendon in the bicipital groove. Flexion and supination against a resistance are often painful (Yerguson test). Resisted forward elevation of the arm with the elbow extended and the forearm supinated also elicits pain (Speed test). A partial rupture of the biceps tendon is indistinguishable from tendinitis by clinical examination, but a complete rupture is clearly manifested by the bulging muscle belly of the long head of the biceps.

Radiographs

Standard radiographic views are unremarkable. Special views of the bicipital groove may show a shallow groove (suggesting subluxation of the biceps tendon) or osteophytes.

Ultrasound

Ultrasound in biceps tendinitis can show broadening and decreased structural density of the biceps tendon. Tenosynovitis is characterized by a hypoechoic halo surrounding the biceps tendon (Fig. 10.5-1). Ultrasound can also demonstrate defects ranging from thinning of the biceps tendon to nonvisualization of the tendon.

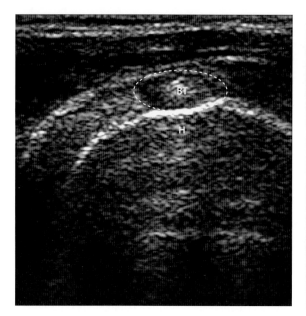

Fig. 10.5-1. Ultrasound appearance of biceps tendinitis (*H* contour of humeral head, *dashed line* peritendinitis, *BT* biceps tendon)

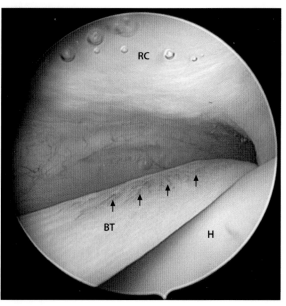

Fig. 10.5-2. Local synovitis (*arrows*) on the biceps tendon (*BT*) (*H* humeral head, *RC* rotator cuff)

MRI

MRI demonstrates the same changes detectable with ultrasound and therefore does not add to the sonographic examination.

Arthroscopic Findings

The normal biceps tendon has a uniform whitish color and is covered by transparent synovium. With biceps tendinitis, the synovium shows prominent vascular markings and varying degrees of redness, which may extend into the bicipital groove (Fig. 10.5-2).

With a partial rupture, arthroscopy may show a displaced tendon flap (Fig. 10.5-3). Fraying that almost completely encircles the tendon is a sign of impending complete rupture. In this case the tendon ends may appear thickened and frayed and may even lead to incarceration.

▶ **Note:** Biceps tendon changes are frequently accompanied by rotator cuff lesions.

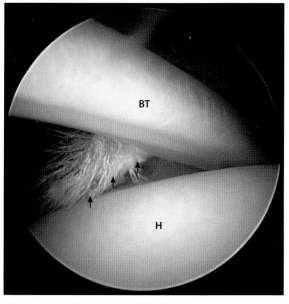

Fig. 10.5-3. Fraying (*arrows*) of the biceps tendon (*BT*) (*H* humeral head)

Therapeutic Management

Clinically diagnosed tendinitis should be managed conservatively (injections). However, rotator cuff lesions should always be excluded or treated as required. It is very common to find tendinitis accompanying a partial-

or full-thickness rotator cuff tear or instability-related impingement.

- **Partial rupture.** With a partial rupture, mobile tendon flaps are debrided if they create a potential or confirmed mechanical obstruction. Again, coexisting rotator cuff lesions should be detected and treated accordingly (see Sect. 10.7).

- **Complete rupture.** Because this frequently occurs in older patients in the wake of chronic degenerative changes, and the patient may show no measurable loss of strength, conservative treatment is an appropriate option. Tendon stumps that repeatedly catch between the articular surfaces should be arthroscopically resected. A surgical procedure on the biceps tendon is indicated in younger, athletically active patients. Fixation of the tendon in the bicipital groove should be considered.

Operative Technique

Debridement of the Biceps Tendon

Mobile, mechanically disruptive tendon flaps and frayed fibers are carefully removed with a synovial resector. Harder portions of the tendon can be partially detached with a small basket forceps or electrocautery probe (hook electrode) and extracted with a grasping forceps. When pronounced degenerative changes are present, the still-"intact" biceps tendon should be preserved to avoid iatrogenic tendon rupture.

Postoperative Care

Following tendon debridement alone without rotator cuff surgery, unrestricted shoulder movements are allowed on the first postoperative day. Immobilization is not required.

▶ **Note:** The patient should be informed about the possibility of an accompanying rotator cuff lesion, as this would increase the likelihood of a subsequent complete biceps tendon rupture.

10.6 Anterior Capsule and Ligaments (Shoulder Dislocation)

Cause

Direct or indirect violence can cause the humeral head to dislocate from the glenoid. A critical factor is whether the dislocation was caused by adequate trauma or a particular movement. Differentiating between a traumatic and nontraumatic etiology has an important bearing on further management (see below).

Classification

Frequency. An initial dislocation is distinguished from recurrent dislocation.

Etiology. The dislocation is classified as having a traumatic or atraumatic etiology. Factors that suggest a traumatic etiology are as follows:

History of an adequate traumatic event
- Lengthy delay between dislocation and reduction
- Shoulder can only be reduced under general anesthesia
- Presence of a bony Bankart lesion
- Presence of a large Hill-Sachs lesion

The following factors are more consistent with an atraumatic etiology:
- Increased ligamentous laxity
- No history of adequate trauma
- Proneness to dislocation
- Spontaneous reduction
- Shoulder can be reduced without general anesthesia
- Absence of a Hill-Sachs lesion

Direction of the dislocation. The humeral head may dislocate anteriorly, posteriorly, or inferiorly.

Multidirectional instability.

Symptoms

In most traumatic initial shoulder dislocations, spontaneous reduction is not possible. The patient describes very severe pain involving the entire shoulder and sometimes the entire arm. Patients with an existing shoulder instability and a history of inadequate trauma or an inciting movement describe less pain. In these cases a helper or even the patient himself can reduce the dislocation by gently pulling on the arm.

Clinical Diagnosis

Given the major therapeutic implications of the etiology, a detailed evaluation is necessary. It must be determined whether the dislocation is traumatic or atraumatic.

- **Acute anterior dislocation.** The arm is held in a position of slight abduction, anteversion, and external rotation. The patient complains of very severe pain. The contour of the shoulder may or may not differ from the unaffected side. In some cases the examiner can palpate the empty glenoid and the dislocated humeral head, which is next to or below the coracoid process.
  Blood flow (radial artery) and sensation (axillary nerve) should always be tested. If tests indicate neurovascular compromise, the shoulder should be reduced immediately after the radiographic examination.

- **Recurrent dislocation.** The patient gives a prior history of an initial dislocation. It is important to establish whether the prior dislocation could be easily reduced (e.g., by a helper pulling on the arm) or whether it required reduction under general anesthesia. The latter indicates a traumatic etiology of the initial dislocation.
  Following recurrent dislocations, the joint is usually found to be in a reduced rather than dislocated position. Often the dislocation is easily reduced with traction applied by a helper or the patient himself. Usually the range of shoulder motion is undiminished. The anterior apprehension test consists of abduction and external rotation of the shoulder. A positive test elicits muscular guarding to keep the shoulder from dislocating or subluxating anteriorly.

General ligamentous laxity should be tested as well. A positive sulcus sign on both sides (inferior displacement of the humerus by downward traction on the relaxed forearm) indicates general ligamentous laxity. Unilateral multidirectional instability results in a unilateral positive sulcus sign.

Radiographs

Dislocated position. Radiographs in two planes (AP view and scapular Y view) document the dislocated position and exclude fractures of the humeral head and glenoid.

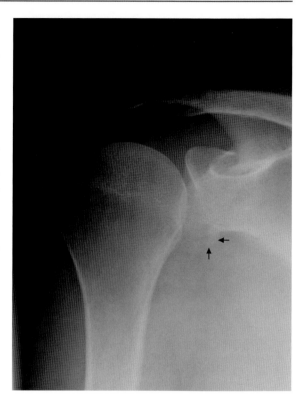

Fig. 10.6-1. Bony avulsion of the inferior glenoid rim (*arrows*) due to shoulder dislocation

Reduced position. Radiographs in the reduced position can demonstrate secondary changes in the glenoid, such as an osseous Bankart lesion, and a Hill-Sachs lesion in the humeral head (Fig. 10.6-1). Avulsion fractures of the greater tuberosity can also be excluded.

Ultrasound

A Hill-Sachs defect can be clearly visualized with ultrasound. The shoulder is also scanned for rotator cuff lesions, since partial and full-thickness tears can accompany shoulder dislocation, especially in patients over 40 years of age. Rotator cuff repairs are of special importance in these cases.

MRI, CT

MRI or double-contrast CT scanning is recommended for preoperative planning, especially if an arthroscopic repair is proposed. These studies are helpful for evaluating the condition of the anterior capsule, glenoid rim, and labrum and excluding preexisting torsional deformity of the humerus.

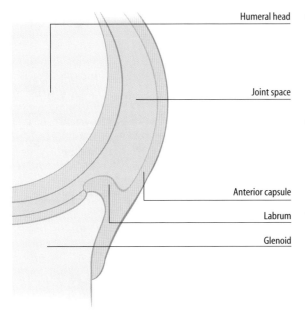

Humeral head

Joint space

Anterior capsule

Labrum

Glenoid

Fig. 10.6-2. Normal anatomy of the intact labrum-capsule complex

Arthroscopic Findings

There are a number of characteristic intraarticular changes that differ from normal findings (Fig. 10.6-2):

- **Bankart lesion.** This lesion involves a detachment of the anterior inferior labrum from the glenoid with involvement of the inferior glenohumeral ligament. The continuity between the cartilage and labrum is disrupted, but the periosteal attachment is intact. Areas of interstitial hemorrhage may be seen after acute injuries, while recurrent dislocations may present with degenerative fraying of the labrum and occasional labral tears.

▶ **Note:** Careful inspection and probing of the anterior inferior labrum is of key importance, because the labrum-glenoid region is subject to many types of lesions in anterior shoulder instability that are not amenable to arthroscopic repair (Fig. 10.6-3).

- **Hill-Sachs lesion.** This lesion consists of a chondral or osteochondral impaction in the posterolateral aspect of the humeral head (Fig. 10.6-4). The Hill-Sachs defect is typically V-shaped. If the dislocation is reproduced during arthroscopy, the configuration of the defect matches the anterior labrum-glenoid complex.

- **Glenoid lesions.** These injuries affect the anterior inferior region of the glenoid. They range from chondral flake fractures to anteroinferior glenoid fractures. Extensive cartilage lesions with degenerative fraying of the labrum signify numerous prior dislocations (chronic anterior instability).

- **Capsular lesions.** Tearing of the inferior glenohumeral ligament may occur, even if the labrum remains firmly attached to the glenoid. Combined injuries involving the anterior inferior labrum can also occur (see Fig. 10.6-4).

- **Associated lesions.** Intraarticular loose bodies may consist of chondral fragments sheared from the glenoid or fragments from a Hill-Sachs lesion. Partial- or full-thickness rotator cuff tears should also be excluded.

- **Finding the dislocation path.** The path of the dislocation should be reproduced under arthroscopic control to establish the direction of the dislocation.

Therapeutic Management

Immediate reduction is indicated, although this can be quite difficult with an initial traumatic dislocation. In a very muscular patient, it may be necessary to perform the reduction under sedation or general anesthesia.

▶ **Tip:** Proceed carefully when reducing an initial dislocation. Adequate analgesia (or general anesthesia) should be provided.

- **Reduction.** In the classic reduction techniques, an effort is made to manipulate the humeral head – which is engaged on the anterior glenoid rim by a Hill-Sachs lesion and fixed by muscular guarding – back into the glenoid fossa. The reduction should be accomplished carefully and "without force." In principle, the humeral head is freed from its dislocated position using traction and an axillary fulcrum, externally rotated, and then reduced in internal rotation. The axillary fulcrum may consist of a heel (Hippocratic technique), fist (Milch technique), or chair back (Arlt technique). In the Stimson technique, the patient lies in a prone position and hangs the affected arm over the edge of the examination table. A weight or manual traction is then placed on the arm to induce gradual muscular relaxation. This is supported by repeatedly telling the patient to relax the muscles throughout the procedure. It may take up to 20–30 min for spontaneous reduction to occur.

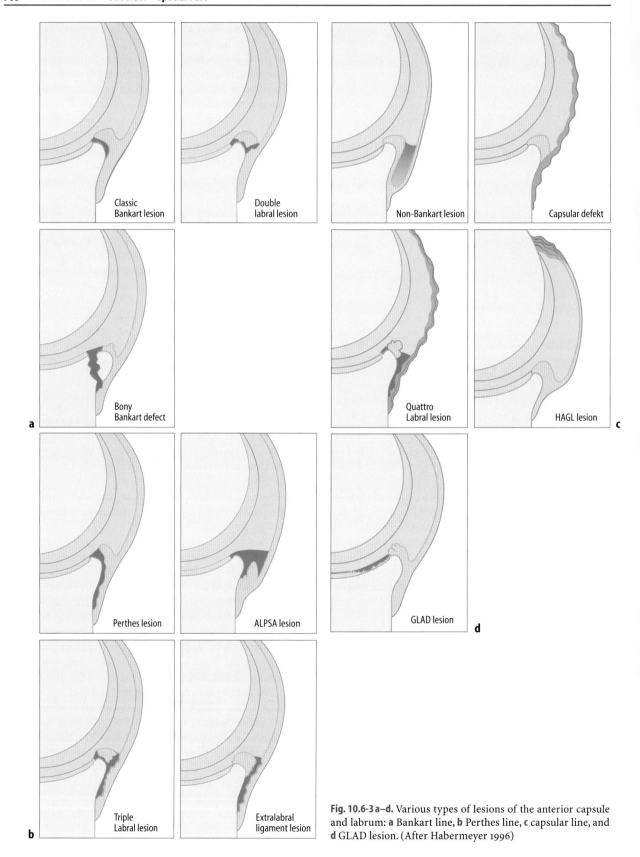

Fig. 10.6-3 a–d. Various types of lesions of the anterior capsule and labrum: **a** Bankart line, **b** Perthes line, **c** capsular line, and **d** GLAD lesion. (After Habermeyer 1996)

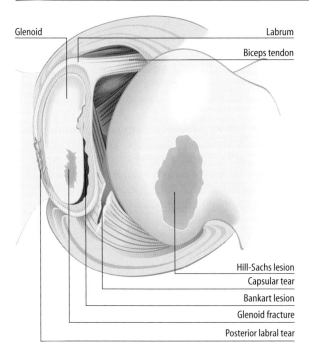

Glenoid — Labrum
— Biceps tendon
— Hill-Sachs lesion
— Capsular tear
— Bankart lesion
— Glenoid fracture
— Posterior labral tear

Fig. 10.6-4. Typical lesions associated with shoulder dislocation: Hill-Sachs lesion, cartilage damage or fracture in the anterior inferior glenoid, Bankart lesion, and a capsular tear in the area of the inferior glenohumeral ligament. Posterior inferior labral tears can also occur (after Esch 1993)

After the dislocation has been reduced, whether under anesthesia or using one of the technique described, blood flow and sensation are again tested and biplane radiographs are obtained. If a glenoid or humeral head fracture is suspected, an extra radiographic view or preferably CT scans should be obtained to document the extent of the fracture.

Conservative Treatment

Following an initial dislocation, the shoulder is first immobilized. It has been found that immobilizing the shoulder for longer than 3 weeks does not decrease the rate of redislocation. Physical therapy is then initiated to increase the range of motion. Rotator- and adductor-strengthening exercises are also performed. Generally this treatment is less successful for posttraumatic insta-bilities than atraumatic instabilities.

▶ **Note:** Young patients with posttraumatic instability are particularly prone to redislocation.

Operative Treatment

Recurrent Anterior Instability

Studies by Bankart proved that a labrum that has been detached by a dislocation will not heal spontaneously in a normal position. The incidence of recurrence after an initial dislocation will vary, depending on the etiology (traumatic atraumatic). Given the complex anatomy of the shoulder joint and the various types of lesions and associated injuries that can occur, more than 150 differ-ent operative techniques have been devised for the treat-ment of recurrent anterior shoulder dislocation.

Two basic types of operative techniques are available (Wiedemann 1996):

1. **Anatomic techniques.** The goal of these techniques is to produce an anatomic reconstruction of the dam-aged structures.
2. **Palliative techniques.** These techniques involve creat-ing or surgically introducing a barrier to prevent recurrent dislocation. Examples are the Putti-Platt capsulorraphy, the Lange bone graft procedure, and the Eden-Hybbinette procedure (bone graft insertion into the anterior scapular neck).

▶ **Note:** In the light of modern discoveries in pathome-chanics, palliative techniques can no longer be rec-ommended.

Indications

An essential criterion in selecting patients for operative treatment is the high incidence of redislocations in the presence of coexisting labral injuries. Redislocation rates of 60 % to 90 % have been reported in the litera-ture.

In selecting a suitable anatomic reconstruction, it must be decided whether to use arthroscopic or open technique. This has become a frequent topic of discus-sion at every scientific conference that deals with shoul-der instability. To date, there have been no randomized prospective studies dealing with this important issue. For the present, therefore, we must weigh the advantages and disadvantages of arthroscopic techniques and draw our own conclusions:

▶ **Advantages**
- **Low invasiveness**
- **No risk to proprioception**

▶ **Disadvantages**
- **Complex operative technique**
- **Increased complication rate when metallic implants are used**
- **Need for a posterior incision when transglenoid fixa-tion is used**
- **Higher incidence of recurrence**

▶ **Tip:** At present we must regard open techniques as the "gold standard." Successful arthroscopic repairs require a precise operating technique and discriminating patient selection.

▶ **Note:** An intact labrum-capsule-ligament complex is essential in arthroscopic repairs, as it will stabilize and protect the reattachment to the anterior glenoid rim.

Contraindications to Arthroscopic Repair

Each of the following factors would contraindicate an arthroscopic procedure:

1. Bony Bankart lesion
2. Hill-Sachs defect
3. Absence or destruction of the labrum-capsule-ligament complex (e.g., Quatro labral lesion, see Fig. 10.6-2).
4. Associated lesions. While technically these lesions would not preclude an arthroscopic repair, their presence would compromise a successful outcome:
   – Complete rupture of the subscapularis tendon
   – Interval lesion with subluxation or dislocation of the long biceps tendon
   – Tear of the subscapularis tendon
   – Multidirectional instability
   – Isolated posterior instability

Basic Principles of Arthroscopic Repair Techniques

The goal is to reattach the anterior inferior labrum-capsule-ligament complex to the glenoid. The various operative techniques can be classified as transglenoid or anterior, depending on whether or not the fixation requires transglenoid drilling.

1. **Transglenoid techniques.** Sutures are passed from anterior to posterior through transglenoid drill holes and are secured with knots on the posterior side of the scapula or on the infraspinatus muscle. The free ends on the anterior side are then tightened and tied to secure the anterior labrum-capsule-ligament complex to the glenoid, as in the three-point labral repair (see below).

2. **Anterior techniques.** The detached complex is fixed to the glenoid on the anterior side using a screw, tack, or staples made of absorbable or nonabsorbable material. The advantage of these techniques is that they do not require a posterior incision or transglenoid drilling. Their disadvantage is the need to introduce implants (screws, staples), which can cause numerous complications such as breakage or loosening of the fixation hardware. Absorbable implants can also be used but may produce lytic areas that would make subsequent revision procedures more difficult. Staple

fixation alone has such high recurrence and complication rates that it is no longer recommended.

Suture anchors and bone anchors can also be placed anteriorly to fix the anterior complex to the glenoid. In these cases as well, the bone implant can compound the difficulty of subsequent revision surgery.

▶ **Tip:** Whenever doubt exists, an open procedure is preferred. If technical difficulties arise or if the lesions found at operation are more serious than expected, do not hesitate to convert to an open procedure. This contingency should be explained to the patient preoperatively and informed consent secured.

Many patients who know about the advances of arthroscopic surgery in recent years and may have already had a different arthroscopic ligament reconstruction (e.g., an ACL reconstruction in the knee) may demand an arthroscopic reconstruction in the shoulder. These patients should be educated about the fundamental differences between instability in the glenohumeral joint and instability in the knee.

Operative Technique

Three-Point Labral Repair: The Habermeyer Technique
(Figs. 10.6-5 through 10.6-8)

This transglenoid technique is a modification of the Morgan repair.

1. **Inspection and probing.** The glenohumeral joint is visualized. The anterior inferior labrum-capsule-ligament complex is carefully palpated with the probe through an anterior inferior portal. Associated lesions (loose bodies, biceps tendon lesions, rotator cuff tears) that might contraindicate an arthroscopic procedure are excluded. If the labrum-capsule-ligament complex is stable and there is no instability in another direction, it is feasible to proceed with arthroscopic repair. The portals are switched (arthroscope to an anterior portal), and the posterior joint region is inspected.

2. **Removal of adhesions.** Adhesions that have formed between the avulsed labrum and the scapular neck are removed with a cautery probe (hook electrode), basket forceps, or synovial resector. If this region is difficult to reach, the hook electrode of the cautery probe can be prebent to facilitate access. Dissection with the cautery probe should not be carried far distally along the scapular neck, as this might injure the axillary nerve. If vision is inadequate, therefore, the adhesions should be removed with a basket forceps

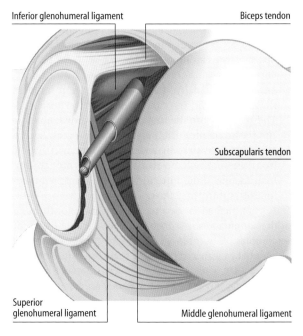

Inferior glenohumeral ligament

Biceps tendon

Subscapularis tendon

Superior
glenohumeral ligament

Middle glenohumeral ligament

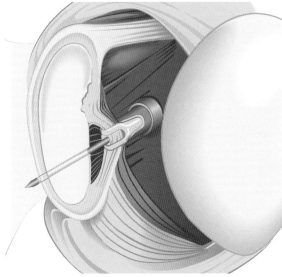

Fig. 10.6-5. The anterior glenoid rim is freshened with a round bur

Fig. 10.6-6. The anterior inferior capsulolabral complex is grasped with a cannulated grasper, and a Kirschner wire is drilled in the posteroinferior direction

or rasp using a combination of blunt and sharp dissection.

3. **Mobilizing the inferior glenohumeral ligament.** This most important ligamentous component of the anterior capsular complex should be mobilized so that it can be raised to the level of the glenoid surface. According to Habermeyer (1996), the mobility of the labrum-ligament complex is critical to the success of this repair.

4. **Freshening the anterior inferior scapular neck.** The scapular neck is decorticated with a curved sharp rasp or small round bur until a cancellous bed is obtained (Fig. 10.6-5).

▶ **Tip:** This exposure is essential for subsequent healing of the reattached capsule and ligaments. Avoid damaging the cartilaginous surface of the glenoid, however.

5. **Placing the fixation sutures and anchor knots.** A cannulated grasper is introduced and is used to grasp, elevate, tighten and shorten the mobilized glenohumeral ligament. At the same time, the labrum is anatomically reduced to the glenoid rim. First the inferior glenohumeral ligament is grasped at its junction with the labrum and brought up to the 4 o'clock position (right shoulder) on the glenoid rim. Care is taken to achieve adequate tensioning the ligament.

Next a pointed wire (1.7 mm in diameter) with an eyelet is introduced through the cannulated grasper and drilled into the glenoid rim at the junction of the cartilage and bone (Fig. 10.6-6). The drilling angle is 30° inferior and 15° posteromedial relative to the scapular plane. The wire should enter the infraspinous fossa and exit the skin posteriorly about 10 cm below the scapular spine. A pair of sutures (PDS) are threaded through the eyelet in the wire, and the wire is pulled out posteriorly, bringing the sutures with it. The sutures are tied together to form an anchor knot approximately 4 mm in diameter. The suture tails protruding from the cannulated grasper are then pulled, drawing the anchor knot back through the skin and against the posterior scapula. The knot on the posterior scapular neck provides a stable posterior fixation point.

▶ **Tip:** It is easier to pull the anchor knots through the skin by first making a small skin incision and spreading the subcutaneous tissue with a small clamp.

The sutures should be pulled firmly to seat the anchor knots securely against the scapular neck. The manual traction may be vigorous enough to pull the scapula and shoulder girdle forward.

The same technique is used to drill a second transglenoid hole, parallel to the first, at the 3 o'clock position on the glenoid (lateral decubitus position). As before, a cannulated grasper is used and the Kirschner wire is brought out posteriorly with the second

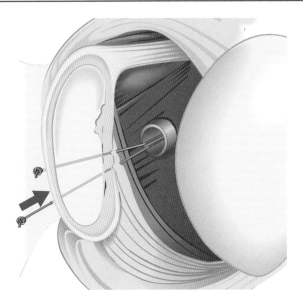

Fig. 10.6-7. The inferior anchor knot (*arrow*) is pulled back against the scapular neck. The course of the drill holes is shown

The advantage of the three-point suturing technique of Habermeyer is that it places stable anchor knots on the posterior scapular neck that will not loosen post-operatively as swelling subsides.

6. **Anterior fixation.** At this point, four sutures pass through the working cannula in the anterior portal. The sutures from the first transglenoid drill hole are clamped to distinguish them from the second suture pair. Under no circumstances should the two sutures from the first hole be tied together on the labrum. Instead, one of the superior sutures is matched to an inferior suture, and those sutures are tied together. A knot pushed is used to advance the knot through the cannula to the reduced labrum-capsule-ligament complex (Fig. 10.6-8). The knot-tying technique should be clean and precise. Because the suture material is PDS, a minimum of five knots should be tied, and preferably six. The suture ends are trimmed with a small punch. The same technique is used to tie the two remaining sutures together and advance the knot.

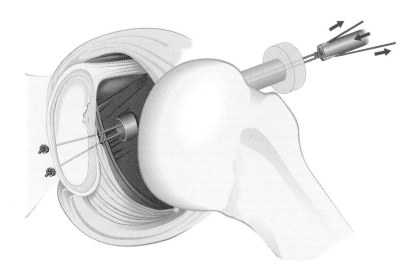

Fig. 10.6-8. After the anchor knots have been placed on the posterior side of the glenoid, the anterior knot is advanced to the capsulolabral complex with a knot pusher

7. **Probing.** The reattached labrum-ligament complex is palpated with the probe to assess the adequacy of the repair. Optimally, the labrum should be positioned over the glenoid rim so that it once again reinforces the anterior inferior glenoid rim and enlarges the articular surface.

pair of sutures. The subcutaneous tissue is spread open, and the anchor knot is pulled back against the posterior scapular neck (Fig. 10.6-7).

▶ **Tip:** In the technique described by Morgan, the two pairs of sutures are brought out posteriorly and tied together, requiring a larger posterior incision. Because the sutures are tied over the infraspinatus muscle, they tend to loosen as the extravasated fluid clears during the hours following surgery. Also, the broad posterior suture line poses a risk to the supraspinatus nerve.

Caspari Technique of Arthroscopic Labral Repair
(Fig. 10.6-9)

1. **Inspection and probing** (see p. 910).

2. **Removal of adhesions.** As in the Habermeyer technique, adhesions between the avulsed labrum and scapular neck are removed (see p. 910).

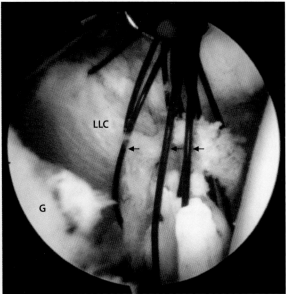

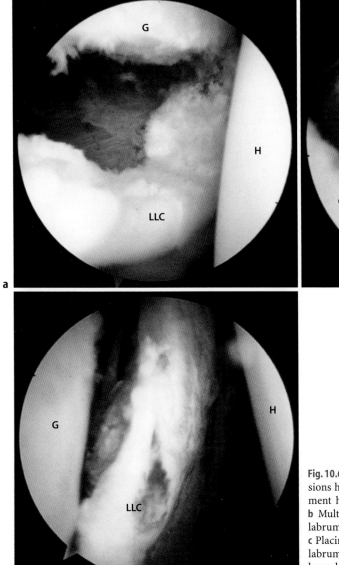

Fig. 10.6-9a–c. Caspari technique of labral repair. **a** After adhesions have been removed and the inferior glenohumeral ligament has been mobilized, the scapular border is freshened. **b** Multiple sutures (*arrows*) are placed through the avulsed labrum-ligament complex (*LLC*) (*H* humeral head, *G* glenoid). **c** Placing tension on the sutures reapproximates the detached labrum-ligament complex to the glenoid. The sutures are brought out posteriorly and tied down over the infraspinatus fascia. (Photos courtesy of Kai-Uwe Jensen, Hamburg)

3. Mobilizing the inferior glenohumeral ligament (see p. 911).

4. Freshening the anterior inferior scapular neck (see p. 911).

5. Placing the fixation sutures. The detached labrum-ligament complex is grasped as far inferiorly as possible with a special suture forceps called a Caspari suture punch. PDS suture material is advanced through the suture punch with a feeder mechanism until it appears within the joint. This technique is very similar to the all-inside technique for meniscal repairs (see Fig. 2.1-17).

A total of 5 to 8 sutures are placed in the avulsed structures and brought out through an anterior instrument portal. Then a transglenoid hole is drilled with a 3.5-mm pin, angling the drill exactly as in the three-point technique (see above). Drilling is started at the 12 o'clock position, however. The sutures are threaded through the eyelet at the end of the pin and passed from anterior to posterior through the transglenoid drill hole. On the posterior side, the sutures are tensioned and tied over the infraspinous fascia.

6. Probing the repair (see p. 912).

▶ **Note:** The main danger is postoperative loosening of the sutures, which are tied over the infraspinatus muscle. After the extravasated fluid has cleared from the soft tissues, some degree of suture loosening will occur.

The advantage of the Caspari technique is that the steps in the procedure are clearly divided into (1) piercing the labrum, (2) transglenoid drilling, and (3) passing the sutures through the drill hole and tying them. The disadvantage is the postoperative loosening that will occur as extravasated fluid clears during the initial hours after surgery. We therefore recommend placing the knots as deeply and as close to the posterior scapular neck as possible.

Suture Anchor System
(Figs. 10.6-10 to 10.6-12)

Instrumentation. Besides specially designed suture anchors (Arthrex), the instrument set includes a special cannulated grasper used both for drilling the guidewire and for inserting the complete suture anchor.

Because this technique is purely anterior and does not require transglenoid drilling, it does not risk injury to structures posterior to the scapular neck (the suprascapular nerve).

1. **Inspection and probing** (see p. 910).

2. **Removal of adhesions** (see p. 910).

3. **Mobilizing the inferior glenohumeral ligament.** As in the transglenoid techniques, mobilization of the inferior glenohumeral ligament is of key importance (see p. 911).

4. **Freshening the anterior inferior scapular neck.** The anterior scapular neck is freshened with a sharp rasp or small round bur (see Fig. 10.6-5).

5. **Fixation of the labrum-ligament complex with the suture anchor.** The grasper is introduced through a working cannula in the anterior superior portal and grasps the detached capsule-ligament complex. The complex should be grasped securely and moved toward the biceps tendon. The grasper remains in place, and the suture anchor – a small self-tapping titanium screw with a suture eyelet – is twisted in through the grasper using a special applicator. The eyelet has been threaded with a No. 2 PDS suture.

▶ **Tip:** Grasp as much of the inferior glenohumeral ligament and labrum with the grasper as possible to achieve optimum capsular plication (Fig. 10.6-10 a).

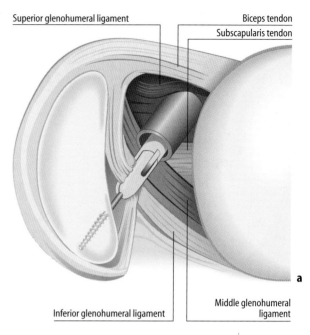

Superior glenohumeral ligament · Biceps tendon · Subscapularis tendon · Inferior glenohumeral ligament · Middle glenohumeral ligament

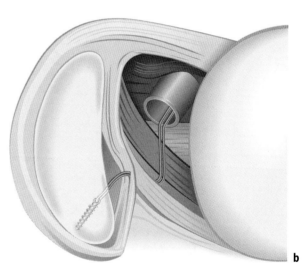

Fig. 10.6-10. a The capsulolabral complex is grasped with a special grasper, and a suture anchor is screwed into the bone. **b** The grasper is withdrawn, leaving the threaded anchor in place. The suture runs from the anchor through the avulsed labrum-ligament complex and through the working cannula to the outside

The grasper is withdrawn, leaving the threaded anchor in place. A single suture loop passes from the anterior scapular neck through the avulsed labrum-ligament complex. From there it passes out of the joint through the working cannula (Fig. 10.6-10 b). After the first suture anchor has been placed at the 4 o'clock position, a second suture anchor is placed at the 3 o'clock position using an identical technique (Fig. 10.6-11).

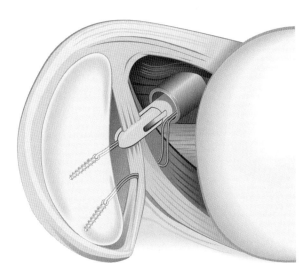

Fig. 10.6-11. A second suture anchor is inserted

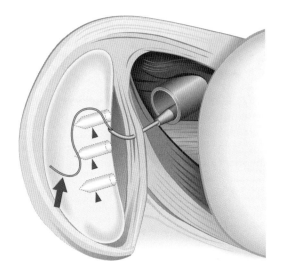

Fig. 10.6-13. After the pilot holes for the Mitek anchors (*arrowheads*) have been drilled, the detached anterior labrum-ligament complex is pierced with a cannulated needle, and the suture material (*arrow*) is advanced through the hook

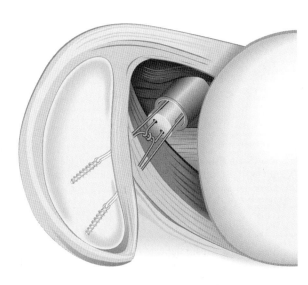

Fig. 10.6-12. One suture tail from the first anchor is tied to a suture tail from the second anchor, and the knot is advanced to the anterior capsule with a knot pusher

Mitek Anchor System
(Figs. 10.6-13 to 10.6-16)

Instrumentation. The instrument set includes a special drill bit matched to the length and diameter of the suture anchor (Mitek system). A special drill sleeve is required along with an inserter for the suture anchor. Also required are a suture passing instrument and suture passing tips with assorted angulations. As an alternative, the all-inside meniscal repair set can be used (see Fig. 2.1-7).

1. **Inspection and probing** (see p. 910).

2. **Removal of adhesions** (see p. 910).

3. **Mobilizing the inferior glenohumeral ligament** (see p. 911).

4. **Freshening the anterior inferior scapular neck** (see p. 911).

5. **Drilling pilot holes for the suture anchors.** A special "shark-mouth" drill sleeve is introduced through the anterior inferior portal and positioned at the bone-cartilage junction of the glenoid. Usually three pilot holes are drilled. The first hole is placed as low on the anterior glenoid as possible, and the second hole is placed as high as possible. The third hole is placed between the first two. The holes should be drilled at a 15°–20° posterior angle relative to the glenoid surface (Fig. 10.6-13).

Next the sutures are tied. The suture tails from the same anchor should not be tied together. This is avoided by tagging the tails from the first anchor with a hemostat or small knot. The knots are advanced to the anterior capsule with a knot pusher (Fig. 10.6-12).
▶ **Tip:** With an extensive anterior detachment, it may be necessary to place a third suture anchor in the 2 o'clock position.

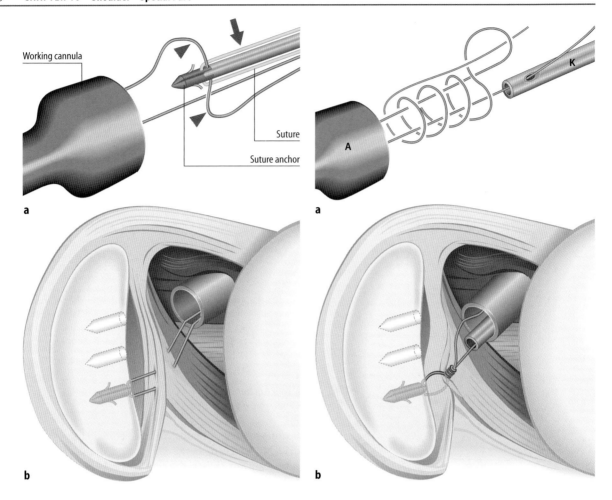

Fig. 10.6-14. a A fixation suture (*arrow*) secures the anchor to the tip of the impaction rod. One end of the intraarticular suture (*arrowhead*) is also passed through the eyelet. **b** The rod is withdrawn, leaving the suture across the detached labrum and capsule

Fig. 10.6-15. a A fisherman's slip knot is tied outside the joint (*K* knot pusher, *A* working cannula). **b** The knot is advanced to the anterior inferior capsulolabral complex with the knot pusher

▶ **Tip:** Avoid damaging the glenoid cartilage. Drilling the pilot holes at too shallow an angle could damage the cartilage during drilling and anchor insertion.

6. **Suturing the capsulolabral complex.** The suture hook is introduced through the working cannula and passed through the capsulolabral complex inferior to the highest of the pilot holes (see above). The suture is advanced through the hook and grasped with a small grasping forceps (Fig. 10.6-13).

▶ **Tip:** Insert the most distal suture anchor first, as this will help tighten the capsule by shifting the anterior inferior capsulolabral complex superiorly.

7. **Inserting the suture anchor.** Before the suture anchor is placed in the inserter, a fixation suture is passed through its eyelet to hold the anchor securely at the tip of the rod. The end of the suture that was placed

through the capsulolabral complex is also threaded through the eyelet. The suture anchor is then passed through the working cannula into the joint space on the tip of the inserter, and the anchor is driven into the pilot hole (Fig. 10.6-14).

▶ **Note:** The barbs on the side of the anchor are oriented parallel to the glenoid surface.

After the anchor has been inserted, the inserter is released and withdrawn without much twisting. The stabilizing barbs will deploy in about 10–15 seconds. The sutures are then pulled gently to secure the anchor in place.

8. **Tying the sutures.** The two suture tails protruding from the working cannula are now tied together, and the knot is advanced into the joint with a knot pusher. The first knot should consist of a fisherman's slip knot (Fig. 10.6-15). Then two square knots are tied

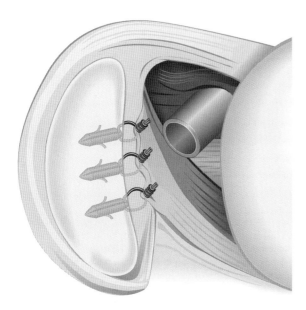

Fig. 10.6-16. Final appearance of the repair using three suture anchors

over the slip knot and advanced to the repair site. Finally the sutures are trimmed.

The same technique is used to insert the remaining anchors (Fig. 10.6-16).

Postoperative Care

The shoulder is immobilized in a Gilchrist bandage for 3 weeks. Mobilization is begun in week 4, but external rotation and forcible abduction should be avoided until week 12. The patient should refrain from sports for 6 months.

10.7 Rotator Cuff Lesions

Cause

Rotator cuff lesions are among the most common shoulder lesions. Traumatic tears are rare except in cases of massive shoulder trauma. Most rotator cuff tears result from extensive degenerative changes based on the very high stresses that act on the cuff and other adverse mechanical factors. The most important of these factors is the very confined space beneath the acromion, due in part to the coracoacromial ligament stretching between the coracoid process and the acromion. This situation predisposes to early degenerative cuff changes, and histologic signs of tendon degeneration can be found in most individuals over 30 years of age. The relatively poor blood supply to the rotator cuff serves to exacerbate this "natural" attrition process.

Mechanically, the tendon degeneration leads to surface irregularities and fraying. Degenerative tears usually start on the undersurface of the rotator cuff near the greater tuberosity. This type of tear, which is located adjacent to the glenohumeral joint, is called an articular-side tear (type A tear). Less commonly the tear starts on the superior surface of the rotator cuff, which forms the floor of the subacromial space. These tears are known as bursal-side tears (type B tears).

The degenerative surface irregularities on the rotator cuff interfere with tendon gliding and promote irritation of the subacromial space (subacromial bursitis).

These changes most commonly affect individuals who do strenuous manual work, especially when it involves repetitive overhead lifting or prolonged periods of abduction (e.g., painters, hairdressers, etc.). Various types of sport (e.g., tennis, squash, volleyball, weightlifting) can also predispose to degenerative cuff changes.

The overall presentation of the disease is on a continuum with subacromial syndrome (see Sect. 10.10 for details).

Symptoms

Patients with rotator cuff lesions typically describe pain during arm movements (especially retroversion and abduction) and also nocturnal pain combined with sleeping difficulties.

Patients with a true traumatic cuff tear give a history of adequate trauma. Some patients claim to have heard the tear or felt a pop in the shoulder accompanied by severe pain. After the tear, which usually involves the full thickness of the rotator cuff, the patient experiences significant weakness in abduction due to tearing of the supraspinatus muscle. There may also be a marked loss

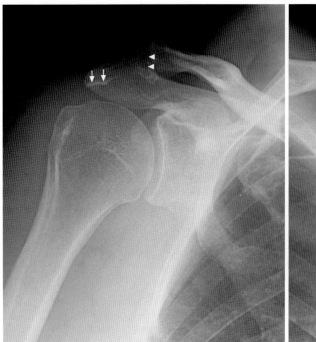
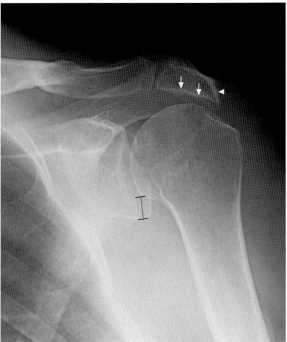

a   b

of external rotation caused by tearing of the infraspinatus muscle.

The symptoms may be severe enough to produce a "pseudoparalysis" condition in which the patient can barely move the arm.

By contrast, full-thickness tears due to degenerative cuff disease are usually marked by a gradual progression of pain and other complaints. Patients occasionally describe a minor traumatic event that led to an exacerbation of preexisting complaints. It is not unusual for acute trauma to enlarge a preexisting cuff tear, causing it to become symptomatic. It should also be noted that shoulder dislocations in patients over 40 years of age are frequently associated with a rotator cuff tear.

Clinical Diagnosis

With a partial-thickness tear, marked tenderness is noted over the greater tuberosity at the insertion of the supraspinatus muscle. This is accompanied by a painful arc and a positive Jobe test.

Full-thickness (complete) tears also lead to tenderness over the greater tuberosity, and often this is accompanied by crepitus on passive rotation of the upper arm. Inspection may reveal atrophy of the supraspinatus and infraspinatus muscles. Acute abduction weakness (pseudoparalysis) is found mainly in cases with a traumatic etiology. It is manifested by a positive Jobe test and positive drop-arm test. In these tests the arm is passively abducted as far as possible and then actively lowered. In

Fig. 10.7-1 a, b. Radiographic features of rotator cuff lesions. **a** This rotator cuff tear (supraspinatus rupture) is marked by subacromial osteophyte formation (*arrows*) and incipient osteoarthritis in the AC joint (*arrowheads*). **b** This film shows superior migration of the humeral head secondary to rotator cuff defect arthropathy. Note the sclerotic margin (*arrows*) and osteophyte formation (*arrowhead*) on the acromion. The amount of humeral head elevation can be measured (*dotted line*)

a positive test, the arm can no longer be held up on reaching approximately 90° of abduction and falls limply to the side. Resistive tensioning tests are negative.

Radiographs

Radiographs may demonstrate sclerotic or lytic areas in the greater tuberosity, but these changes do not necessarily correlate with clinical findings. A full-thickness tear is often associated with superior migration of the humeral head suggesting a torn rotator cuff.

The acromiohumeral distance (distance between the undersurface of the acromion and the top of the humeral head) is determined on the AP view with the arm in the neutral position (Fig. 10.7-1). The normal distance is between 7 and 14 mm. The critical value is 7 mm; a distance less than 7 mm implies that rotator cuff repair will not yield a favorable result. A value of 5–7 mm means that surgical closure of the cuff defect will be technically demanding, and 4.5 mm means that the cuff

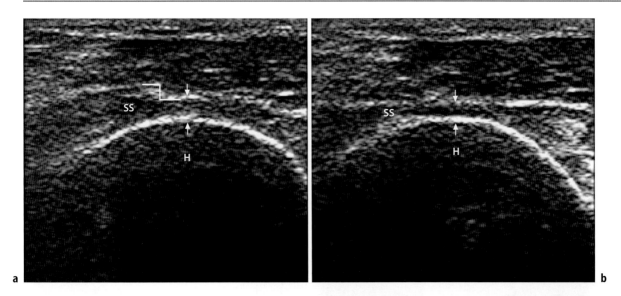

Fig. 10.7-2 a, b. Ultrasound scans of a rotator cuff tear. **a** Scan of a partial-thickness tear shows thinning of the supraspinatus tendon (*SS, arrows*) with a stepoff in the bursa (*line*) (*H* humeral head contour). **b** Narrowing (*arrows*) of the supraspinatus tendon (*SS*) (transducer position I described by Hedtmann and Fett)

defect probably cannot be completely closed. Thus, the radiographic acromiohumeral distance is a very useful index for predicting the efficacy of a rotator cuff repair (Habermeyer 1996).

Ultrasound

Ultrasound has a special role in evaluating the rotator cuff and acromial bursa (Fig. 10.7-2). The deltoid muscle and humeral head contour can also be evaluated. The sensitivity of ultrasound in the diagnosis of full-thickness rotator cuff tears is 97% (Hedtmann and Fett 1995), which is equivalent to that of contrast arthrography. Because ultrasound can also define structural changes, it is superior to any other technique for detecting partial-thickness tears, especially intratendinous tears located on the bursal side. This capability makes ultrasound the modality of first choice in the diagnosis of rotator cuff lesions.

MRI

The condition of the rotator cuff can also be evaluated with MRI. Because tissue defects are often indistinguishable from degenerative areas by MRI, however, this modality ranks second to ultrasound in the evaluation of partial-thickness tears.

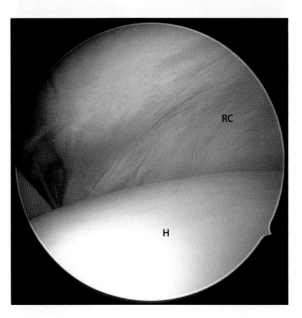

Fig. 10.7-3. Intact rotator cuff (*RC*) with a smooth surface (*H* humeral head)

Arthroscopic Findings

The normal rotator cuff is smooth and covered by synovium (Fig. 10.7-3).

- **Partial tear.** Degenerative partial-thickness rotator cuff tears usually start at the insertion of the cuff on the greater tuberosity, where degenerative fraying can be found. In later stages, numerous fibers become separated and present the features of an articular-side partial tear (type A tear) (Fig. 10.7-4). Palpation with the probe is necessary to determine whether the tear is partial or full-thickness. Most partial-thick-

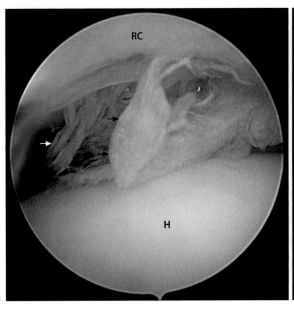
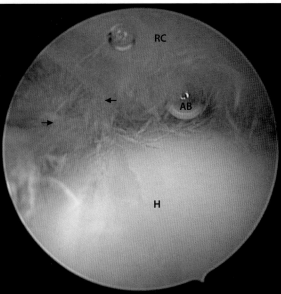

a   b

Fig. 10.7-4a,b. Partial-thickness rotator cuff tear. Numerous fronds of torn cuff (*arrows*) are visible in the joint (*RC* rotator cuff, *H* humeral head, *AB* air bubble)

ness tears occur in zone B (Fig. 10.7-5). Endoscopy of the subacromial space can demonstrate bursal-side (type B) tears.

- **Complete tear.** With a complete rotator cuff tear, the subacromial space can be visualized from the glenohumeral joint. The quality of the torn tendon edge is evaluated arthroscopically, as this will have a bearing on the operative procedure. With an acute, usually traumatic cuff tear, the tear margin is covered with blood. If the tendon edge is thinned, has a soft consistency, or is indurated or even atrophic, repair will be technically more difficult. The location of the tear is also assessed (Fig. 10.7-5).

Tear localization is aided by subdividing the rotator cuff into zones:

Zone A: anterior zone (subscapularis tendon, rotator interval, and long biceps tendon)
Zone B: superior zone (supraspinatus tendon)
Zone C: posterior zone (infraspinatus and teres minor tendons)

A line drawn along the axis of the scapular spine separates zones B and C (Fig. 10.7-5).

The size of the tear (greatest width of the defect) is defined as follows in the Batemann classification:

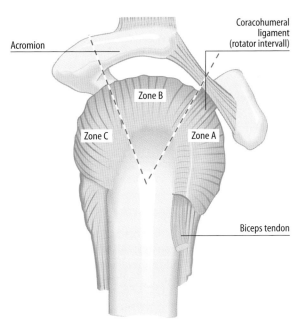

Fig. 10.7-5. Zonal classification of rotator cuff lesions (see text for explanation). (After Habermeyer 1996)

- **Small tear (< 1 cm)**
- **Medium-size tear (1–3 cm)**
- **Large tear (3–5 cm)**
- **Massive tear (> 5 cm)**

Cuff tears can also be classified by their shape: longitudinal, transverse, stellate, or massive.

Because the biceps tendon is in close relation to the rotator cuff, its condition should always be evaluated along with the rotator cuff. It is determined whether the biceps tendon is torn (partial or complete), whether it is dislocated or subluxated, and whether (as in tendinitis) it is covered by synovitis.

Therapeutic Management

Partial Tear

Partial rotator cuff tears can be treated symptomatically with corticosteroid injections to reduce the irritation of the subacromial bursa.

> **Caution:** Do not inject a cortisone preparation into the rotator cuff, as this can exacerbate the tissue defect and make subsequent repair surgery far more difficult.

Meanwhile an intensive physical therapy program is initiated to strengthen the rotators and adductors, as these muscles will bring the humeral head downward (depressors) and thus restore dynamic equilibrium between the deltoid muscle and rotator cuff. Distal movement of the humeral head will also expand the narrowed subacromial space. If conservative treatment does not yield the desired result, endoscopic subacromial decompression (ESD) should be performed. Mobile tags of rotator cuff that are causing mechanical problems are carefully debrided. If the partial tear involves more than 50 % of the tendon thickness and there is a history of an acute event, rotator cuff repair may be considered.

Controversy continues to surround not just the technique and timing of surgery but also the possible prognostic factors. Conservative treatment is also an option for rotator cuff tears.

The decision whether to treat a cuff tear operatively or nonoperatively depends on various factors:

- Patient age
- Patient activity level
- Concomitant lesions (e.g. shoulder dislocation)
- Range of joint motion
- Symptoms
- Tear location

There are other factors that imply a favorable or unfavorable prognosis.

> **Unfavorable factors are:**
- **Advanced age**
- **Large cuff defect**
- **Passive limitation of shoulder motion**
- **Small acromiohumeral distance**
- **Unstable tendon tissue**

- **Cuff tears in zone A or in all three zones**
- **Biceps tendon lesion**
- **Multiple cortisone injections** (perhaps even in the rotator cuff) prior to surgery
- **Obesity?**

Conservative Treatment

The following factors suggest a favorable response to nonoperative treatment:

1. Gradual onset of complaints
2. Degenerative lesion
3. Sedentary patient
4. Advanced age
5. Lack of motivation
6. Concomitant limitation of motion (e.g., frozen shoulder)

Conservative treatment includes analgesic therapy combined with nonsteroidal anti-inflammatory medication. A brief period of immobilization can be beneficial in the acute stage. Subacromial corticosteroid injection will reduce acute pain symptoms but should not be done more than three times, as this would compromise the prognosis of a subsequent operative repair.

> **Note:** Appropriate physical therapy is essential to restore passive joint mobility and achieve specific muscle strengthening, particularly of the muscle groups that depress the humeral head.

Additionally, the patient must learn how to cope with the lesion through the modification of daily activities.

Operative Treatment

The following are considered contraindications to nonoperative treatment (Habermayer 1996):

- **Acute trauma**
- **Active, working patient**
- **Previous shoulder dislocation in a patient over 40 years of age**
- **Patient younger than 50 years of age**

The indication for operative treatment also depends critically on shoulder pain. Loss of strength and function are less important concerns. A significant criterion is the demands placed by the patient on his or her arm and shoulder, which influences motivation. Every surgical repair must be followed by adequate rehabilitation.

The various surgical options, particularly arthroscopic rotator cuff repairs, are still a matter of contro-

Table 10.7-1. Lesion-specific indications for operative treatment (SSP supraspinatus tendon, ISP infraspinatus tendon, SCP subscapularis tendon, LBS long biceps tendon, AC arthroscopy, AHD acromiohumeral distance, OSD open subacromial decompression, ESD endoscopic subacromial decompression). (From Habermeyer 1996)

Type of lesion	Operative treatment
Partial-thickness tear	
SSP grade II°a (articular side)	AC shaving + ESD
SSP grade III°a (articular side)	AC repair + ESD or open repair + OSD
SSP grade II°b (acromial side)	AC shaving + ESD
SSP grade III°b (acromial side)	AC shaving + ESD or open repair + OSD
SCP	(Combined with dislocation: severe capsular damage, open repair SCP, deltopectoral approach)
Full-thickness tear	
SSP	• Athletes < age 40, AS repair, defect < 2 cm • ESD + mini-open repair, defect 2–3 cm • OSD + open repair, defect > 3 cm
SSP + ISP	• Transosseous repair + OSD, AHD ≥7 mm • Transosseous repair + OSD + Mumford, AHD 5–7 mm • Latissimus transfer, < age 45, AHD 5–7 mm • Deltoid flap, < age 45, AHD 5–7 mm
SSP + SCP	• Transosseous (Cofield) repair + OSD • Deltoid flap, AHD 5–7 mm
SCP	• Open transosseous repair, no OSD, deltopectoral approach • Transosseous repair + OSD (possible only in acute cases)
SSP + ISP + SCP (massive tear)	• (Neviaser flap + OSD + Mumford, AHD 5–7 mm) • Deltoid flap + OSD + Mumford, AHD 5–7 mm • Burkhart equatorial partial repair • AS debridement + tuberculoplasty
Rotator cuff defect arthropathy	• Hemiprosthesis (ESD or OSD not indicated), AHD < 5 mm

versy. It is reasonably clear that arthroscopic repair is feasible only for acute traumatic tears, as this requires little or no tendon mobilization. With an old tear or large traumatic tear, open treatment is advised.

Habermeyer (1996) devised a system of indications for operative treatment based on the types and combinations of tendon lesions (Table 10.7-1).

The following arthroscopic surgical techniques are available for the treatment of rotator cuff lesions:

- **Rotator cuff debridement.** The therapeutic efficacy of tendon debridement is still unclear at present due to a lack of studies in large clinical series.

- **Endoscopic subacromial decompression** (see Sect. 10.10). This appears to have much greater value than debridement, even when done as an open procedure.

- **Rotator cuff repair.** Various repair techniques are in the clinical testing stage, but there is still a lack of intermediate- and long-term results in large case numbers.

▶ **Note:** Because the rotator cuff is easily accessible through a mini-arthrotomy, open techniques are generally preferred.

When a partial tear is treated by debridement alone, it is very likely that the lesion will progress to a full-thickness tear. The patient should be informed of this prior to surgery.

Operative Technique

Endoscopic Subacromial Decompression (ESD)
(see pp. 933–940, Figs. 10.10-5 to 10.10-10)

Rotator Cuff Debridement

1. **Inspection and probing.** The frayed tendon area is visualized and then probed to determine the depth of the lesion.

2. **Debridement.** Projecting or mechanically obstructive tags of cuff tissue are carefully debrided with a syn-

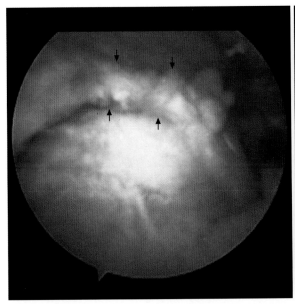

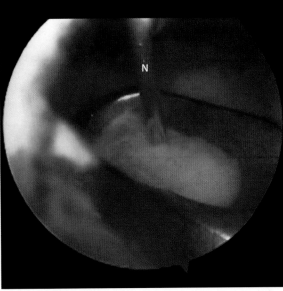

Fig. 10.7-6. Endoscopic rotator cuff repair. Initial appearance of the cuff tear. The free edge (*arrows*) is markedly thickened. (Photo courtesy of Peter Habermayer, Heidelberg)

Fig. 10.7-7. Endoscopic rotator cuff repair (continued from Fig. 10.7-6). The optimum portal site is determined with a percutaneous needle (*N*). (Photo courtesy of Peter Habermayer, Heidelberg)

ovial resector or fine basket forceps. This should be done with extreme care to avoid converting a partial rotator cuff tear into a full-thickness tear.

Rotator Cuff Repair

Various suture anchor systems (Mitek anchor, Ethicon; corkscrew anchor, Arthrex) are available for arthroscopic rotator cuff repairs. Each of these techniques can be performed endoscopically or through a mini-arthrotomy. The technique for endoscopic cuff repair with the corkscrew anchor is described below.

Instrumentation. Besides the implant (corkscrew anchor) preloaded with nonabsorbable sutures, a special grasper is required.

1. **Inspection and probing.** The size, location, and pattern of the supraspinatus tear are evaluated from the glenohumeral joint. Medial retraction and quality of the rotator cuff are also assessed (Fig. 10.7-6).
   Note: Large, extensive tears with degenerative changes in the cuff tissue are not suitable for arthroscopic repair.

2. **Visualizing the subacromial space, subacromial decompression.** After adhesions in the subacromial space have been cleared, ESD is performed (see Sect. 10.10 for technique). The instrument portal for subacromial decompression should be placed about 4 cm lat-

eral to the acromial border, as this portal will also be used for the rotator cuff repair.

3. **Rotator cuff debridement** (see above).

4. **Making a bony trough in the greater tuberosity.** After adhesions have been removed, a bone trough approximately 4–5 mm wide is made at the junction of the humeral head and greater tuberosity using a round bur through the previously placed lateral subacromial portal. The trough is located beneath the rotator cuff tear.

5. **Cuff mobilization.** The grasper is introduced through the lateral portal. The torn portion of the cuff is grasped and pulled laterally over the preplaced bony trough. If the cuff cannot be mobilized far enough medially, it may be necessary to make a capsulotomy along the superior glenoid rim.
   If the cuff can be adequately mobilized to cover the defect, the suture anchor (corkscrew) is introduced.
   Tip: If pulling the retracted edge of the cuff back to its insertion creates tension, it is better to convert to an open procedure so that the cuff can be adequately mobilized.

6. **Placing the suture anchor.** The cuff is held in the reduced position with the grasper, and a percutaneous needle is inserted to locate the optimum portal site for introducing the suture anchor (Fig. 10.7-7). The anchor should be introduced at an angle of

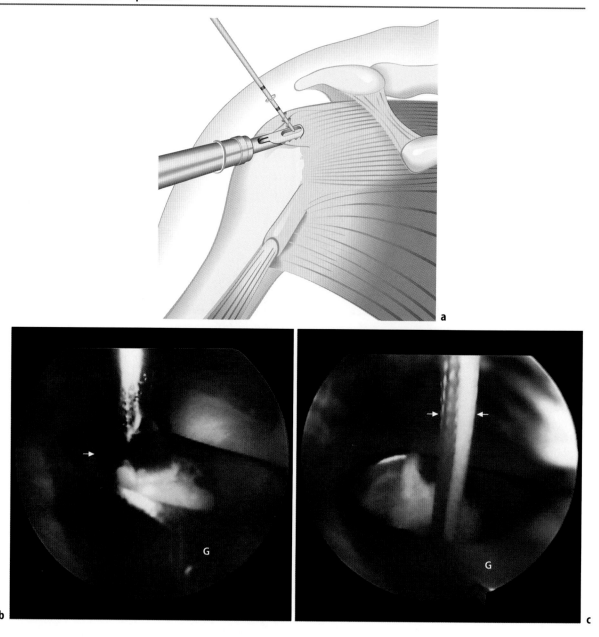

70°–80°. If the needle confirms optimum access to the reduced cuff, the skin at the needle entry site is incised and the subcutaneous tissue carefully spread open. The corkscrew anchor is advanced through the stab incision on its inserter. It is passed through the window in the grasper, through the reduced tendon edge, and is screwed directly into the bony trough in the humerus (Fig. 10.7-8). With its auger type thread and thin 2.0-mm core diameter, the anchor makes only a very small hole when penetrating the tendon. The insertion depth is indicated by two marks on the inserter (see Fig. 10.7-8 b). When the grasper jaw is in direct contact with the greater tuberosity, the anchor is screwed in until the second mark on the

Fig. 10.7-8a–c. Endoscopic rotator cuff repair (continued from Fig. 10.7-7). **a** The cuff is held in position with the grasper, and the corkscrew anchor is inserted. Two marks are visible on the inserter. **b** The anchor is screwed in until the second mark (*arrow*) reaches the upper jaw of the grasper (*G*). **c** The inserter is withdrawn. The sutures (*arrows*) pass through the grasper. (Photos courtesy of Peter Habermayer, Heidelberg)

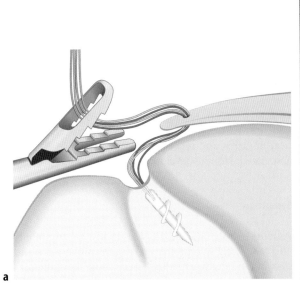

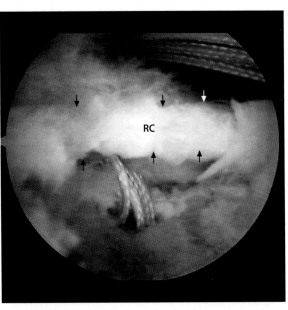

a

b

Fig. 10.7-9a,b. Endoscopic rotator cuff repair (continued from Fig. 10.7-8). **a** The grasper is designed so that when it is withdrawn, it automatically brings the sutures out through the instrument portal. **b** Arthroscopic view: free edge of the rotator cuff (*RC, arrows*). The green and white suture ends are visible. (Photo courtesy of Peter Habermayer, Heidelberg)

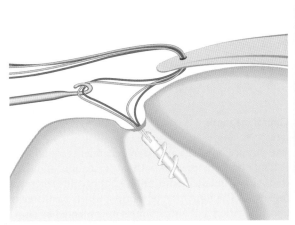

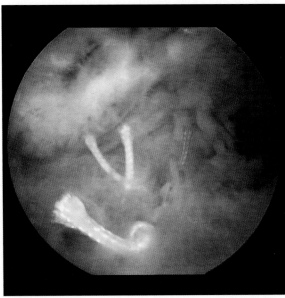

Fig. 10.7-10. A crochet hook is used to retrieve one suture pair

Fig. 10.7-11. Endoscopic rotator cuff repair (continued from Fig. 10.7-10). Final appearance of the cuff repair. (Photo courtesy of Peter Habermayer, Heidelberg)

inserter reaches the window in the closed grasper (Fig. 10.7-8 b). If the lower jaw is not in contact with the bone, the anchor is inserted only as far as the first mark.

7. **Suture retrieval and knot tying.** Because the corkscrew anchor is preloaded with two sutures of contrasting colors, two white and two green suture strands are seen after the grasper is withdrawn (Fig. 10.7-8 c). Since the lower jaw of the grasper is fork-shaped while the upper jaw is rounded, withdrawing the grasper automatically transports the sutures out of the joint and through the instrument portal (Fig. 10.7-9 a, b).

With all four suture strands passing through the rotator cuff (Fig. 10.7-9 b), one white and one green suture end are separated and pulled out with a small crochet hook (Fig. 10.7-10). At this point one suture end runs directly out of the joint from the bone trough while the other end runs from the trough through the rotator cuff before passing to the outside. Before the first suture (e. g., the green suture) is tied, the white suture is held under tension to retain the position of the cuff over the bone trough. When the knot has been tied, it is advanced through the working cannula to the rotator cuff with a knot pusher. The second suture is tied using the same technique. The tissue bridge between the two sutures should be as large as possible. Therefore the second suture should be positioned with the probe such that the second knot will be anterior or posterior to the first knot. This ensures that a sufficiently strong tissue bridge will be maintained between the two knots (Fig. 10.7-11).

▶ **Tip:** If the rotator cuff tear is more than 1 cm wide, a second suture anchor is required. It is inserted using the same technique. When a second anchor is used, one suture pair from each anchor can be placed as a vertical stitch. The other sutures can then be placed between the anchors in mattress fashion. Sutures of contrasting colors are tied together, i. e., the green suture from the first anchor is tied to the white suture of the second anchor. The two remaining suture ends are also tied together.

Postoperative Care

If the cuff has been repaired without tension, the arm is immobilized in a Gilchrist bandage for 6 weeks. If the cuff was repaired under tension, a shoulder abduction splint may have to be worn for 4–6 weeks.

10.8 Frozen Shoulder (Adhesive Capsulitis)

Cause

Frozen shoulder is a separate disease entity and does not denote shoulder stiffness due to subacromial pathology. The cause is poorly understood but may be multifactorial. Trauma, cervical syndromes, autoimmune processes, Pancoast tumor, thyroid disorders, Parkinson disease, head injuries, and myocardial infarction have all been associated with the development of adhesive capsulitis.

Symptoms

Patients between 40 and 70 years of age are commonly affected. Early symptoms consist of night pain and sleeping difficulties. As the disease progresses, the predominant symptoms are increasing limitation of glenohumeral motion and pain with overhead arm use or when reaching behind the back (e. g., to tie an apron). With passage of time, these movements cause excruciating pain and eventually cannot be performed at all. The natural history consists of three phases:

Phase I (pain phase). Duration: 2–9 months. The patient complains of acute pain that worsens at night and interferes with sleep. The predominant symptoms are pain and increasing limitation of motion (freezing phase).

Phase II (frozen phase). Duration: 4–12 months. Symptoms consist of pain with increasing motion loss and secondary muscular atrophy.

Phase III (thawing phase). Duration: 6–9 months. This phase is characterized by a gradual return of motion.

Clinical Diagnosis

The physical findings are stage-dependent (see above). Patients typically present with a very painful shoulder that initially retains some motion but becomes increasingly stiff. The limitation of motion, which particularly affects rotation and abduction, is documented by clinical examination.

Frozen shoulder requires differentiation from other conditions that cause restriction of shoulder motion: rotator cuff tears, old shoulder dislocations, calcifying rotator cuff tendinitis, and osteoarthritis. Differentiation from subacromial syndrome is also required (see Sect. 10.10).

Radiographs, Ultrasound

Radiographic and ultrasound findings in frozen shoulder are usually normal. Local osteopenia is sometimes noted.

Arthroscopic Findings

The arthroscopic findings vary with the stage of the disease. Phase I is characterized by massive synovial hypertrophy and phase II by a marked decrease in joint volume (capsular contraction), obliteration of the axillary recess by adhesions, and marked induration of the joint capsule.

Therapeutic Management

Reports on the natural history of this disease are contradictory. Several years ago, frozen shoulder was thought to be a self-limiting disease in which complete recovery of shoulder function occurred in 1–2 years on average. Long-term studies have shown, however, that recovery of motion can be greatly prolonged and that significant motion deficits may persist. Despite considerable experience with the disease, current treatment options do not offer satisfactory success rates.

Conservative Treatment

Primary treatment is symptomatic, consisting of nonsteroidal anti-inflammatory agents and analgesic medications. Sedatives and calcitonin are beneficial in some cases. Intraarticular corticosteroid injections combined with physical therapy may also be tried. The goal of physical therapy is to improve pain and motion by stretching the muscles and capsule.

Operative Treatment

If conservative measures are unsuccessful or if the patient is unwilling to wait for the disease to run its course, distention of the joint capsule can be performed under arthroscopic control. Arthroscopic synovectomy and, if necessary, arthrolysis should be performed along the inferior circumference of the capsule to create a "point of least resistance" for subsequent manipulation under anesthesia.

Manipulation under anesthesia should be done extremely carefully due to frequent reports of complications such as humeral fractures, labral avulsion with instability, rotator cuff tears, and nerve injuries.

Operative Technique

1. **Arthroscope portal.** Sheath insertion can be difficult in a frozen shoulder due to the restricted joint play and indurated capsule. The operation should be reserved for experienced surgeons, therefore. When the sheath is intraarticular, the joint is distended with fluid. A normal degree of expansion is not obtained because of the contracted capsule. However, the fluid distention itself provides a therapeutic effect by stretching the capsule.

2. **Instrument portal.** Given the frequently tight confines in a frozen shoulder joint, particular care must be exercised when creating the anterior inferior instrument portal. The Wissinger rod technique should be used.

3. **Partial synovectomy.** It is common to find diffuse synovitis, adhesions, and contracted tissue in the anterior part of the joint. In this case a partial synovectomy should be performed, and adhesive bands should be removed as required. If diffuse synovitis is found in the inferior part of the joint, a partial synovectomy should be performed with a synovial resector.

4. **Capsulotomy.** The inferior circumference of the capsule is carefully incised with electrocautery (hook electrode) to create a point of least resistance for subsequent, gentle manipulation under anesthesia.
   > **Tip:** The close proximity of the axillary nerve to the inferior recess warrants extreme caution. If doubt exists, the capsulotomy should be omitted.

5. **Subacromial bursectomy.** The arthroscope is advanced into the subacromial space, which is cleared of scar tissue and adhesions. If possible, subacromial decompression is not performed.

6. **Manipulation under anesthesia.** The patient's arm is grasped just below the elbow, and the other hand is placed in the axilla to obtain the shortest possible lever arm. The arm is now passively anteverted at the shoulder joint. The hand in the axilla can feel a decrease in soft-tissue resistance accompanied by snapping and tearing sounds, usually between 80° and 120°. Next the arm is gently externally rotated and simultaneously abducted to 90°.
   > **Tip:** Proceed very carefully and gently when manipulating the arm. Overvigorous manipulation can cause fractures, massive tears, or other injuries to anatomically intact structures.

7. **Arthroscopic inspection.** The final condition of the joint is evaluated arthroscopically. In most cases a

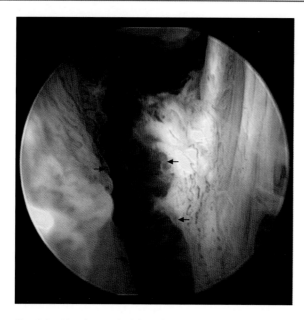

Fig. 10.8-1. Tear (*arrows*) of the inferior recess following manipulation of a frozen shoulder under anesthesia

tear will be found in the previously small axillary recess (Fig. 10.8-1). Local bleeding sites are controlled with electrocautery (ball-tipped electrode).

8. **Steroid injection.** An intraarticular corticosteroid injection can be administered under arthroscopic control to reduce the synovitis.

Postoperative Care

An intensive exercise program is essential and should include manual therapy to improve joint mobility (distraction, translation, and separation exercises). Plexus anesthesia (Winnie block) is helpful in the postoperative period. Continuous passive motion is started on the first postoperative day.

A cold therapy pad (e. g., Polar Care) can be used to reduce pain and swelling.

10.9 Infection

Cause

Percutaneous aspiration, injection, previous arthroscopy, or hematogenous spread are the most frequent causes of joint infection. As in other joints, the main causative organism is Staphylococcus aureus.

Symptoms

Patients present with typical inflammatory signs such as redness, swelling, pain, and limited motion. Elevation of body temperature may also be found.

▶ **Note:** Intraarticular cortisone injection can mask the symptoms of infection, causing a delay in diagnosis and treatment.

Clinical Diagnosis

Joint infection can be diagnosed clinically from the overt signs and from laboratory findings (ESR, CRP). A faster way to confirm or exclude an intraarticular infection suspected from the history or physical findings is by determining the WBC in joint aspirate. If the count is higher than 35,000 cells per mL, or if unequivocal clinical symptoms are present, appropriate treatment for joint infection should be instituted without delay. It is desirable to obtain culture results whenever possible, however.

▶ **Caution:** Waiting for lab results (e. g., CRP) or a positive culture should not delay the surgical treatment of infection.

Radiographs

Radiographic changes such as joint space narrowing, articular surface destruction, or local cyst formation indicate that the joint infection has been present for several weeks.

Ultrasound

Ultrasound can demonstrate intraarticular effusion and may show paraarticular fluid collections.

MRI

MRI can demonstrate intraarticular changes and reactive synovial changes (thickening of the synovial membrane).

Arthroscopic Findings

Arthroscopy reveals typical infection-related changes like those found in other joints (see Sect. 2.18).

Therapeutic Management

▶ **Note:** Intraarticular infection constitutes an emergency indication for treatment.

If the infection has developed as a result of injection, percutaneous aspiration, prior arthroscopy, or hematogenous spread, it should be treated arthroscopically. Arthroscopic treatment is not indicated for an infection that has spread to extraarticular tissues. These cases are managed by the open treatment of all affected areas.

As in other joints, treatment includes intensive arthroscopic lavage with removal of necrotic and infiltrated tissues. Fibrin clots and hematomas are also removed, as they provide an excellent culture medium for bacteria. Synovitis is managed by partial or complete synovectomy. Surgical treatment may conclude with the intraarticular placement of absorbable antibiotic-impregnated material (e.g., gentamicin), as in other joints. This is a controversial measure, however, because the antibiotic can cause cartilage damage by altering the local pH.

▶ **Caution:** Never irrigate the joint with antiseptic solution, as this can produce deep cartilage lesions (Fig. 10.9-1).

If the patient's condition does not improve significantly within two days after arthroscopic treatment (lavage, synovectomy, etc.) and the CRP remains elevated, arthroscopic lavage should be repeated and combined if necessary with further synovectomy and the implantation of antibiotic-impregnated material.

The patient should be informed preoperatively about the possible need for arthroscopic reintervention or the potential for permanent functional deficits in the shoulder, with ankylosis being the worst-case scenario.

Postoperative Care

Early but gentle mobilization is indicated to prevent severe motion loss. The postoperative regimen is conducted in close cooperation with the physical therapist. If any new signs of inflammation appear (pain, swelling, redness), the physical therapist should contact the surgeon at once if the patient is already in an ambulatory setting.

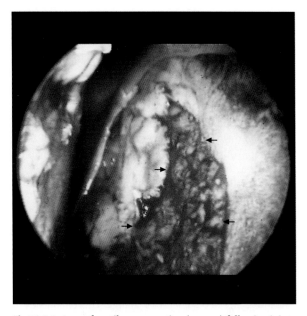

Fig. 10.9-1. Area of cartilage separation (*arrows*) following joint irrigation with an antiseptic solution (Lavasept). (Photo courtesy of André Gächter, St. Gallen)

10.10 Subacromial Space

The subacromial space is considered a functionally separate anatomic unit. Because it is occupied by the subacromial bursa, endoscopic procedures in the subacromial space are more accurately described as bursoscopy or endoscopy rather than arthroscopy.

Lesions of the subacromial space were formerly referred to as "humeroscapular periarthropathy." Today the preferred term is "subacromial syndrome," which better reflects our functional understanding of subacromial pathology.

Cause

Subacromial irritation results from rotator cuff tendinopathy due to vascular insufficiency combined with a local "crowding" of the cuff and limitation of the subacromial space superiorly by the acromion and coracoacromial ligament. The causes of rotator cuff lesions are reviewed in Sect. 10.7.

Bigliani and Levine (1997) distinguish between intrinsic and extrinsic causes.

Intrinsic factors are:
- Muscle weakness
- Overuse of the shoulder
- Rotator cuff degeneration

Extrinsic factors are:

- Glenohumeral instability
- Osteoarthritis of the AC joint
- Impingement on the coracoacromial ligament
- Impingement on the coracoid process
- Os acromiale (unfused epiphysis in the distal articular cartilage)
- Impingement on the posterior superior glenoid. When the arm is extended, abducted, and externally rotated during throwing, the rotator cuff impinges on the posterior superior corner of the glenoid. This inherently "normal" impingement can assume pathologic significance in throwing athletes.

Classification

Various forms of subacromial syndrome can be distinguished radiographically and sonographically based on various types of degenerative change. This enables us to classify the forms based on their pathomorphologic features:

- **Simple subacromial syndrome.** Mechanical irritation of the bursa and rotator cuff in the less vascularized zone in front of the tendon insertion produces an inflammatory condition that leads to edematous swelling. This further narrows the already tight anatomic confines of the subacromial space. Even a small degree of arm abduction uses up the available space (impingement), resulting in pain. If there are no structural changes in the soft tissues and there is still a normal range of shoulder motion, a "simple subacromial syndrome" is present.

- **Calcifying subacromial syndrome.** Foci of chondroid metaplasia (fibrocartilaginous transformation) develop within a still-viable tendon. Ultrasound shows nonhomogeneity of the tendon echoes. Calcium salt deposition may occur in the transformed areas. These variable-sized deposits are often found in the critical zone of diminished blood flow (about 0.5–1.5 cm in front of the tuberosity). This form of the subacromial syndrome can be diagnosed radiographically and sonographically.

- **Adhesive subacromial syndrome.** Chronic inflammation caused by frictional wear of the tendon surface and/or the release of calcium salt crystals leads to fibrin exudation and adhesion formation in the subacromial space (Fig. 10.10-1).

- **Rotator cuff tearing.** Adverse mechanical factors acting on the tendon, combined with decreased vascularity, can cause degenerative rotator cuff tears ranging to a complete avulsion of the cuff (see Sect. 10.7

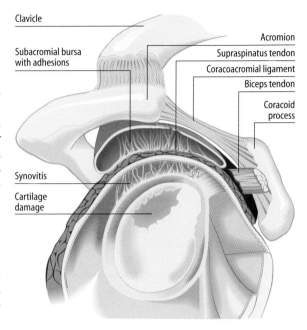

Fig. 10.10-1. Lesions found in adhesive subacromial syndrome. Synovitis and adhesions are most pronounced in the subacromial space (after Esch 1993)

for details). Older patients are predominantly affected.

- **Rotator cuff defect arthropathy.** Tearing of the rotator cuff leads to superior migration of the humeral head (decreased acromiohumeral distance). The operative or conservative treatment of this condition often leads to unsatisfying results.

- **Biceps tendon syndrome.** Because of the close functional relationship of the biceps tendon to the rotator cuff, associated lesions of the biceps tendon (tendinitis, partial or complete rupture) must be taken into consideration (see Sect. 10.5).

Symptoms

The clinical hallmark of subacromial syndrome is shoulder pain during abduction of the humeral head (painful arc). Usually the pain is greatest between about 80° and 110° of elevation and decreases beyond that point. Rest pain and night pain are common, causing patients to awaken when they lie on the affected shoulder. Often the most severe subjective pain is not localized to the subacromial space itself but to the lateral side of the upper arm.

The symptoms depend greatly on the type of subacromial syndrome that is present. For example, patients

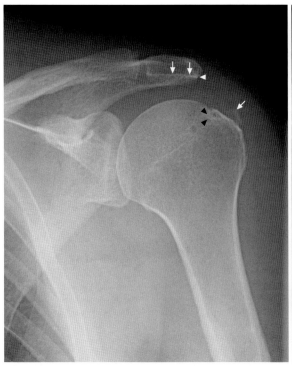 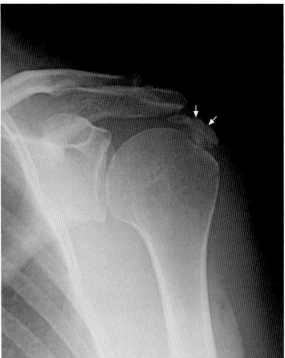

with rotator cuff defect arthropathy may be virtually free of complaints, and their condition is diagnosed entirely from the history and radiographic examination. Other patients with this type of syndrome may have very severe pain but no significant radiographic changes.

Irritative conditions and pronounced rotator cuff defects are usually associated with limitation of active shoulder motion. This is based on proprioceptive inhibition and an inability to retain the humeral head in the glenoid during abduction. Because this condition resembles a "paralyzed arm," it is commonly referred to as pseudoparalysis.

Clinical Diagnosis

Clinical inspection reveals atrophy, bursal swelling, or biceps tendon abnormalities ranging from irritation to tearing or dislocation. Palpation elicits subacromial crepitus, due for example to a rotator cuff tear or cuff defect arthropathy. Sites of maximum tenderness may be located at the front of the subacromial space, over the greater tuberosity, and/or over the long biceps tendon. Function testing includes tests of active and passive motion (painful arc). Limitation of active and passive motion is indicative of subacromial adhesions or secondary capsular contraction.

The following special tests are performed to help differentiate the pathogenesis and site of involvement:

Fig. 10.10-2 a, b. Calcifications in the supraspinatus tendon. **a** AP view shows a small, localized calcification (*arrow*) with volcano cysts (*arrowheads*) in the humeral head. Other findings are subacromial sclerosis (*arrows*) and a small osteophyte (*arrowhead*). **b** Extensive calcification (*arrows*) in the supraspinatus tendon

- **Impingement signs** (Neer test, Hawkins sign)
- **Jobe supraspinatus test**
- **Speed test**
- **Drop-arm sign**
- **Resistive tensioning tests**

The injection of a local anesthetic into the subacromial bursa (Neer test) is helpful for confirming the diagnosis of a subacromial syndrome. If shoulder pain is significantly reduced or relieved by the injection, the diagnosis is confirmed. Otherwise a different cause of the pain should be sought. The Neer test is also useful in predicting the efficacy of operative treatment (subacromial decompression).

Instabilities of the glenohumeral joint (see Sect. 10.6) should also be excluded.

Radiographs

Calcifications or bony changes may be seen as evidence of chronic impingement (Fig. 10.10-2). Thus, radiographs may show sclerotic changes, spurring on the

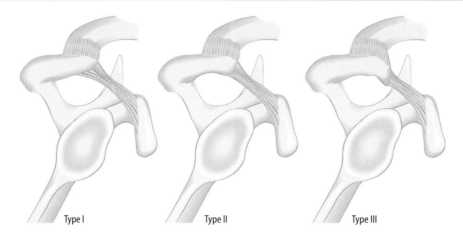

Type I   Type II   Type III

Fig. 10.10-3. Types of acromion morphology, as described by Bigliani

undersurface of the acromion, and contour irregularities on the greater tuberosity. Degenerative changes in the glenohumeral and AC joint should be excluded. Anatomic variants and changes in the acromion (Bigliani types of acromion morphology) can be visualized (Fig. 10.10-3).

Ultrasound

Ultrasonography is the modality of choice for investigating changes in the rotator cuff and subacromial bursa (Fig. 10.10-4). Additionally, ultrasound can define the contour of the humeral head and structural changes in the deltoid muscle.

MRI

If a soft-tissue lesion is presumed but cannot be demonstrated with other techniques, MRI should be performed. CT is useful for evaluating bony lesions.

Arthroscopic Findings

Glenohumeral Joint

Local synovitis may provide evidence of a rotator cuff lesion if a partial or complete tear cannot be found (see Sect. 10.7). Most of these lesions involve the anterior or anterosuperior portion of the rotator cuff and are more characteristic of shoulder instability than a subacromial syndrome. Therefore the joint is also inspected for instability-related changes (see Sect. 10.6).

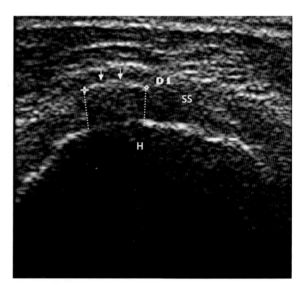

Fig. 10.10-4. Ultrasound features of subacromial syndrome: calcification (*arrows*) of the supraspinatus tendon (*SS*) with a posterior acoustic shadow (*dotted lines*) (*H* humeral head contour). Transducer position I described by Hedtmann and Fett

Subacromial Space

Normally the subacromial bursa is free of vascular congestion. Irritation of the bursa is characterized by synovitis. The anatomic structures of the subacromial space (acromion, coracoacromial ligament, and rotator cuff) often cannot be adequately evaluated until a partial synovectomy has been performed.

Radiographically visible calcifications are often difficult to verify at arthroscopy. Extensive calcium deposits appear as surface irregularities in the rotator cuff. The examiner may attempt to "lance" these foci with a thin needle. The needled focus may release calcium crystals or a pasty whitish material representing the calcium deposit.

Therapeutic Management

Conservative Treatment

Conservative treatment should be tried first in cases where significant mechanical causes, such as large osteophytes in the AC joint, have been excluded. Treatment consists of symptomatic measures, local measures (maximum of three subacromial steroid injections), and systemic measures (nonsteroidal anti-inflammatory agents, analgesic medication in the acute stage), and particularly physical therapy. The aim of physical therapy is to strengthen the adductor and rotator muscles so that they can pull the humeral head downward. All the shoulder muscles should be conditioned in a hyperlax joint.

During conservative treatment, the patient is told to avoid prolonged arm abduction and overhead movements.

Operative Treatment

Following at least a 6-month trial of unsuccessful conservative treatment, subacromial decompression is indicated. This procedure consists of:

1. Division and partial resection of the coracoacromial ligament.
2. The Neer anterior acromioplasty.

Once it has been decided to proceed with subacromial decompression, it must be decided whether to use open or arthroscopic technique. Arthroscopic decompression can be performed through two portals and is preferred in young patients (under age 50) and in females. Adequate visualization of the subacromial space is an important concern. Because open subacromial decompression is performed through a 3-cm-long skin incision, the surgeon can always convert to that procedure if doubt exists or if endoscopic visualization becomes too difficult. The patient should be told of this possibility ahead of time. Thus, measures to improve visualization in the subacromial space (see Sect. 9.12) are of critical importance.

Operative Technique

Endoscopic Subacromial Decompression (ESD)

1. **Arthroscopy of the glenohumeral joint.** As a prelude to every ESD, the glenohumeral joint is inspected and examined for concomitant pathologic changes (synovitis, rotator cuff tears, signs of instability).

2. **Entering the subacromial bursa.** The arthroscope is withdrawn from the glenohumeral joint. Then the blunt obturator is inserted, and the sheath is advanced into the subacromial space (see Sect. 9.11.7 for technique).

3. **Orientation and inspection.** The sheath with blunt obturator is swept from medial to lateral to lyse adhesions and create room in the subacromial space. Visualization is improved by inserting the synovial resector through a lateral portal and removing adhesive bands and portions of the synovium (Fig. 10.10-5a, b). Bleeding sites are controlled with electrocautery (Fig. 10.10-5c).

4. **Dividing the coracoacromial ligament.** First a needle is inserted to mark the position of the acromion and its junction with the coracoacromial ligament (Fig. 10.10-5d). Then the coracoacromial ligament is carefully divided in layers with an electrocautery (hook or ball-tipped electrode) (Fig. 10.10-6).

   ▶ **Tip:** Do not divide the ligament with "one cut," as this can provoke bleeding from the coracoacromial artery or its side branches, making the rest of the procedure far more difficult.

   Particular care is taken to adequately transect the medial band of the ligament.

   If a shaver (round bur or acromionizer) is introduced right away and used on the acromion, bleeding from the ligament stump can obscure the field. Consequently, bleeding should be meticulously controlled after dividing the ligament (Fig. 10.10-6). All "red spots" on the cut surface are cauterized with the ball electrode. If doubt exists, the inflow is reduced or turned off to determine whether larger vessels have been opened.

5. **Visualizing the undersurface of the acromion.** Before the acromioplasty is performed, portions of the coracoacromial ligament that attach to the acromion are released from the acromial undersurface with the shaver (Fig. 10.10-7). This tissue is carefully cauterized to reduce the risk of bleeding and make the tissue easier to resect. The undersurface of the anterior and anterolateral acromion is then examined for bone spurs.

   ▶ **Note:** Exposing the bony undersurface of the acromion is a sine qua non for performing an acromioplasty.

6. **Acromioplasty.** The undersurface of the acromion is resected in layers with a motorized bur (Fig. 10.10-8). It is advantageous to use a conical bur ("acromionizer") rather than a round bur. The resection should create a smooth, flat acromial surface while eliminat-

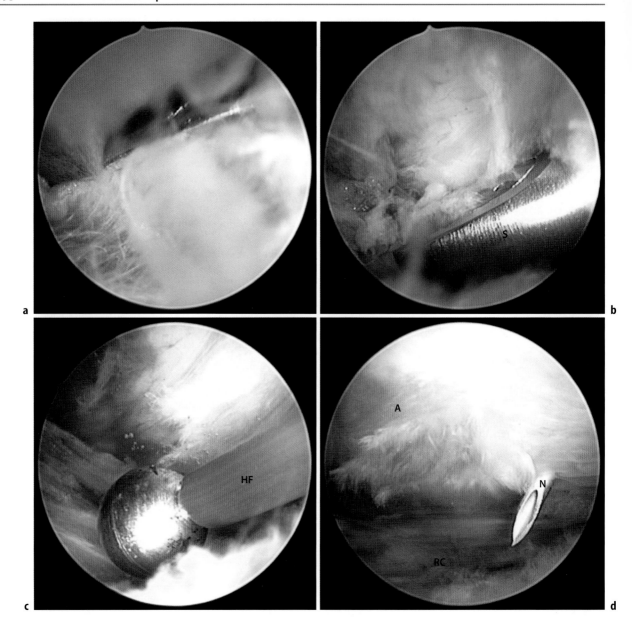

Fig. 10.10-5 a–d. ESD. **a** First, it is necessary to remove adhesive structures to obtain a better view. **b** Partial synovectomy is performed with a shaver (*S*). **c** Local bleeding sites are selectively coagulated with a ball-tipped cautery probe (*HF*). **d** A needle (*N*) is inserted at the anterior border of the acromion to facilitate orientation (*A* acromion, *RC* surface of rotator cuff)

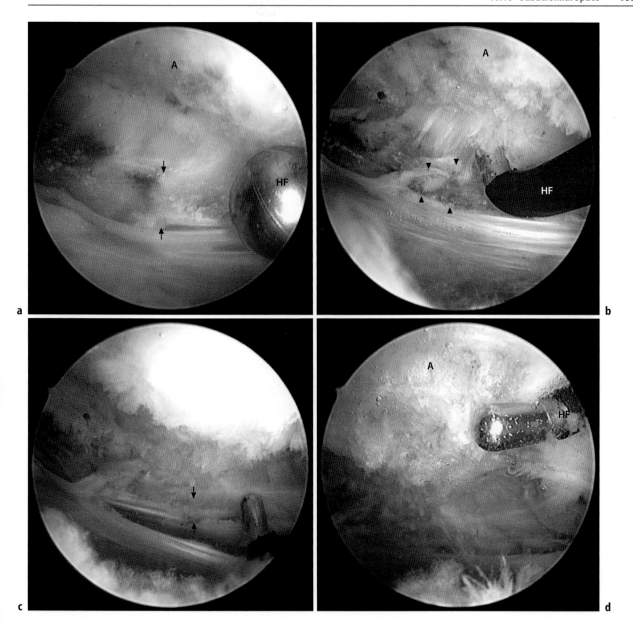

Fig. 10.10-6a–d. ESD (continued from Fig. 10.10-5). **a** The coracoacromial ligament is released from the acromion with a ball-tipped cautery probe (*HF*). The cut edges (*arrows*) are clearly visible. **b** Division of the ligament is continued with a hook electrode (*arrowheads* cut edge). **c** Bleeding points on the cut edges are selectively cauterized to maintain a clear view within the small space. **d** Removal of subacromial soft tissues

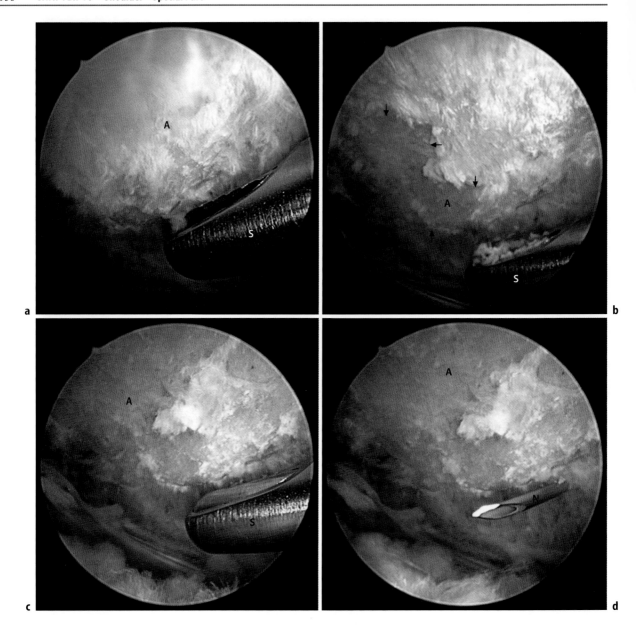

Fig. 10.10-7 a–d. ESD (continued from Fig. 10.10-6). **a** The undersurface of the acromion (*A*) is cleared of soft tissues with a shaver (*S*). **b** At first only a portion of the bone is exposed (*arrows*). **c** Finally the entire subacromial bony surface is cleared of soft tissues. **d** A marking needle (*N*) is inserted at the anterior edge of the acromion so help gauge the extent of the subacromial resection (*A* undersurface of acromion)

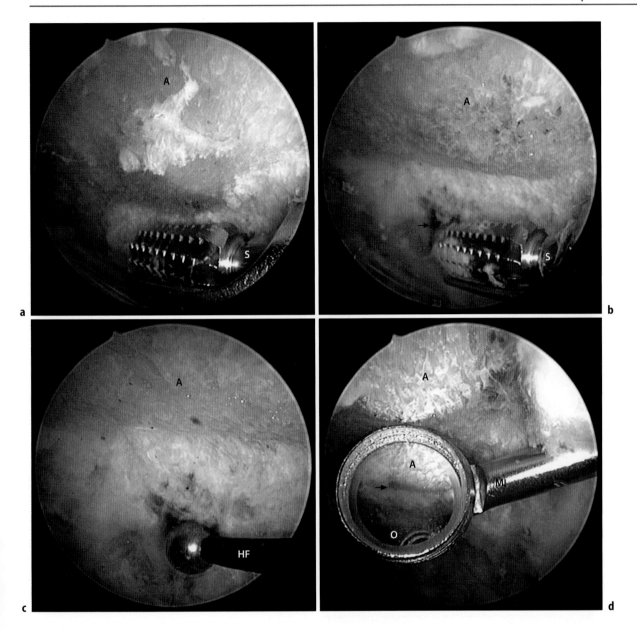

Fig. 10.10-8a–d. ESD (continued from Fig. 10.10-7). **a** The subacromial surface is resected with a conical bur (*S*). **b, c** Local bleeding sites (*arrow*) are coagulated with the ball-tipped cautery probe (*HF*) to maintain a clear view. **d** A mirror (*MI*) can be used to check for remaining bony prominences in the lateral part of the subacromial space or below the AC joint (*O* tip of arthroscope)

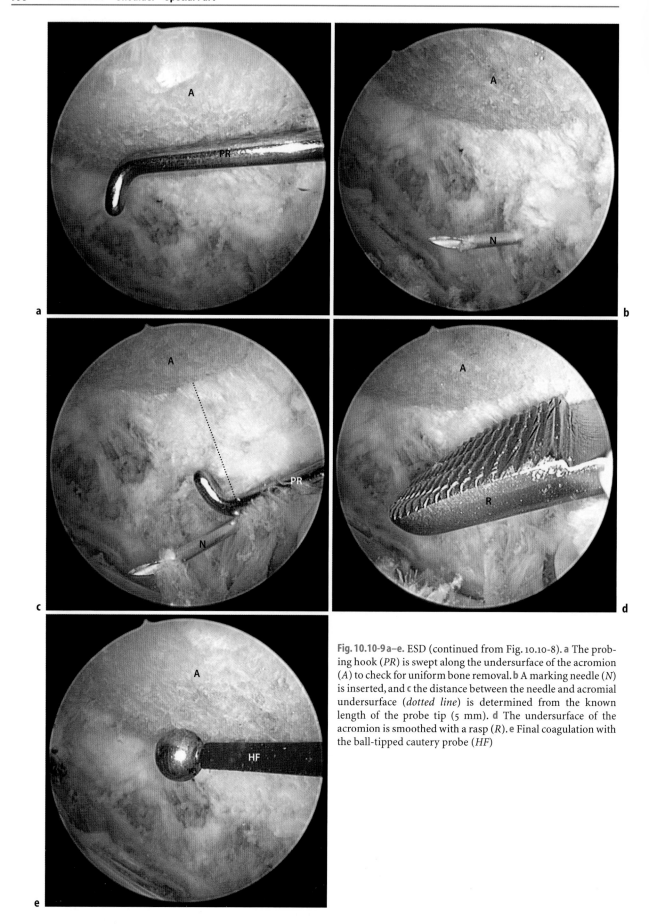

Fig. 10.10-9 a–e. ESD (continued from Fig. 10.10-8). **a** The probing hook (*PR*) is swept along the undersurface of the acromion (*A*) to check for uniform bone removal. **b** A marking needle (*N*) is inserted, and **c** the distance between the needle and acromial undersurface (*dotted line*) is determined from the known length of the probe tip (5 mm). **d** The undersurface of the acromion is smoothed with a rasp (*R*). **e** Final coagulation with the ball-tipped cautery probe (*HF*)

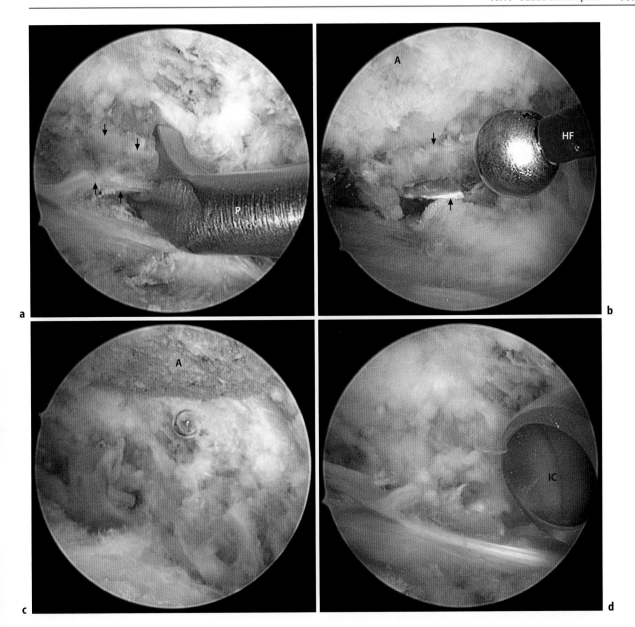

Fig. 10.10-10 a–d. ESD (continued from Fig. 10.10-9). **a** After the acromioplasty is completed, the cut edge of the coracoacromial ligament (*arrows*) appears much thicker. It is therefore resected with a punch (*P*). **b** Meticulous hemostasis is maintained with the ball-tipped cautery probe (*HF*). **c** Final appearance after subacromial decompression (*A* undersurface of acromion). **d** Adequate hemostasis can be confirmed by introducing an irrigation cannula (*IC*) and starting the outflow. The reduced intraarticular pressure may disclose bleeding sites requiring selective electrocoagulation

ing the anterior hook. A mirror can be used to inspect the result (Fig. 10.10-8 d). It is usually sufficient to thin the anterolateral edge of the acromion by 6–9 mm. Bleeding from the anterior tissues or residual ligament during the resection can be controlled with electrocautery (ball-tipped electrode). The undersurface of the acromion is palpated with the arthroscopic probe to confirm a uniform resection (Fig. 10.10-9 a).

The marking needle is used to determine the extent of the resection from the anterolateral undersurface of the acromion (Fig. 10.10-9 b, c).

After the undersurface of the acromion has been adequately thinned, it is smoothed with a rasp (Fig. 10.10-9 d) and then cauterized with the ball-tipped electrode to reduce the risk of postoperative bleeding from the opened cancellous bone (Fig. 10.10-9 e).

7. **Ligament resection.** Completion of the acromioplasty may leave a thick, projecting stump of the divided coracoacromial ligament. This residual stump is resected with a basket forceps (Fig. 10.10-10 a). Bleeding from the cut edges is controlled with electrocautery (Fig. 10.10-10 b).

8. **Final inspection.** Division of the ligament has considerably enlarged the subacromial space (Fig. 10.10-10 c). A final inspection is made for additional bleeding sites, and the rotator cuff is evaluated (Fig. 10.10-10 d). It is scrutinized for any calcium deposits that were detected by preoperative imaging (technique, see below). The cuff is also evaluated for tears, which are managed by debridement or repair (see Sect. 10.7).

Postoperative Care

To prevent adhesions, passive mobilization of the shoulder is initiated as early as possible. Active exercises can be started at about 2 weeks, but rotator cuff strengthening should not be started before weeks 6–8 to avoid irritating the subacromial tissues.

Removal of Calcium Deposits

1. **Inspection.** Because calcium deposits in the rotator cuff are usually associated with narrowing of the subacromial space, ESD is performed first (see above). Then the surface of the rotator cuff is scrutinized. Local irregularities or foci of whitish discoloration may indicate a calcium deposit. The probe can also locate deposits by their hard consistency.

2. **Needling.** The calcium deposit is pierced with a needle.

This may yield individual calcium crystals or a pasty white matter containing calcium.

3. **Debridement.** The calcium deposit is incised and carefully debrided with a sharp spoon or small synovial resector. The shaver should be used with caution to avoid removing too much cuff tissue.

4. **Lavage of the subacromial space.** After a calcium deposit has been opened and debrided, the entire subacromial space should be copiously irrigated. This is essential for reducing postoperative pain, as liberated crystals can incite a massive synovitis leading to severe pain.

5. **Probing.** The debrided site of the calcium deposit is carefully probed to exclude small rotator cuff tears and residual calcium.

Postoperative Care

The debridement of calcium deposits may require gentler and more prolonged rehabilitation, as there may be some residual crystals that will incite a synovitis if the shoulder is exercised too vigorously in the early phase. The patient should be informed of this prior to surgery, and of the fact that residual calcifications may still be visible on postoperative radiographs.

10.11 Acromioclavicular Osteoarthritis

Acromioclavicular separations (Tossy grades I and II) can lead to posttraumatic osteoarthritis of the AC joint. This condition is less common after Tossy grade III injuries. Acromioclavicular osteoarthritis can also develop in the absence of trauma.

Symptoms

Common symptoms are pain during overhead work, local tenderness, and night pain during recumbency on the affected shoulder.

Clinical Diagnosis

Tenderness is usually noted in the area of the AC joint. Axial compression of the AC joint and arm elevation past the horizontal can also cause pain. Crepitus in the AC joint can often be elicited by crossing the arms.

As in the subacromial space, the intraarticular injection of a local anesthetic is helpful in determining the cause of the pain. The differential diagnosis should include postural defects in the shoulder girdle and pain secondary to spinal pathology.

Radiographs

Osteoarthritic changes (joint space narrowing, osteophytes) are often demonstrated. As in other joints, osteoarthritis of the AC joint may be of a hypertrophic or atrophic (lytic) form.

With hypertrophic disease, osteophytes may project from the AC joint into the subacromial space and incite pronounced subacromial symptoms.

With atrophic disease, it is not uncommon to find cystic changes in the lateral portion of the clavicle.

MRI

MRI is of some value in assessing the condition of the articular disk.

Ultrasound

Ultrasound can add a small amount of information (capsular swelling, effusion, etc.) to other modalities.

Arthroscopic Findings

The AC joint can be visualized directly, but more often it is inspected via the subacromial space. Osteophytes cause the joint capsule to bulge toward the subacromial space at the clavicle and acromion. Removing the capsule and osteophytes usually reveals extreme attrition of the articular disk accompanied by deep cartilage lesions.

Therapeutic Management

The recommended treatment for hypertrophic osteoarthritis is ESD combined with osteophyte removal. Portions of the lateral clavicle and acromion can also be arthroscopically resected. It is desirable to preserve the stability of the AC joint, but this is difficult to achieve when the articulating surfaces have been resected.

When extensive changes are present, open resection and interpositional grafting, perhaps combined with a Weaver-Dunn transposition of the coracoacromial ligament, is an option that can preserve some degree of joint stability. Arthroscopic resection of the lateral end of the clavicle (Mumford procedure) has frequently been described but remains undocumented by substantial case numbers.

Subtalar Joint

11.1 Historical Development

Parisien and Vangsness first reported on arthroscopy of the subtalar joint in 1985. They inspected the posterior subtalar joint and recommended a posterolateral portal. Most of the posterior articular surface of the calcaneus and the synovial lining could be evaluated through this portal. Just three years later, Parisien described the first results of arthroscopic operations on the subtalar joint.

Since then, Lundeen (1987, 1994), Frey et al. (1994), Demaziere et al. (1991), and Jerosch (1996) have published articles on the arthroscopy of this difficult-to-reach joint.

11.2 Instrumentation

Subtalar arthroscopy should not be performed with a standard 30° oblique arthroscope (4 mm diameter). In this small joint a smaller-diameter scope (2.4 mm) should be used (see Fig. 5.2-1). A short-barreled scope is recommended, as this makes it easier for the surgeon to brace the arthroscope hand against the patient.

The rest of the instruments (sheath, light source, light cable) are the same as those used in wrist arthroscopy (see Sect. 5.6).

11.3 Video System

A standard video system is used as in knee arthroscopy (see Sect. 1.3).

11.4 Probe

A shorter probing hook should be used in the subtalar joint to permit gentler and more precise probing within the small joint.

11.5 Operating Instruments

"Standard" operating instruments are not usefull (see Sect. 1.6.1). Smaller instruments like those used in wrist arthroscopy (see Sect. 5.6) should be available.

A shaver (see Sect. 1.6.2) is helpful. Besides the standard attachments, which may be somewhat cumbersome because of their length, smaller attachments like those used in the wrist should be available (see Sect. 5.6.2).

Electrocautery is useful for point hemostasis and dividing adhesions (see Sect. 1.6.3). Again, the smaller attachments used in wrist arthroscopy should be available (see Sect. 5.6.3).

A laser can be useful in very tight joint spaces or for removing marginal osteophytes (see Sect. 1.6.4).

11.6 Anesthesia

General anesthesia is preferred, as it provides excellent muscular relaxation. Spinal block or epidural anesthesia can also be used, however (see Sect. 1.7).

11.7 Positioning

The supine or lateral decubitus position can be used. The position should allow access for image intensification fluoroscopy of the operative site.

- **Supine position.** As in ankle arthroscopy, the supine position is preferred. Access to the subtalar joint is facilitated by flexing the operative leg at the knee, internally rotating the thigh at the hip, and tilting the operating table to the opposite side (side rests on the contralateral side).

- **Lateral decubitus position.** In this position the knee is slightly flexed and the lower leg is supported on a role or cushion to facilitate access to the subtalar joint.

- **Distraction.** The joint is distracted manually by an assistant or the scrub nurse. Noninvasive sling systems for subtalar distraction have also been described (Ferkel 1986).

11.8 Tourniquet

All operations are performed using a thigh tourniquet or exsanguinating wrap. The advantage of a tourniquet is that the short saphenous vein on the lateral side of the leg can be identified intraoperatively, reducing the risk of injury.

11.9 Draping

The draping technique is the same as that used for ankle arthroscopy (see Sect. 3.10). The foot is draped only as far as the metatarsus, however.

11.10 Distention Medium

As in other joints, a nonelectrolytic irrigating solution is used. The distention pressure is regulated by adjusting the height of the reservoir bag. A roller pump can be helpful but should be used at a low pressure setting.

11.11 Setup and Preparations for Arthroscopy

The same principles apply as in arthroscopy of the ankle joint (see Sect. 3.12).

11.12 Portal Placement

Since all subtalar portals are placed on the lateral side, the lateral anatomy of the foot and ankle must be well known. The portals are either anterolateral or posterolateral, i.e., located anterior or posterior to the tip of the lateral malleolus.

11.12.1 Anatomy

The lateral malleolus, palpable in all patients, is the principal landmark for identifying the posterior facet of the subtalar joint. The sinus tarsi is also palpable even in obese patients. Pronation and supination movements are helpful in locating the sinus. The inferolateral portion of the talus can also be palpated.

The sural nerve runs approximately 2 cm posterior and 2 cm inferior to the lateral malleolus. The peroneal tendons run along the posterior border of the fibula (Fig. 11.12-1).

On its lateral aspect the subtalar joint is covered anteriorly and laterally by the anterior talofibular ligament and farther laterally by the calcaneofibular ligament, which is an important lateral stabilizer of the joint.

The posterior subtalar joint is in close relation to the posterior compartment of the ankle joint, owing to the sharp posterior taper of the talus. This must be considered during placement of the posterior portals. The posterior subtalar joint is difficult to palpate because of the overlying Achilles tendon.

The subtalar joint is divided into anterior and posterior articulations separated by the sinus tarsi and tarsal canal. The tarsal canal is formed by sulci on the under-

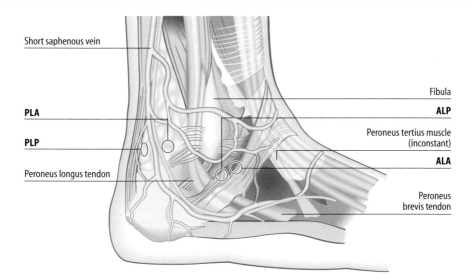

Short saphenous vein

PLA

PLP

Peroneus longus tendon

Fibula

ALP

Peroneus tertius muscle
(inconstant)

ALA

Peroneus
brevis tendon

Fig. 11.12-1. Portals for accessing the subtalar joint (lateral aspect) and their relationship to anatomic structures (*ALA* anterolateral anterior portal, *ALP* anterolateral posterior portal, *PLA* posterolateral anterior portal, *PLP* posterolateral posterior portal)

surface of the talus and the superior surface of the calcaneus. The lateral opening of the tarsal canal is called the sinus tarsi. The anterior subtalar joint is formed by the anterior talus, the posterior surface of the navicular bone, the anterior surface of the calcaneus, and the powerful calcaneonavicular ligament (spring ligament).

The posterior subtalar joint is composed of the posterior facet of the calcaneus and the posterior inferior facet of the talus. This articulation is convex on the calcaneal side and concave on the talar side. The longitudinal axis of the joint forms about a 40° posterior angle with the lateral border of the foot.

Between the anterior and posterior portions of the subtalar joint is the interosseous talocalcaneal ligament, which interconnects the talus and calcaneus.

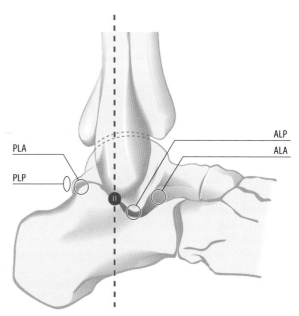

PLA

PLP

ALP

ALA

Fig. 11.12-2. Anterior and posterior subtalar portals in relation to the tip of the lateral malleolus (*ALA* anterolateral anterior portal, *ALP* anterolateral posterior portal, *PLA* posterolateral anterior portal, *PLP* posterolateral posterior portal)

11.12.2 Anterolateral Portals

These portals are located anterior to the long axis of the fibula (Fig. 11.12-2).

Anterolateral Anterior Portal (ALA Portal)

This portal is located approximately 2–3 cm anterior and 5 mm distal to the tip of the lateral malleolus. It serves as the primary arthroscope portal.

The ALA portal is located just posterior to the anterior process of the calcaneus. Structures at risk during placement are the posterior cutaneous branches of the superficial peroneal nerve, the lateral dorsal cutaneous nerve (continuation of the sural nerve), the peroneus tertius tendon (if present), and perhaps portions of the short saphenous vein.

Anterolateral Posterior Portal (ALP Portal)

Located 10 mm anterior to the long axis of the fibula, this portal gives direct access to the sinus tarsi. The anterior malleolar artery is at risk during portal placement.

11.12.3 Posterolateral Portals

The posterolateral portals – one anterior and one posterior – are located posterior to the fibula (Fig. 11.12-3).

Posterolateral Anterior Portal (PLA Portal)

This portal is located just posterior to the peroneal tendon compartment, approximately 5–8 mm proximal to the tip of the lateral malleolus. The peroneal tendons are at risk and can interfere with instrument manipulations.

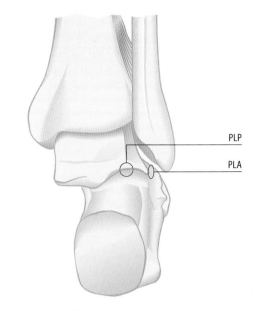

Posterolateral Posterior Portal (PLP Portal)

This portal is placed directly lateral and anterior to the Achilles tendon about 25 mm posterior and 6 mm proximal to the tip of the lateral malleolus. The sural nerve and short saphenous vein are at risk during portal placement.

> ▶ **Caution:** When establishing the PLP portal, bear in mind its proximity to the posterior compartment of the ankle joint. This distance is so small that one can easily enter the posterior aspect of the talocrural joint by mistake.

Fig. 11.12-3. Location of the posterolateral subtalar portals (*PLA* posterolateral anterior portal, *PLP* posterolateral posterior portal)

11.12.4 Creating the Arthroscope Portal: Technique

A standard technique is followed in creating the arthroscope portal:

1. **Palpation.** Key anatomic landmarks such as the tip of the fibula, the calcaneus, the talus, and the peroneal tendons are palpated.

2. **Needle test.** A needle is inserted lateral to the Achilles tendon (PLP portal) and advanced into the posterior subtalar joint. The needle is moved medially and laterally to determine whether the needle tip has entered the joint or is still in subcutaneous or capsular tissue.

3. **Distention.** The joint is distended with 5–10 mL of irrigating fluid. Backflow confirms an intraarticular injection.
> ▶ **Tip:** Do not empty too much of the fluid. The joint should remain well distended.

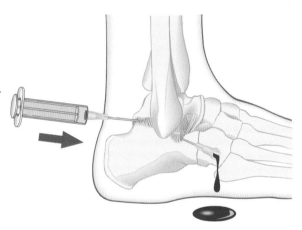

Fig. 11.12-4. The subtalar joint is distended through a posterior needle. Outflow through a needle inserted anterior to the tip of the lateral malleolus confirms joint entry

4. **Locating the anterolateral portal.** A needle is inserted 3 cm anterior to the tip of the lateral malleolus and advanced toward the posterior subtalar joint at about a 45° angle. Fluid outflow from the hub confirms that the needle has entered the joint (Fig. 11.12-4).
> ▶ **Tip:** If there is a danger of losing access to the joint, the needle can initially be left in the posterolateral portal. Then, with the joint maximally distended, a three-way stopcock can be connected to the needle to provide a way of maintaining joint distention if problems arise in creating the arthroscope portal.

5. **Skin incision.** A skin incision 4–6 mm long is made at the site of the anterior needle insertion, and the needle is removed. It is important to note the angle and orientation of the needle, as the sheath will be introduced in the same direction.

6. **Spreading the subcutaneous tissue.** A fine, blunt clamp is used to spread the subcutaneous tissue down to the capsule. The joint is not yet entered.

7. **Inserting the sheath.** The sheath with blunt obturator and open spigot is advanced into the joint (in the same direction as the anterior needle). Fluid outflow from the open spigot confirms joint entry. The blunt obturator is then withdrawn, and the arthroscope is inserted.

11.12.5 Creating the Instrument Portal: Technique

The first instrument portal to be established is the PLP portal. It is placed under visual control following a standard technique:

1. **Needle test.** The needle is inserted at the posterolateral site (about 20–25 mm posterior and 6 mm proximal to the tip of the lateral malleolus) until it appears within the joint.

2. **Skin incision.** A 2-mm skin incision is made at the needle site.

3. **Spreading the subcutaneous tissue and joint capsule.** A fine, blunt clamp is used to spread the subcutaneous tissue and enter the joint. The skin incision is enlarged by spreading it open with the clamp.

4. **Inserting the probe and operating instruments.**

11.12.6 Switching Portals

A switching rod is used to interchange the portals for viewing and instrumentation (see Sect. 1.13.6 for technique).

11.13 Examination Sequence

The first structures visualized from the anterolateral portal are the calcaneus, talus, and lateral recess (Fig. 11.13-1). The arthroscope is then retracted to view the posterior facet of the subtalar joint. Anteriorly, the part of the anterior capsule with the ligament bounding the tarsal canal can be visualized. After the anterior portion of the joint has been inspected, the posterolateral portal is established under visual control.

By switching portals (placing the arthroscope in the posterolateral portal), the posterior part of the lateral recess and the posterior portion of the joint can be inspected. While maneuvering the arthroscope, the examiner should keep in mind the convexity of the calcaneus and the concavity of the talus in the posterior subtalar joint.

11.14 Complications

In theory, any of the complications encountered in other joints may arise during subtalar arthroscopy (see Sect. 1.15).

- **Fluid extravasation.** This is not classified as a true complication, as the fluid should clear within 12 hours.

- **Vascular injury.** The short saphenous vein and its tributaries are at risk during placement of the anterolateral portals.

- **Reflex sympathetic dystrophy.**

11.15 Documentation

Documentation in subtalar arthroscopy should meet the same requirements as in arthroscopy of the knee (see Sect. 1.16).

11.16 Outpatient Arthroscopy

Subtalar arthroscopy can be performed on an ambulatory basis (see Sect. 1.17), but more complex procedures such as arthrodesis should be performed in an inpatient setting.

11.17 Indications

As experience with subtalar arthroscopy has grown, its indications have expanded. The spectrum of indications for subtalar arthroscopy cover the following conditions:

- Loose bodies
- Subtalar joint stiffness (arthrofibrosis)
- Degenerative changes
- Synovitis
- Osteochondral lesions of the talus
- Osteoarthritis
- Refractory pain of unknown cause

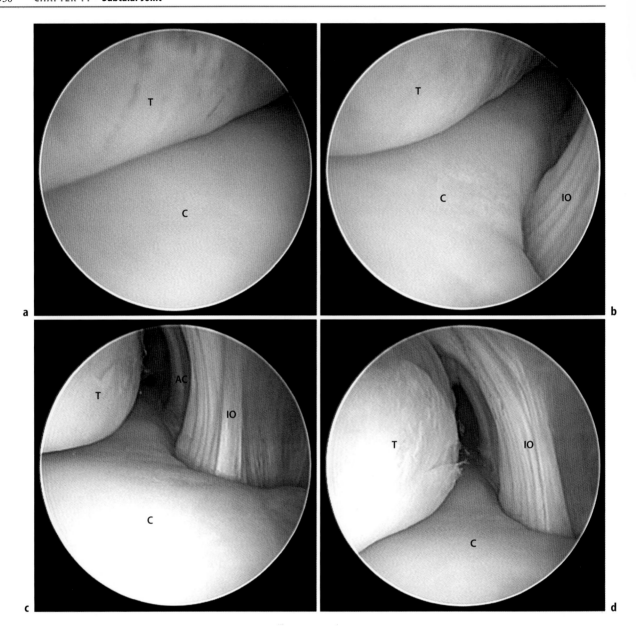

Fig. 11.13-1 a–d. Inspection of the anterior part of the subtalar joint. **a** The arthroscope has been passed through the antero-lateral portal, and its tip is in the anterolateral recess (*T* talus, *C* calcaneus). **b** The arthroscope is carefully swept anteriorly to survey the anterior part of the joint. The interosseous talocal-caneal ligament (*IO*) inserts on the anterior circumference of the talus. **c, d** The interosseous talocalcaneal ligament, which forms the dominant portion of the anterior capsule (*AC*), is visible for its full extent

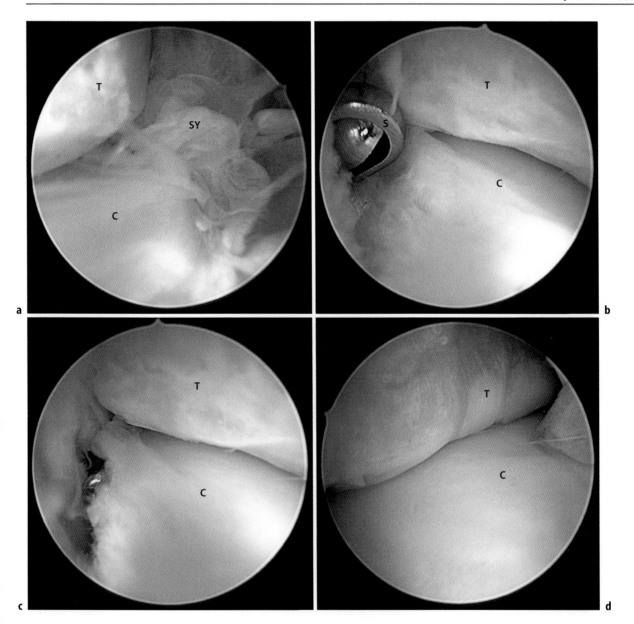

a

b

c

d

11.18 Synovitis

A partial synovectomy is often necessary to improve intraarticular vision. It is performed with a small synovial resector (from the small-joint set) (Fig. 11.18-1 and 11.18-2).

Fig. 11.18-1a–d. Synovitis in the subtalar joint. **a** Vision is markedly obscured by synovitis (*SY*) (*C* calcaneus, *T* talus). **b** Synovectomy is performed with a shaver (*S*) through a posterolateral portal. **c, d** The synovectomy has improved visualization of the calcaneus and talar articular surfaces

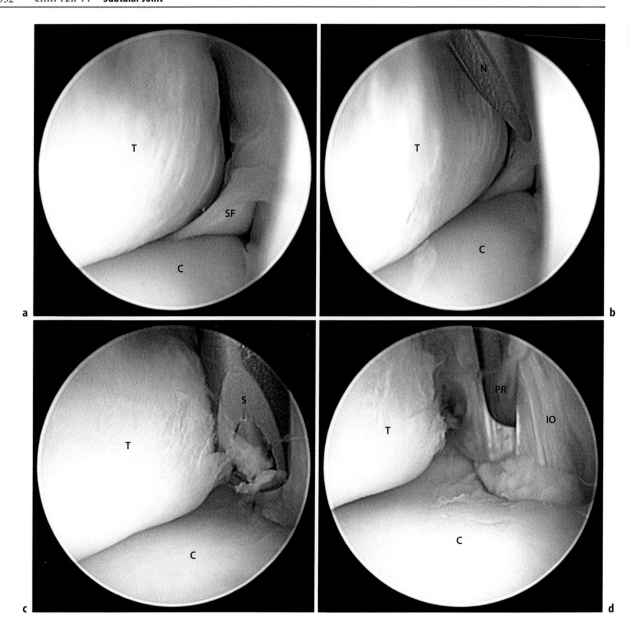

Fig. 11.18-2a–d. Synovectomy in the subtalar joint. **a** The anterior part of the joint is obscured by a synovial frond (*SF*) (*T* talus, *C* calcaneus). **b** A needle (*N*) is passed through an accessory anterior portal to determine the optimum site for placing the instrument portal. **c** A shaver (*S*) is introduced through this portal to remove the synovial frond. **d** With the front removed, the interosseous talocalcaneal ligament (*IO*) can be identified and palpated with the probe (*PR*) to check for laxness or disruption

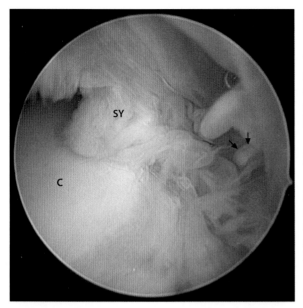

Fig. 11.19-1. Loose body in the subtalar joint. The patient, a 47-year-old man, presented with intermittent locking (*SY* local synovitis, *arrows* small loose body). Partial synovectomy was performed with a shaver, and the loose body was removed (*C* calcaneus)

11.19 Loose Bodies

When loose bodies are found in the subtalar joint (Fig. 11.19-1), they are removed using the technique described for other joints (see Sect. 2.9). A small grasper should be available, and accessory portals may be required.

11.20 Cartilage Lesions

As in other joints, varying degrees of cartilage pathology may be found in the subtalar joint. Numerous procedures are available, ranging from the debridement of fibrillated lesions to subchondral abrasion. Given the substantial loads on the subtalar joint, it is very unlikely that these treatments will be of much benefit if the changes are advanced. The principles of arthroscopic evaluation and treatment are the same as in the knee joint (see Sect. 2.2).

11.21 Symptomatic Os Trigonum

The os trigonum is an accessory bone that may cause symptoms due to its fibrous union with the talus. A symptomatic os trigonum can be excised arthroscopically. The technique is the same as for removing a fixed loose body (see Sect. 2.9).

11.22 Adhesions

Sprains and other injuries can lead to pain and limited motion. Adhesive bands in the subtalar joint can be visualized and divided arthroscopically. This treatment should improve symptoms unless significant cartilage lesions have developed.

11.23 Arthroscopic Arthrodesis

Arthrodesis of the subtalar joint can be performed as an arthroscopically assisted procedure. While the joint is distracted, the cartilage is resected from the articular surfaces, and cannulated lag screws are inserted from the anterior side through the talus (Jerosch 1996) or from the posterior side through the tuber calcanei (Ferkel 1996). The advantage of arthroscopic arthrodesis is the sparing bone resection, which allows favorable positioning of the bony surfaces.

11.24 Outlook and Personal Experience

Arthroscopic surgery of the subtalar joint is still in an early stage of development. Only a few case reports have been published to date. Our own statistics document the relative infrequency of subtalar arthroscopy compared with ankle arthroscopy: while ankle arthroscopy was performed in 922 patients at our center from 1992 to 1999, only 23 patients had arthroscopic surgery of the subtalar joint. During the last two years subtalar arthroscopy becomes more common in our department.

Joints of the Toes

Arthroscopic surgery has found its way into the smallest of the human joints. Even the metatarsophalangeal joints of the toes have become accessible to arthroscopic examination and treatment.

12.1 Historical Development

Watanabe et al. reported in 1986 on 22 arthroscopic examinations of the metatarsophalangeal and interphalangeal joints of the toes. In 1987, Lundeen described his initial experience with arthroscopy of the metatarsophalangeal joints of the toes.

12.2 Instrumentation (Arthroscopy System)

Small-diameter arthroscopes are necessary for arthroscopy of the toe joints. A scope diameter of 1.9 mm is recommended for the metatarsophalangeal joints of the second through fifth toes and the interphalangeal joints. Either that instrument or a 2.4-mm scope can be used in the metatarsophalangeal joint of the big toe (see Sect. 5.2). Even the small scopes should provide an image of adequate size. Advances in fiberoptic technology have made it possible to reduce the scope diameter to just 1 mm (Fig. 12.2-1).

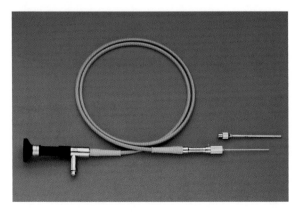

Fig. 12.2-1. Fiberoptic arthroscope 1 mm in diameter (Karl Storz, Tuttlingen, Germany)

12.3 Video System

The video system is the same as that used for knee arthroscopy (see Sect. 1.3). A light source of sufficient intensity should be available. Very small-diameter scopes may offer limited image size, and therefore it is very useful to have a video camera with zoom capability (see Sect. 1.3.1).

12.4 Probe

The probe is the same type used in arthroscopy of the wrist (see Sect. 5.4).

12.5 Operating Instruments

The operating instruments are like those used in wrist arthroscopy (see Sect. 5.6). A small-joint shaver system is particularly useful for resecting tissues and applying suction in tiny joint spaces.

12.6 Anesthesia

The anesthetic options for toe arthroscopy are spinal block, epidural anesthesia, regional anesthesia, as well as general anesthesia. General anesthesia is recommended, as it allows for optimum joint distraction.

12.7 Positioning

The patient is positioned supine with the operative foot on the operating table. The foot does not extend past the end of the table as in ankle or subtalar arthroscopy (see Sect. 3.8).

12.8 Tourniquet

Because any degree of bleeding can obscure visualization, the surgery should be performed in an exsanguinated field with a pneumatic tourniquet on the thigh (350–500 mm Hg).

12.9 Draping

The draping technique is like that used for ankle arthroscopy (see Fig. 3.10), except that the foot is draped free.

12.10 Distention Medium

The joint is distended with a nonelectrolytic solution (e.g., Purisole SM, Fresenius) to permit the use of electrocautery.

12.11 Setup and Preparations for Arthroscopy

These are the same as for ankle arthroscopy (see Sect. 3.12)

12.12 Portal Placement

12.12.1 Anatomy of the Metatarsophalangeal Joint of the Big Toe

This joint is formed by the head of the first metatarsal bone and the base of the proximal phalanx. One medial and one lateral sesamoid bone are embedded in the plantar joint capsule. These bones are components of the sesamoid complex, which includes the two sesamoids in addition to eight ligaments and seven muscles (Alvarez et al. 1984). This underscores the complex plantar structure of the metatarsophalangeal joint and accounts for the many types of pathology that occur in this area.

On the dorsal side, the extensor hallucis longus tendon passes over the center of the joint. Just plantar and somewhat lateral to it is the tendon of extensor hallucis brevis. Expansions from the brevis tendon also reinforce the capsule and ligaments that stabilize the joint on the extensor side. The medial part of the capsule is reinforced by a medial collateral ligament and by the abductor hallucis longus tendon. The lateral part of the capsule is less reinforced than on the medial side, being stabilized only by expansions from the oblique and transverse heads of the adductor hallucis muscle. The powerful medial collateral ligament and somewhat thinner lateral collateral ligament is each composed of two parts: one from the metatarsal to the proximal phalanx and one from the metatarsal to the sesamoid.

The skin on the plantar side is supplied by a blood vessel on the medial and lateral sides and by the terminal branches of the medial plantar nerve. The skin on the dorsal side is supplied by fine medial and lateral neurovascular bundles that must be spared during portal placement. The nerve branches arise from the superficial peroneal nerve.

12.12.2 Anatomy of the Metatarsophalangeal Joints of the Second through Fifth Toes

The anatomy of these joints is comparable to that of the metatarsophalangeal joint of the big toe. There are no sesamoid bones on the plantar side and consequently no sesamoid complex. Medial and lateral capsular reinforcements are less well developed than in the metatarsophalangeal joint of the big toe. On the dorsal side, the capsule is covered by the extensor digitorum communis tendon and reinforced by its expansions.

12.12.3 Portal Sites

Two portals can be placed on the extensor side of each toe joint, one medial and one lateral to the extensor tendon (dorsomedial and dorsolateral portals) (Fig. 12.12-1). The metatarsophalangeal joint of the big toe can be accessed through a medial portal placed at the level of the joint space on the medialmost side.

12.12.4 Creating the Arthroscope Portal: Technique

A standard technique is recommended for creating the arthroscope portal:

1. **Palpation.** While the metatarsophalangeal joint is manually distracted, the joint line and extensor tendon are identified by palpation and marked on the skin.

2. **Needle test.** While constant distraction is maintained, a percutaneous needle is inserted just medial to the extensor tendon and advanced into the joint space. By moving the needle medially and laterally, the surgeon can confirm that the needle has entered the joint.

3. **Distention.** The joint is distended with irrigating fluid. Backflow from the needle confirms intraarticular distention (Fig. 12.12-2). To keep the joint fully distended, pressure is maintained on the plunger as the needle is withdrawn.

4. **Skin incision.** An incision 2–3 mm long is made through the skin only.

5. **Spreading the subcutaneous tissue.** The subcutaneous tissue is spread with a small, blunt mosquito clamp, sparing the small dorsal neurovascular bundle that runs just medial to the portal site. The joint is not entered at this stage, as this would cause loss of distention.

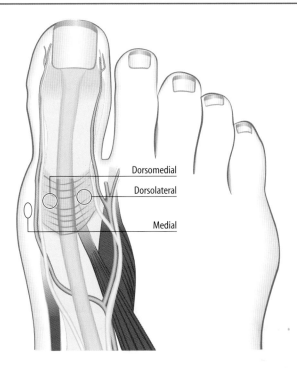

Fig. 12.12-1. Portal sites for metatarsophalangeal arthroscopy of the big toe

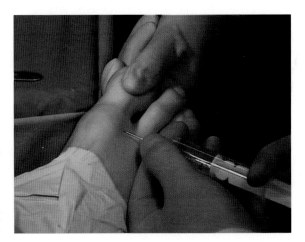

Fig. 12.12-2. Distending the metatarsophalangeal joint of the big toe

6. **Inserting the sheath.** The direction of sheath insertion is an important concern. The sheath cannot be advanced into the center of the joint, as the overall convexity of the joint space would risk iatrogenic cartilage damage. Therefore, when the sheath has pierced the capsule it is advanced laterally on the plantar side of the extensor tendons. Initially, then, the sheath is in the posterior part of the joint.

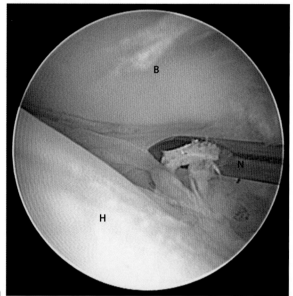

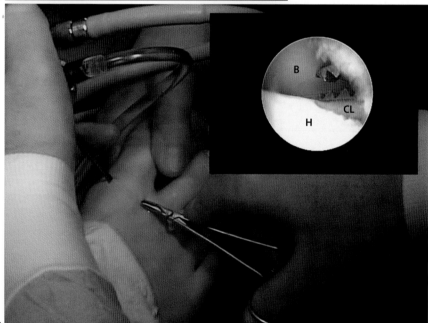

12.12.5 Creating the Instrument Portal: Technique

The instrument portal is placed under arthroscopic control.

1. **Needle test.** A needle is inserted into the joint, and its tip is visualized (Fig. 12.12-3 a).

2. **Skin incision.** A 3-mm incision is made through the skin only.

3. **Perforating the capsule.** After the subcutaneous tissue

Fig. 12.12-3 a, b. Creating the instrument portal for the metatarsophalangeal joint of the big toe. **a** The portal location is determined with a percutaneous needle (*N*) (*B* base of proximal phalanx, *H* head of first metatarsal). **b** After spreading the subcutaneous tissue, a clamp (*CL*) is advanced into the joint space and opened to develop the portal

has been spread, a small mosquito clamp is passed through the capsule and opened to create access for inserting a probe (Fig. 12.12-3 b). An identical technique is used for arthroscopy of the other metatarsophalangeal joints (Fig. 12.12-4).

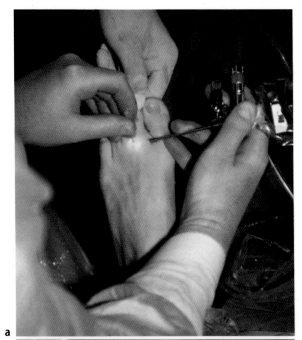

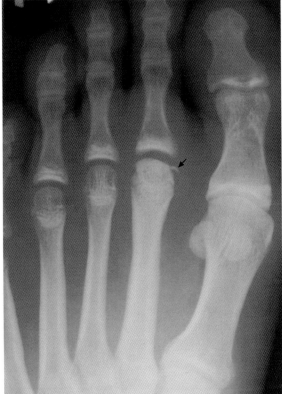

Fig. 12.12-4a,b. Arthroscopy of the second metatarsophalangeal joint of the second toe. **a** Locating the lateral instrument portal. **b** Arthroscopy was performed for an osteochondral fracture (*arrow*) in the head of the second metatarsal in a 19-year-old female gymnast. The displaced fragment was removed arthroscopically

12.12.6 Switching Portals

Complete inspection and surgical treatment always require interchanging the instrument and arthroscope portals. This is done with a switching rod that conforms to the diameter of the sheath (see Sect. 1.13.6 for technique).

12.13 Examination Sequence

The posterior part of the joint is examined first, followed by the lateral recess. When distraction is applied, the base of the proximal phalanx and the head of the metatarsal can be inspected. The portals are switched to allow visualization of the medial part of the dorsal capsule and the medial recess. The plantar joint region can be inspected only in the metatarsophalangeal joint of the big toe in patients with hyperlax ligaments. In most cases the ligaments of the toe joints are more lax than one might assume. The plantar portion of the metatarsophalangeal joint of the big toe can be inspected through a medial portal. This instrument portal is placed under vision and can be used for viewing by inserting a switching rod and then the arthroscope. This allows inspection of the plantar joint structures including the sesamoid bones

12.14 Complications

Given the small case numbers described in the literature and documented in our own records, we know of no complications relating specifically to toe arthroscopy. Patients should, however, be informed of the general complications that can arise in any arthroscopic procedure (see Sect. 1.15). Structures at risk are the extensor tendons and the neurovascular bundles that run medial and lateral to the tendons.

12.15 Documentation

As in other joints, both written and visual documentation are required (see Sect. 1.16).

12.16 Outpatient Arthroscopy

All arthroscopic surgical procedures on the metatarsophalangeal joints of the toes can be performed on an outpatient basis.

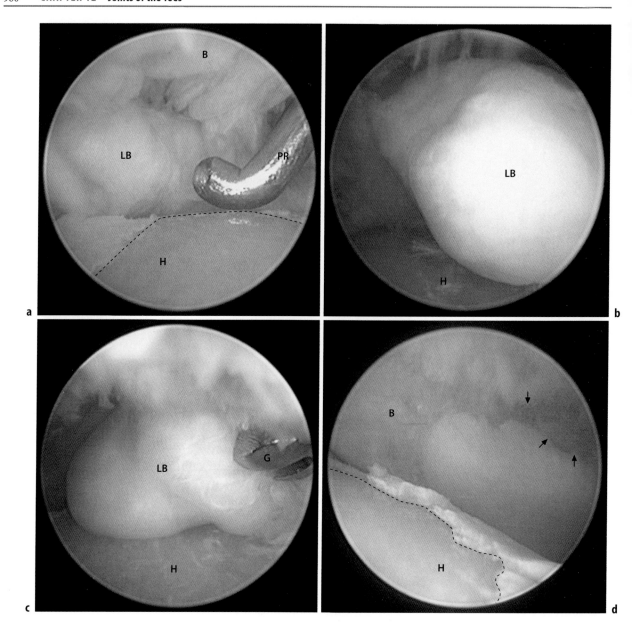

12.17 Indications

To date there has been no experience with toe arthroscopy in large clinical series. The technically demanding nature of this surgery calls for a discriminating approach to patient selection. The indications are as follows:

- **Chronic pain**
- **Chronic swelling**
- **Joint locking**
- **Free or fixed loose bodies**
- **Osteochondritis dissecans**

For the symptom-based indications, all other available diagnostic techniques should be employed to narrow the diagnosis. Arthroscopy is indicated only if a definitive diagnosis, such as a loose body or osteochondritis dissecans, can be established.

12.18 Contraindications

The contraindications are analogous to those in the large joints (see Sect. 1.19).

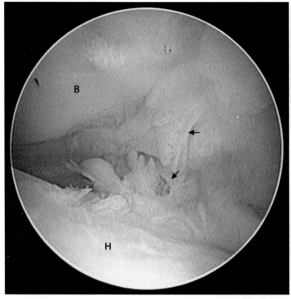
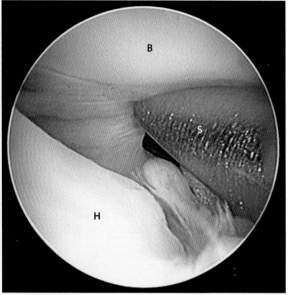

a b

◀ **Fig. 12.19-1 a–d.** Loose body in the metatarsophalangeal joint of the big toe in a 42-year-old patient with intermittent locking. **a** The loose body (*LB*) is located with a probe (*PR*) (*B* base of proximal phalanx, *H* head of first metatarsal, *dashed line* exposed bone). **b** While the joint is distracted, the probe is used to bring the loose body forward. **c** The object is grasped with a forceps (*G*) and extracted. **d** Postextraction view shows exposed bone areas on the head of the first metatarsal (*dashed line*) and the base of the proximal phalanx (*arrows*)

Fig. 12.20-1 a, b. Synovitis. **a** Vision is obscured by synovitis (*arrows*) (*B* base of proximal phalanx, *H* head of first metatarsal). **b** Synovectomy is performed with a shaver (*S*)

12.19 Loose Bodies

Intermittent locking and pain signify a free or fixed loose body, which can be treated by arthroscopic removal. Once the loose body has been located within the joint, it is grasped with a grasping forceps and extracted (Fig. 12.19-1).

12.20 Synovitis

As in other joints, chronic synovitis in the metatarsophalangeal joints of the toes can lead to recurring pain and functional deficits. Evaluation of the synovium follows the same principles as in the knee joint (see Sect. 2.3).

The altered synovium is removed with a small synovial resector (Fig. 12.20-1). A very small grasping forceps can be used to obtain a synovial biopsy.

12.21 Osteophytes

Symptomatic osteophytes may develop at the base of the proximal phalanx due to degenerative disease. These bone spurs can cause capsular irritation and limited motion. The extent of the osteophytes is determined radiographically (Fig. 12.21-1). Osteophytes in the metatarsophalangeal joint of the big toe are first visualized and then excised with a small round bur or laser.

12.22 Cartilage Lesions

Cartilage lesions are found predominantly on the convex articular surfaces (metatarsal heads). A cartilage lesion at the center of the metatarsal head in the metatarsophalangeal joint of the big toe is considered evidence of incipient hallux valgus.

Treatment options are the same as in large joints (see Sect. 2.2) and include debridement and subchondral abrasion. The constant loads on the toe joints compromise the prospects for successful fibrocartilage repair, however.

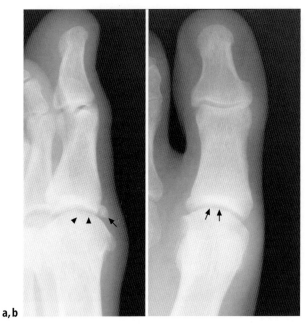

a, b

Fig. 12.21-1 a, b. Osteochondritis dissecans. **a** OCD lesion in the head of the first metatarsal (*arrowheads*) and a dorsal osteophyte (*arrow*) on the base of the proximal phalanx. **b** AP projection of the OCD lesion (*arrows*)

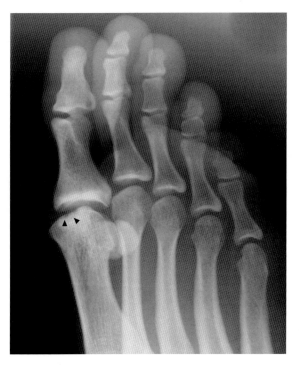

Fig. 12.23-1. Osteochondritis dissecans of the head of the first metatarsal (*arrowheads*)

12.23 Osteochondritis Dissecans

Pain of unknown cause, pain on axial compression, and/or intermittent locking may signify osteochondritis dissecans, which can be confirmed radiographically and by MR tomography (Fig. 12.23-1).

With a separated osteochondral fragment or cartilage fracture, the unstable areas are removed (Fig. 12.23-2). Fibrocartilage induction (subchondral abrasion, microfracture technique) is an option for residual defects (Fig. 12.23-3).

Postoperative Care

The operated joint is kept non-weightbearing for 1–2 weeks. If subchondral abrasion was performed on the head of the first metatarsal, a 5-cm heel lift is prescribed for 8 weeks. The sole on the opposite side is raised by 5 cm to prevent pushing off on the metatarsophalangeal joint of the big toe.

12.24 Summary and Personal Experience

Between 1994 and 2000, we performed metatarsophalangeal arthroscopy in 19 patients at our center. Thirteen cases involved the big toe and one the second toe. Five of the patients were operated for unexplained pain, five for osteochondritis dissecans, and four for intraarticular loose bodies, which were removed.

Metatarsophalangeal arthroscopy of the second toe was performed for a suspected osteochondral fracture of the metatarsal head in a competitive female gymnast. A bony ligament avulsion was found at operation, and the bone fragment was arthroscopically removed. Arthroscopy also revealed massive, localized cartilage swelling consistent with Kienböck disease.

Besides a special small instrument set, arthroscopy of the toe joints requires a meticulous operating technique. Initial encouraging results have been published, but studies in larger series have not yet been reported. There is no question that arthroscopic resections (e.g., for treatment of hallux valgus or hammertoe) are technically feasible. It remains to be seen whether they will produce the desired clinical results. The development of smaller optical systems in particular should lead to the broader utilization of this arthroscopic technique (see Fig. 12.2-1).

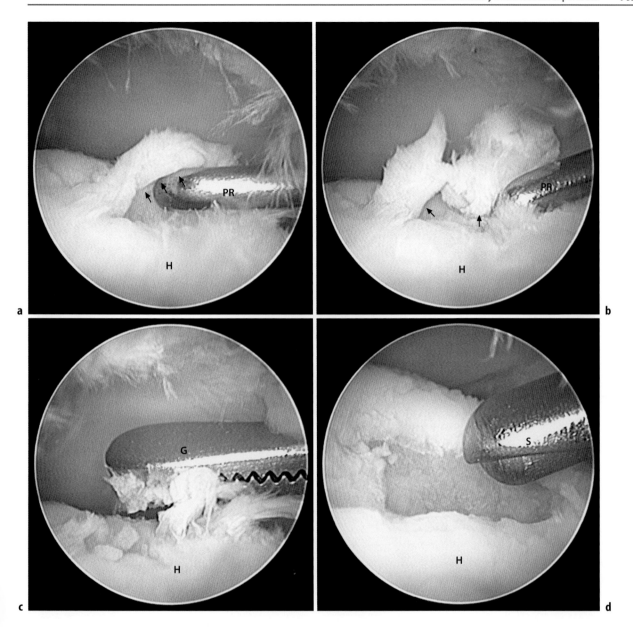

Fig. 12.23-2 a–d. Osteochondritis dissecans of the head of the first metatarsal. **a** The lesion is palpated with a probe (*PR*), and unstable fragments are elevated (*arrows*) (*H* head of first metatarsal). **b, c** Additional unstable fragments (*arrows*) are grasped and removed with a grasping forceps (*G*). **d** The resection site is smoothed with a shaver (*S*)

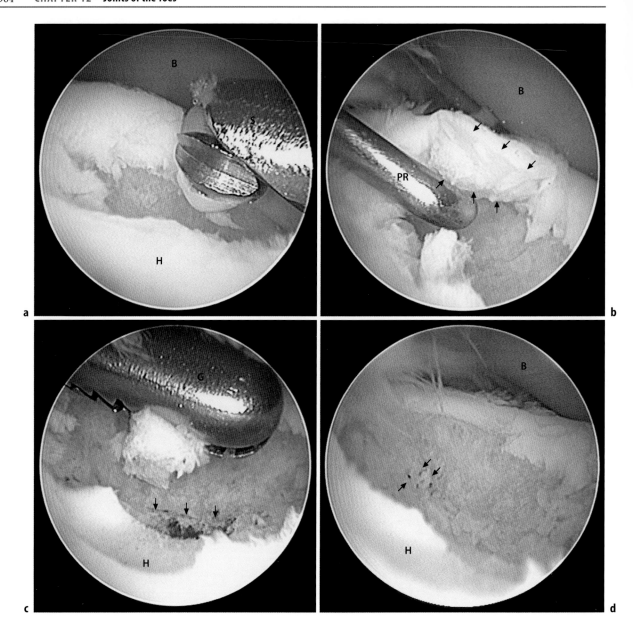

Fig. 12.23-3 a–d. Osteochondritis dissecans of the head of the first metatarsal (continued from Fig. 12.23-2). **a** The subchondral defect is abraded with a round bur (*S*) to induce fibrocartilage formation (*B* base of proximal phalanx, *H* head of first metatarsal). **b** Another unstable osteochondral fragment (*arrows*) is mobilized with the probe (*PR*). **c** This fragment is removed with a grasping forceps (*G*) (*arrows* hemorrhagic areas). **d** Final appearance of the treated bed, with bleeding points (*arrows*)

Joints of the Fingers

The metacarpophalangeal and interphalangeal joints of the fingers, like the joints of the toes (see Chap. 12), have become accessible to arthroscopic examination and treatment.

13.1 Historical Development

In 1979, Chen reported on arthroscopies of the wrist and finger joints that he performed in 34 clinical cases between 1973 and 1978 using a No. 24 arthroscope. Most of his cases were patients with rheumatoid arthritis of the metacarpal, proximal interphalangeal and distal interphalangeal joints. Dorsal portals were used exclusively to avoid flexor tendon injury. Watanabe (1986) also reported on arthroscopies of the finger joints.

13.2 Instrumentation

The operating instruments, arthroscope, probe, and video system must satisfy the same requirements as in arthroscopy of the toe joints (see Sections 12.2–12.5).

13.3 Anesthesia

Local anesthesia and various forms of regional anesthesia are available, but general anesthesia is recommended for optimum distraction and painless positioning. Also, since finger arthroscopy is still in the developmental stage, general anesthesia eliminates the problem of a patient overhearing uncertainties voiced by the operating surgeon.

13.4 Positioning

As in wrist arthroscopy, a traction tower is used to distract the finger joints (Fig. 13.4-1) (see Sect. 5.8). Only one finger trap is used, however, leaving the uninvolved metacarpophalangeal joints freely mobile.

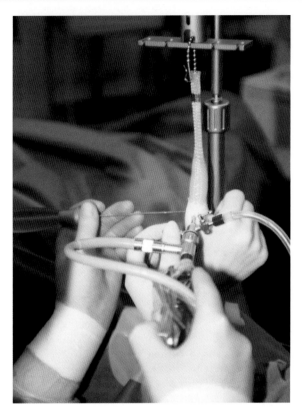

Fig. 13.4-1. Distraction of the metacarpophalangeal joint of the thumb using a finger trap and traction tower

> ► **Problem:** It can be difficult to hold a very thin finger securely in a plastic finger trap, which can easily slip off. The finger trap may require additional fixation with small strips of adhesive tape.

13.5 Tourniquet

All procedures are performed in a bloodless field. An exsanguinating wrap is placed on the arm, and a pneumatic tourniquet on the upper arm is inflated to 250 mm Hg.

13.6 Draping

The draping technique is like that used for wrist arthroscopy (see Sect. 5.10).

13.7 Distention Medium

The joint is distended with fluid, which may consist of Ringer lactate or a nonelectrolytic solution (to permit electrocautery use).

13.8 Setup and Preparations for Arthroscopy

The setup is the same as in wrist arthroscopy (see Sect. 5.12).

13.9 Portal Placement

Portal placement requires a knowledge of hand anatomy. We recommend palpating the extensor tendons and, if desired, marking them on the skin. The joint space can be entered radial and ulnar to the extensor tendon with virtually no risk of neurovascular injury. Volar portals should be avoided.

13.9.1 Arthroscope Portal

A standard routine is followed in creating the arthroscope portal:

1. **Palpating the joint space.** The joint line is palpated in the distracted condition. It is identified by the slightly flared bone margins at the base of the proximal phalanx.

2. **Needle test.** A needle is inserted radial or ulnar to the extensor tendon and advanced into the joint space. By moving the needle medially and laterally, the surgeon can determine whether the needle tip has entered the joint.

3. **Distention.** The joint space is distended with fluid. When the joint is fully distended, the needle is withdrawn while pressure is maintained on the plunger.

4. **Skin incision and subcutaneous dissection.** A 2- to 3-mm longitudinal incision is made through the skin, and the subcutaneous tissue is carefully spread in the longitudinal and transverse directions with a fine, blunt clamp without perforating the joint capsule.

5. **Inserting the sheath.** The sheath with blunt obturator is carefully introduced. A decrease in resistance indicates perforation of the capsule. The sheath is not directed toward the center of the joint but into its dorsal expansion (dorsal recess) on the radial or ulnar side.

13.9.2 Instrument Portal

The instrument portal is established under arthroscopic control.

1. **Guide needle.** A needle is inserted into the joint space on the other side of the extensor tendon until the needle tip can be seen with the arthroscope (Fig. 13.9-1).

2. **Skin incision.** A 2- to 3-mm longitudinal skin incision is made.

3. **Spreading the subcutaneous tissue and capsule.** The subcutaneous tissue is spread with a fine mosquito clamp, which also perforates the capsule. The jaws of the clamp are then opened to spread the perforation site for the insertion of a probe or motorized instrument.

13.9.3 Switching Portals

Standard switching-rod technique is used to interchange the viewing and instrumentation portals (see Sect. 1.13.6).

13.10 Examination Sequence

The dorsal part of the metacarpophalangeal joint and the metacarpal head are inspected first. When viewing through a primary radial portal, the surgeon next visualizes the ulnar recess and the ulnar half of the base of the proximal phalanx. Then the portals are switched (arthroscope to the ulnar side) to view the radial base of the proximal phalanx, the radial recess, and the radial half of the metacarpal head.

13.11 Complications

The complications are the same as those encountered in the toes and wrist (see Sect. 12.14).

13.12 Documentation

Standard written and visual documentation are required (see Sect. 1.16).

13.13 Outpatient Arthroscopy

All arthroscopic procedures on the finger joints can be performed on an ambulatory basis.

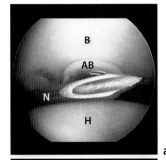

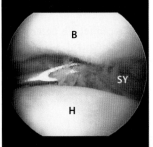

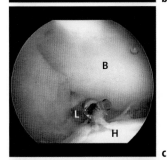

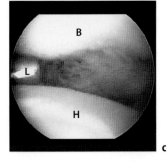

Fig. 13.9-1a–d. Synovitis in the metacarpophalangeal joint of the thumb. **a** A needle (*N*) is used to determine instrument portal location. The air bubble (AB) is aspirated to establish a clear field of view (*B* base of proximal phalanx, *H* head of first metacarpal). **b** Pronounced dark synovitis with villous proliferation (*SY*). **c, d** Because the joint space is so small, synovectomy is performed with a laser fiber (*L*)

13.14 Indications

Arthroscopy of the small finger joints is still in the developmental stage and therefore its indications are limited. The following indications are recognized:

- **Loose bodies**
- **Joint locking** (loose bodies, detached cartilage fragments)
- **Chronic effusions in a patient with known or suspected rheumatoid disease**
- **Unresolved pain whose cause cannot be determined with conventional diagnostic techniques** (radiographs, MRI, radionuclide scans)

13.15 Contraindications

The contraindications are analogous to those in wrist arthroscopy (see Sect. 5.19).

13.16 Synovitis

Synovitis in the finger joints may be reactive or may have a rheumatoid cause. Arthroscopic synovectomies have been reported in rheumatoid patients (Chen 1979).

Synovectomy can be performed with a small-joint shaver or laser fiber, whose small dimensions are advantageous in the very small joints of the fingers (Fig. 13.9-1).

13.17 Loose Bodies

Small loose bodies, whether synovial or chondral (posttraumatic) in origin, can be removed arthroscopically. The technique is basically the same as for removing a small loose body from other joints.

13.18 Cartilage Lesions

Posttraumatic or degenerative cartilage lesions are treated according to the standard principles of cartilage therapy (removal of unstable fragments, fibrocartilage induction).

13.19 Summary and Outlook

Arthroscopic procedures on the small finger joints have sophisticated requirements in terms of surgical instrumentation and arthroscopic technique. The results published to date have been encouraging, but studies in larger clinical series are needed before the therapeutic efficacy of finger arthroscopy can be evaluated.

Our own experience is based on finger arthroscopies in five patients: the first MP joint in three patients, the second MP joint in one patient, and the third MP joint in one patient. Three of the patients had unexplained locking, and two had recurrent effusions. A partial synovectomy was performed in all of the joints. We did not find loose bodies as the cause of the locking, but we did discover synovitis with villous hypertrophy.

14.1 Historical Development

Burman, after trying to arthroscope cadaveric hips in 1931, declared it "manifestly impossible to insert a needle between the head of the femur and the acetabulum." He was only able to visualize portions of the femoral neck and capsular pouch. In 1977, Gross reported on the use of arthroscopy in adolescent hips. The indications were congenital hip dislocation, Perthes disease, slipped capital femoral epiphysis, and previous empyema of the hip. Vakili et al. (1980) removed bone cement arthroscopically after a failed total hip replacement. Hogersson et al. (1981) obtained arthroscopic synovial biopsies in juvenile arthritis, and in 1983 Parisien described the treatment of osteochondritis dissecans of the femoral head.

The beginnings of hip arthroscopy were marred, however, by problems of poor joint distention and inadequate instrumentation.

14.2 Instrumentation

A 30° and 70° wide-angle arthroscope (4 mm diameter) are required. If the working length of the arthroscope barrel is too short, problems can arise in very large or obese patients due to the large distance from the skin to the hip capsule.

14.3 Video System

Hip arthroscopy employs the same video equipment used in other joints (see Sect. 1.3).

14.4 Probe

Because of the thickness of the tissues overlying the hip joint, the angled part of the probing hook should be small to facilitate insertion. A longer probe should be used in very large patients.

14.5 Surgical Instruments

Grasping forceps, basket forceps, and a power shaver should be available (see Sect. 1.6.1). The "deep location" of the hip joint can make instrument insertion difficult. Few problems arise in small, thin patients, but the sheath length may be barely adequate in some obese patients.

14.6 Anesthesia

General anesthesia is preferred, as it can provide the complete muscular relaxation necessary for optimum joint distraction.

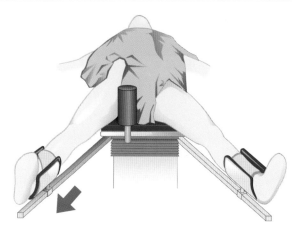

Fig. 14.7-1. Supine position for hip arthroscopy

14.7 Positioning

Positioning is of key importance, as it must allow for hip distraction and provide access for image intensification fluoroscopy. The supine position is more commonly used than the lateral decubitus position.

It must be decided preoperatively whether it is necessary to inspect the interior of the joint or whether it is sufficient to view the anterior hip structures. If the procedure is limited to a synovial biopsy, the latter will be sufficient and joint distraction is not strictly necessary. However, the patient should still be positioned so that the joint can be distracted if required. The hip can be distracted by 1–2 cm without tearing the ligamentum teres of the femur.

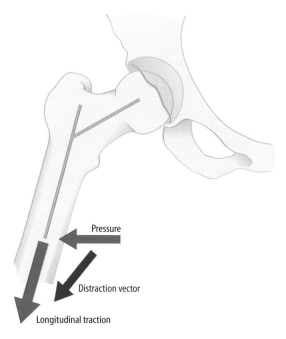

Fig. 14.7-2. Forces acting on the hip joint during distraction

- **Supine position.** The patient is placed on a traction table with the contralateral leg in maximum abduction. The hip is distracted by longitudinal traction combined with pressure from a perineal post (Fig. 14.7-1).

▶ **Caution:** The post should be well padded to avoid pressure injuries in the genital region.
The advantages of the supine position are easier placement of the anterior portal and better X-ray protection of the genital region (lead apron).

- **Lateral decubitus position.** This position requires a special hip distractor and a well-padded perineal bar. Combining 25 kg of longitudinal traction with lateral pressure from the perineal bar causes a resultant pull that is approximately parallel to the femoral neck axis. Villar (1992) stresses the advantages of this type of traction in the arthroscopic debridement of degenerative joint changes. Another advantage of the hip distractor is that the rotational position of the femur and the degree of hip abduction can be adjusted during the operation. Despite this capability, intraoperative position adjustments can be cumbersome.

14.8 Draping

For arthroscopy in the supine position, the contralateral leg, abdomen, and chest are draped first, followed by the lower leg and foot on the operative side. An area measuring approximately 30×40 cm over the hip is left exposed.

14.9 Distention Medium

The hip joint is distended with a nonelectrolytic solution (e.g., Purisole) (see Sect. 1.11).

Adequate inflow is necessary to keep the field clear of blood and maintain adequate visualization. An inflow cannula or roller pump is recommended, therefore (Fig. 1.11-2).

14.10 Setup and Preparations

The same principles apply as in knee arthroscopy (see Sect. 1.12). The operative field should be accessible to an image intensifier, which is used for accurate portal placement (Fig. 14.10-1).

14.11 Portal Placement

The two most commonly used portals are anterior and lateral. A posterior portal has also been described; it requires preliminary open release of the piriformis, obturator internus, and gemelli muscles.

The distance between the skin and joint capsule is greater in the hip than in any other joint. As a result, every portal requires the perforation of numerous structures. A detailed knowledge of anatomy is absolutely essential.

14.11.1 Anatomy

Important bony landmarks about the hip are the anterior superior iliac spine and the greater trochanter, which is palpable even in obese patients.

Muscles

The joint capsule of the hip is covered by muscles on all sides. The anterior structures from medial to lateral are the pectineus muscle, which is attached to the capsule of the hip joint, and the vascular bundle of the femoral artery and vein. Farther laterally are the femoral nerve, iliopsoas muscle, and iliac fascia. Superficial to these

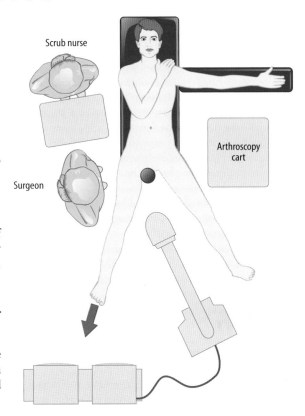

Fig. 14.10-1. Patient position and operating room layout (image intensifier, arthroscopy cart, surgical staff)

structures are the rectus femoris and sartorius muscles. Lateral and superficial to the iliofemoral ligament are the gluteus minimus, gluteus medius, and the tensor fasciae latae with its attachment to the iliotibial tract. The posterior muscles are the piriformis, gemellus superior, obturator internus, gemellus inferior, and obturator externus. The sciatic nerve runs below the piriformis; at the level of the femoral head, it is accompanied distally by the gluteal artery and vein and the inferior gluteal nerve. These structures are covered by the gluteus maximus.

Joint Capsule

The capsule of the hip joint is very powerful, being more stout anteriorly than posteriorly. Its proximal attachment to the acetabular rim is located very close to the acetabular labrum and transverse acetabular ligament. The capsule inserts anteriorly on the intertrochanteric line and posteriorly about 1.5 cm proximal to the intertrochanteric crest. The capsule is reinforced by four ligaments: the iliofemoral, pubofemoral, and ischiofemoral ligaments and the zona orbicularis. The ligaments are taut in extension and internal rotation and lax in flexion, abduction, and slight external rotation.

The femoral head is intraarticular, the epiphyseal zone in children being located within the joint capsule. The femoral head is covered with hyaline cartilage except for the fovea, which marks the insertion of the ligamentum teres. This structure appears as a thickened synovial tube between the fovea and acetabular notch. The ligamentum teres is taut in adduction and lax in abduction. It is traversed by a small artery that anastomoses with the arteries supplying the posterior portion of the femoral head.

The acetabulum is lined with hyaline cartilage except for an anteroinferior area covered by the transverse acetabular ligament. The acetabulum is horseshoe-shaped and its central portion, the acetabular fossa, is covered by synovial tissue. The acetabular labrum is composed of fibrocartilage; it arises from the acetabular rim and forms a ring around the femoral head that extends the articular surface.

14.11.2 Lateral Portal (Supratrochanteric)

This portal is placed just above the greater trochanter. It is directed toward the lateral acetabular rim in the abducted hip.

14.11.3 Anterior Portal

This portal is located at the intersection of a vertical line tangent to the anterior superior iliac spine and a horizontal line tangent to the tip of the greater trochanter (Fig. 14.11-1).

14.11.4 Technique for Creating the Portals

Because the hip joint is so deeply situated, it is important to follow a standard and precise technique when establishing the portals.

1. **Positioning.** Correct positioning of the anesthetized patient is essential. The surgeon should always check personally to see that the patient has been correctly positioned.
   ▶ **Note:** Complete muscular relaxation, adequate joint distraction, and sufficient padding of the genital region are essential!
   The abducted hip is imaged with the image intensifier.

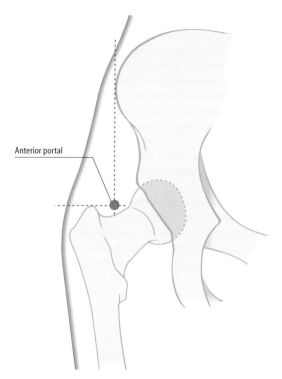

Fig. 14.11-1. Location of the anterior portal for hip arthroscopy

2. **Marking the skin.** The following landmarks are outlined on the skin:
   - Anterior superior iliac spine
   - Tip of the greater trochanter
   - Course of the femoral artery
   When the hip is distracted under image intensification, widening of the joint space should be evident in relation to the undistracted joint position.

3. **Passing a needle into the joint.** After the patient has been draped and the skin aseptically prepared, a long spinal needle is inserted percutaneously into the hip joint. It is inserted about 2 cm superior to the tip of the greater trochanter under fluoroscopic control until it enters the hip joint. Hempfling (1995) recommends injecting contrast medium to opacify the joint space (arthrography). Villar (1992) uses 1–2 mL of air as a radiographic contrast medium.

4. **Distention.** The joint is distended with irrigating fluid. The injection also breaks the vacuum in the joint, allowing the joint to be distracted more efficiently. Up to 40 mL of fluid may be needed to fully distend the joint. The fluid should not escape into the periarticular soft tissues, as this would make the rest of the procedure much more difficult.

5. **Skin incision.** A 5-mm skin incision is made.

6. **Inserting the sheath.** The sheath with blunt obturator is advanced in the direction of the hip joint, making certain that the hip is in an abducted position. If the blunt obturator cannot penetrate the joint capsule, it may have to be replaced with a sharp trocar. One spigot on the sheath is left open so that fluid outflow will confirm joint entry.

7. **Inserting the arthroscope.** A 30° or 70° wide-angle scope is recommended. The 30° scope is inserted first, as arthroscopists are already familiar with its use in other joints.

The rest of the procedure is like that for the lateral portal.

14.12 Examination Sequence

The anterior portal gives access to the inferior part of the joint, which is a common hiding place for loose bodies. Access to the posterior part of the joint is limited unless the hip can be well distracted.

The femoral head and superior part of the joint are inspected through the lateral portal. If the hip has been optimally distracted, the fovea and ligamentum teres can be seen. The 70° scope can be used to obtain a wider field of view. Approximately 90 % of the acetabulum can be visualized arthroscopically (Villar 1992), but this requires maximum hip distraction.

14.13 Complications

Typical complications can arise as in any arthroscopic procedure (see Sect. 1.15). Inadequate distraction can result in injury to the acetabular labrum.

14.14 Documentation

Documentation in hip arthroscopy should meet the same requirements as in any other joint (see Sect. 1.16).

14.15 Outpatient Arthroscopy

Because of the apparatus needed for positioning, distraction, and image intensification during placement of the portals, hip arthroscopy should always be performed in an inpatient setting.

14.16 Indications

Although hip arthroscopy is rarely performed, there are several indications that can justify an arthroscopic procedure:

- **Unexplained pain**
- **Labral lesions**
- **Foreign body removal**
- **Loose body removal**
- **Synovectomy (synovial biopsy)**

Hip arthroscopy in patients with unexplained pain is appropriate only if imaging procedures have been unable to establish the cause and there has been lack of response to conservative treatment.

14.17 Lesions of the Acetabular Labrum

Labral lesions can cause hip pain and intermittent locking. Patients under 35 years of age are predominantly affected. Treatment consists in arthroscopic removal of the avulsed portion of the labrum.

14.18 Loose Bodies

Loose body removal can be very tedious due to the difficulty of manipulating arthroscopic grasping instruments in the deeply situated joint (Fig. 14.18-1).

In patients with synovial chondromatosis, arthroscopic removal of the loose bodies provides a beneficial treatment with low morbidity.

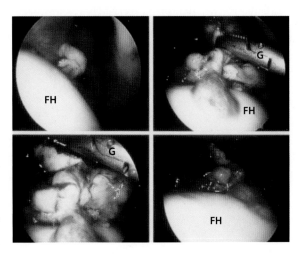

Fig. 14.18-1 a–d. Bony avulsion of the ligamentum teres. **a** Initial appearance (*FH* femoral head). **b, c** The bone fragment is grasped and extracted with a grasping forceps (*G*). **d** Final appearance (Photos courtesy of André Gächter, St. Gallen)

14.19 Removal of Foreign Material

Bone cement residues following a total hip replacement can cause intermittent locking. These fragments can be removed arthroscopically.

14.20 Synovitis

Synovial biopsy and partial synovectomy can be performed arthroscopically. Pigmented villonodular synovitis is accessible to arthroscopic diagnosis.

14.21 Degenerative Changes

It has been shown that arthroscopic irrigation and the removal of cellular debris can reduce complaints in osteoarthritis of the hip (Fig. 14.21-1). This is similar to the lavage effect achieved in other joints with degenerative changes.

14.22 Osteochondritis Dissecans of the Femoral Head

Osteochondritis dissecans, which usually affects the anterolateral portion of the femoral head, can be visualized arthroscopically. The lesion can be treated by drilling the base from a lateral portal under image intensifier control. Unstable fragments can be arthroscopically removed.

14.23 Avascular Necrosis

Avascular necrosis of the femoral head is a controversial indication for hip arthroscopy. Glick (1991) claims that arthroscopy can even worsen the condition as a result of instrument manipulations and prolonged distraction.

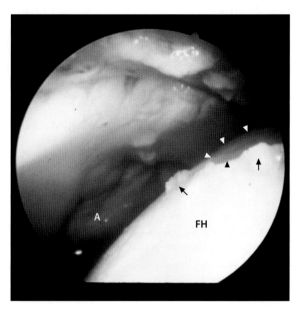

Fig. 14.21-1. Osteoarthritis of the hip. Arthroscopy shows areas of cartilage separation (*arrows*) and exposed bone (*arrowheads*) on the femoral head (*FH*). Less pronounced changes are found in the acetabulum (*A*). The joint was distended with gas (photo courtesy of André Gächter, St. Gallen)

He describes two cases of avascular necrosis in which the femoral head collapsed within three months of arthroscopic surgery.

14.24 Outlook

It is clear that progress in hip arthroscopy has been constrained by difficulties in handling the operating instruments. This is certainly the major factor limiting arthroscopic surgery of the hip. Because the indications are so limited, there are only a few centers at which surgeons are acquiring experience with hip arthroscopy.

CHAPTER 15

Carpal Tunnel Syndrome

Cause

Carpal tunnel syndrome is the most common peripheral compression neuropathy. Various factors can lead to carpal tunnel syndrome (Table 15-1). Women are predominantly affected.

Table 15-1. Possible causes of carpal tunnel syndrome

Anatomic causes
- Bony malalignment (e.g., after a distal radial fracture)
- Congenital deformity
- Space-occupying lesions such as a ganglion, lipoma, or neuroma (rare)
- Tenosynovitis of the flexor tendons (very frequent cause)
- Osteophytes (e.g., due to osteoarthritis or distal radial fracture)
- Posttraumatic compartment syndrome

Neurologic causes
- Peripheral neuropathy (e.g., in diabetes mellitus, chronic alcohol abuse, or hemophilia)
- Proximal nerve lesions

Hormonal causes
- Hyperthyroidism
- Pregnancy
- Menopause
- Acromegaly

Inflammatory synovial causes
- Rheumatoid diseases
- Scleroderma
- Gout

Chronic overuse
- Heavy manual labor that involves repetitive, maximum flexion and extension of the wrist
- Prolonged holding of the wrist in a strained position, e.g., during cycling, typing, or sleeping ("paw position")

Symptoms

Patients describe intermittent or persistent numbness and paresthesias mainly affecting the three radial fingers and the radial half of the ring finger. Pain occurs chiefly at night, causing many patients to awaken in the early morning hours. They may wring the hands or immerse the hands and forearms in cold water to relieve the discomfort. Often the symptoms start on the middle finger and then spread to involve the first three digits and the radial side of the ring finger, including the extensor surfaces (subungual pain). Many patients report a tendency to drop objects held in the hand (loss of grip strength) or an inability to unlock doors with a key (loss of pinch strength). Some patients have difficulty with fine motor activities such as fastening buttons, darning, and knitting.

Clinical Diagnosis

In the Phalen test, the wrist is held at maximum flexion to elicit or exacerbate numbness and paresthesias. Percussion of the median nerve at the wrist can evoke pain that radiates into the fingers (Hoffmann-Tinel sign). Sensory testing demonstrates hypoesthesia in the distribution of the median nerve. This is accompanied by decreased sweat secretion (dry skin) due to concomitant involvement of the autonomic part of the median nerve. Atrophy of the thenar muscles, which may be associated with motor weakness, can be detected by inspection, palpation, and function testing.

The differential diagnosis should include more central causes of neurologic dysfunction:

- Pronator syndrome
- Thoracic outlet syndrome
- Scalenus syndrome
- Cervical syndrome
- Cervical rib

Neurologic Examination

It is helpful to determine the sensory nerve conduction velocity and distal motor latency. Usually this involves comparison of the two sides and comparison with the ulnar nerve. With significant compression of the median nerve, the motor latency to the abductor pollicis brevis is usually longer than 4.5 ms. The sensory nerve conduction velocity between the wrist and the three radial fingers is slower than 40 ms. In advanced stages, tests may show polyphasic or decreased nerve action potentials. Electromyography may show evidence of acute or chronic denervation of the thenar musculature.

Radiographs

Biplane radiographs can be obtained to eliminate bony anomalies. A spot view of the carpal tunnel (Gaynor-Hart projection) may also be obtained. In patients with significant limitation of wrist motion or a previous distal radial fracture, biplane views of the wrist are essential.

MRI

The clinical examination is sufficient. MRI is indicated only if there is good reason to suspect an indeterminate space-occupying lesion in the carpal tunnel.

Therapeutic Management

The treatment of carpal tunnel syndrome depends on the cause, severity, and duration of the complaints.

Conservative Treatment

Conservative management includes local measures to relieve pain and inflammation (ointment dressings) and the use of oral nonsteroidal anti-inflammatory agents (NSAR). A wrist splint can be worn at night to keep the wrist in the neutral position. Some patients may benefit from physical and physiotherapeutic measures on the cervical spine and shoulders to reduce muscle tone. A three-month trial of conservative treatment is advised.

▶ **Caution:** Do not inject a steroid compound into the carpal tunnel, as this can cause nerve and tendon damage.

Operative Treatment

If conservative treatment is unsuccessful or if clinical symptoms are severe, operative treatment should be considered even if complaints have been present only a short time. If thenar atrophy has developed, median

nerve decompression should be combined with exposure of the motor branch. When surgery is elected, it must be determined which anatomic structure requires treatment.

1. **Transverse carpal ligament.** Division of the transverse carpal ligament (synonyms: flexor retinaculum, carpal roof) is the cornerstone of operative treatment. The carpal ligament is completely transected. An incomplete release can lead to a recurrence or persistence of complaints.

2. **Neurolysis of the motor branch.** Exposure and neurolysis of the motor branch is indicated when thenar atrophy is present.

3. **Neurolysis of the median nerve.** Perifascicular neurolysis can no longer be recommended, as clinical studies have shown no significant difference with or without neurolysis (Lowri 1991).
▶ **Note:** Interfascicular neurolysis is strictly contraindicated.

4. **Synovectomy.** If the median nerve compression is based on massive synovitis (e.g., in a patient with underlying rheumatoid disease), surgical reduction of the synovial structures is recommended. If the cause of the synovitis is unclear, synovial biopsy should be performed.

Selection of Operative Technique

Since numerous endoscopic techniques have been added to the traditional open techniques of carpal tunnel release, a very controversial debate has arisen as to the most suitable techniques.

Open Techniques

Techniques for open carpal tunnel release (OCTR) are standardized, have been practiced for many years, and yield reproducible results. Nevertheless, it is important to consider the relative advantages and disadvantages of the open techniques.

▶ **Advantages**
- **Exposure of the median nerve.** It is essential to avoid surgical injury to the median nerve. For many surgeons, the main argument in favor of OCTR is that it enables the median nerve to be clearly exposed at minimal risk ("you can see what you're doing").
- **Neurolysis of the median nerve.** When perineural scarring and adhesions are present, a perineural neurolysis can be performed safely and easily without endangering the nerve.
- **Neurolysis of the motor branch.** Neurolysis of the motor branch is recommended when thenar atrophy is present. If thenar atrophy is severe and nerve func-

tion appears permanently compromised, an opposition transfer such as the palmaris longus transfer (Camitz transfer) can be performed to restore opposition to the thumb.

- **Exposure of the motor branch.** The motor branch (thenar branch) of the median nerve is selectively exposed and identified to avoid surgical injury. The variable course of this nerve (see below) is yet another argument for OCTR.
- **Reduction of synovial tissue.** Synovectomy of the flexor tendons can be performed in patients with rheumatoid disease or chronic tenosynovitis of the flexor tendon sheaths, which is a very common finding.
- **Resection of bony projections.** If bony anomalies are causing or contributing to the nerve compression, the offending projections can be exposed and removed.

▶ **Disadvantages**

- **Long scars.** In the past, skin incisions approximately 14 cm long were not uncommon in open releases. Even today, some standard textbooks of hand surgery continue to describe long incisions. Newer techniques show that an approximately 5-cm skin incision placed parallel and ulnar to the thenar crease is sufficient for dividing the transverse carpal ligament under vision.
- **Longer absence from work.** Numerous studies have documented the longer disability time associated with OCTR.
- **Slower recovery of hand strength.** Complete division of the transverse carpal ligament and palmar fascia in OCTR deprives the median nerve and flexor tendons of palmar support during flexion (loss of the annular-ligament function of the retinaculum). This had led some surgeons to advocate reconstruction of the carpal roof after OCTR. This is done by approximating the radial edge of the carpal ligament to the ulnar cut edge of the palmar fascia to restore the palmar support structures while also protecting the median nerve from scar tissue ingrowth under the skin incision.
- **Lower complication rate.** A frequent argument in favor of OCTR is its lower complication rate compared with endoscopic techniques. Palmer and Toivonen (1995) surveyed the members of the American Society for Hand Surgery on complications in their patients following OCTR and endoscopic release (ECTR); 708 colleagues answered the questions on OCTR and 616 on ECTR. The surprising results are summarized in Table 15-2.

Endoscopic Techniques

Previously described techniques of endoscopic carpal tunnel release (ECTR) offer many advantages:

Table 15-2. Complications of ECTR and OCTR. (After Palmer and Toivonen 1995)

Lesions/complications	ECTR	OCTR
Median nerve	100	147
Complete	17	23
Motor branch	17	117
Ulnar nerve	88	29
Digital nerve	77	54
Tendons	69	19
Complete	62	13
Partial	7	6
Superficial palmar arch	86	21
Ulnar artery	34	11

- **Small scar.** Endoscopic release requires only an 8- to 10-mm skin incision.
- **Excellent cosmetic result.** The small, transverse skin incision in the wrist crease results in a very inconspicuous scar.
- **Rapid recovery of hand strength.** Numerous studies have shown that hand strength is recovered earlier after ECTR than after open surgery.
- **Earlier return to work.** This is a major advantage of ECTR. Palmer et al. (1993) found that endoscopic patients returned to work an average of 29.2 days after an Agee release and 34.6 days after a Chow release, compared with 56.1 days following OCTR. It should be noted, however, that studies vary considerably in their return-to-work data. Nagle et al. found that patients who worked with their hands returned to work 57 to 65 days after ECTR. Chow found an average disability time of 34.6 days following endoscopic release.
- **Lower morbidity.** Mild pain and the advantages listed above account for the lower morbidity of ECTR compared with open techniques.

These advantages of ECTR must be weighed against some highly controversial disadvantages:

- **Higher complication rate.** There have been repeated reports of significant complications following ECTR (Fig. 15-1):
  1. Incomplete release of the transverse carpal ligament
  2. Iatrogenic nerve injuries (partial or complete transection):
     - Median nerve
     - Palmar cutaneous branch
     - Ulnar nerve
     - Digital nerves

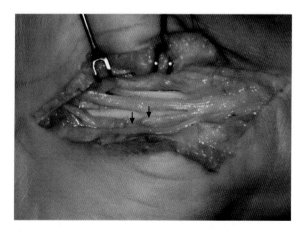

Fig. 15-1. Incomplete division of the median nerve (*arrows*) following ECTR using the Chow technique. (Photo courtesy of Jörg Grünert, Erlangen)

3. Vascular injuries:
   – Ulnar artery
   – Superficial palmar arch
4. Hematomas
5. Flexor tendon injury
5. Reflex sympathetic dystrophy
7. Entry into Guyon's canal
8. Fracture of the hamate hook

Complications can arise during or after any operation, whether open or endoscopic. But the complications in open techniques are clearly attributable to the surgeon, whereas the majority of complications in ECTR are method-related (Table 15-3). The complication rate in the Chow technique, for example, varies considerably. While Chow (1994) reported an almost unbelievably low complication rate of 0.5 % in more than 1000 patients, Kelly et al. (1994) reported complications in 38.1 % of their patients, 9.6 % of whom required a revision procedure (Table 15-3).

Open techniques have also been associated with numerous iatrogenic lesions, even when the operations were performed by qualified hand surgeons or under their supervision (Table 15-2). The study by Palmer and Toivonen (1996) does not specify how many of the total operations were open and how many were endoscopic. Because the number of open releases performed over the years must be substantially higher than the number of endoscopic releases, perhaps a more critical attitude should be taken toward the complications that have been associated with endoscopic releases.

- **Limited visualization or nonvisualization of the median nerve.** None of the endoscopic techniques described to date provides adequate visualization of the median nerve.
- **Nonvisualization of the motor branch.** None of the endoscopic techniques allows visualization of the motor branch. This is necessary, however, in order to release the motor branch in patients with thenar atrophy.
- **Dilation of the carpal tunnel.** The narrowed carpal tunnel must be dilated to create a path for inserting the endoscopic release instruments. This leads to further, albeit transient, compression of the median nerve.
- **Limited visualization or nonvisualization of the superficial palmar arch.** Like the median nerve and its

Table 15-3. Complications of various techniques of ECTR. The complication rate (*CR*) and reoperation rate (*ReOP*) are stated in %

Author	Operative technique	n	CR	ReOP
Okutsu 1989	Okutsu technique	54	7.4	–
Agee 1991	Agee technique	82	4.9	2.4
Brown 1992	Agee technique	149	6.0	0
McDohough 1993	Agee-Chow technique	57	15.8	2
Palmer 1993	Agee-Chow technique	169	14.8	3.1
Arner 1994	Chow technique	53	18.9	5.7
Chow 1994	Chow technique	1154	0.5	0.3
Kelly 1994	Chow technique	97	38.1	9.6
Menon 1994	Agee technique	100	10	1
Nagle 1994	Chow technique	278	5.4	–
Roth 1994	Chow technique	108	10.2	1
Mirza 1995	Uniportal technique	280	1.8	0.4

motor branch (see above), the superficial palmar arch cannot be visualized in ECTR. The portals must be positioned in a way that avoids injury to essential anatomic structures with the operating instruments and minimizes the risk of iatrogenic lesions.

- **Poor visualization after cutting the ligament.** When the carpal ligament is divided, the fatty tissue located between the carpal ligament and palmar fascia herniates into the cut and obscures vision, making it more difficult to complete the cut. This is one reason for an incomplete release when endoscopic techniques are used.

- **Inadequate anatomic dissection during the procedure.** One of the main reasons why endoscopic techniques are criticized is the limited capacity for tissue dissection during the procedure. As a result, it can be difficult to distinguish structures that are to be divided from structures that should be preserved. This marks a fundamental difference between endoscopic and open techniques. In OCTR, the surgeon can use a fine dissecting scissors, for example, to positively identify a questionable structure and determine with confidence whether the structure should be sectioned or preserved. By contrast, cutting in many endoscopic techniques is done according to an "all-or-none principle."

A particular drawback is the use of retrograde knifes for cutting the carpal ligament. If a flexor tendon or nerve is "picked up" on a retrograde knife, it will inevitably be cut when the knife is drawn toward the skin incision. Antegrade cutting is preferred, as the instrument (e. g., a scissors) tends to push nerves and tendons away from the cutting zone as the cut proceeds. Often this effect is intentionally utilized in open procedures to achieve a particular result.

- **Need for special instruments.** ECTR requires the use of specialized instruments such as endoscope holders (Agee technique), dilators, and slotted cannulas for inserting the scope and knife down the carpal tunnel. Because the knives dull rapidly, they are usually available as disposable instruments.

- **High cost.** Deune and Mackinnon (1996) found that the average cost for an endoscopic release was $3468, compared with $2977 for an open procedure. The procurement cost of the special endoscopic equipment must also be taken into account. Mirza and King (1996) calculated the cost of endoscopic release instruments and found that disposable instruments (e. g., knives) cost from $126 to $187 per operation, depending on the technique.

- **Limited field of view.** A major reason why many surgeons, including highly experienced hand surgeons, criticize or reject endoscopic techniques is the limited visualization of the operative site. Because purely endoscopic techniques employ a slotted cannula that is inserted into the carpal tunnel and positioned directly beneath the carpal ligament, the endoscope is located just a few millimeters (1–3 mm) from the site where the ligament will be cut. This results in a tiny field of view, comparable to advancing the arthroscope very close to a femoral condyle in the knee joint. It is impossible to establish anatomic orientation in this situation, let alone perform effective surgery. As a result, the classic surgical activities of dissecting, mobilizing, and retracting anatomic structures are difficult or impossible to accomplish in an endoscopic release. In many cases the carpal ligament is identified purely by feel (washboard effect), whereupon the surgeon makes the cut and "hopes for the best." This was a major factor that prompted us to develop our own minimally invasive technique (see p. 984).

Despite the disadvantages listed above, endoscopic techniques are becoming increasingly popular because, when viewed uncritically, the advantages appear to outweigh the drawbacks. The "learning curve" has often been blamed for problems and complications in ECTR. This should not be considered a valid excuse for complications, however. We share the opinion of Brug (1996), who noted that "a surgeon who cuts the median nerve in an endoscopic release cannot blame the learning curve any more than an airline can claim that the pilot's learning curve was responsible for a plane crash."

Contraindications to Endoscopic Techniques

The guidelines of the German Society for Hand Surgery list the following contraindications to ECTR:

1. Lack of proficiency in OCTR
2. Lack of training in anatomic specimens
3. Thenar atrophy
4. Hypertrophic or rheumatoid synovitis
5. Recurrence
6. Previous local operations
7. Previous soft-tissue injury with adhesions
8. Malunited distal radial fracture
9. Osteoarthritis of the wrist
10. Limitation of wrist motion
11. Space-occupying lesions

Requirements of an Endoscopic or Minimally Invasive Operative Technique

Before deciding which operative technique to use, the surgeon should not only compare the advantages and disadvantages of the various techniques but also consider the requirements that a minimally invasive technique should satisfy:

1. **Good visualization, making it possible to dissect and identify structures that should be preserved.** If necessary, it should be possible to identify the median

nerve, the deep palmar arch, and the thenar motor branch by dissection. Another advantage of dissection is the ability to perform neurolysis of the motor branch, for example, or divide scar tissue surrounding the median nerve.

2. **Small scars.** The scars should be no larger than those resulting from endoscopic techniques. The length of the skin incision should not exceed 1 cm.

3. **Low morbidity.** The procedure should permit the early recovery of hand strength and an early return to work, with a minimum of postoperative pain.

4. **Synovial biopsy.** It should be possible to obtain a synovial biopsy if suspicious synovial changes are found.

5. **Ability to confirm a complete release.** At the end of the operation, it should be possible to determine whether the transverse carpal ligament has been completely divided. Studies in cadaver hands have shown that an incomplete release occurs in up to 61.5% of endoscopic releases using the Chow technique (Deune 1996).

6. **Instrument versatility.** The instrument set should not be so specialized that it cannot be used for other types of surgery.

7. **Minimal use of disposable instruments.** Disposable instruments significantly increase the cost of each operation. Also, an inventory system must be set up for replenishing disposable instrument supplies.

Once the surgeon has opted for a minimally invasive or endoscopic procedure, the patient should be educated about the advantages and disadvantages of the various techniques. The patient should also be told that, regardless of whether an endoscopic or open technique is used, the results at six months are statistically equivalent. The patient should understand that, in the event that unforeseen problems or anatomic variants are encountered intraoperatively, the surgeon may convert to an open release.

Anatomy

A detailed knowledge of anatomy is of fundamental importance, regardless of which operative technique is used.

Boundaries of the carpal tunnel. The carpal tunnel is formed by the carpal bones on the radial, dorsal, and ulnar sides and by the undersurface of the transverse carpal ligament on the palmar side. On the radial side, the transverse carpal ligament is attached distally to the tuberosity of the trapezium and proximally to the tubercle of the scaphoid and the styloid process of the radius. On the ulnar side, the ligament is attached to the hook of the hamate distally and the pisiform proximally. It is continuous proximally with the thin antebrachial fascia. Distally, the transverse carpal ligament ends just proximal to the superficial palmar arch.

Contents of the carpal tunnel. The carpal tunnel is traversed by nine flexor tendons, the median nerve, and the flexor tendon sheaths. While passing through the canal, the median nerve divides into its sensory terminal branches.

Motor branch (thenar branch). The median nerve gives off a motor branch that has variable branching patterns. Lanz (1977) described three different patterns in relation to the transverse carpal ligament:

1. **Extraligamentous (46%):** The motor branch arises past the distal edge of the transverse carpal ligament and turns proximally (recurrent course).
2. **Subligamentous (31%):** The motor branch arises while still under the transverse carpal ligament, so that it accompanies the median nerve in the distal part of the carpal tunnel.
3. **Transligamentous (23%):** The motor branch arises under the transverse carpal ligament and pierces the ligament directly.

A variety of branching patterns may be found. For example, the motor branch may arise from the radial or ulnar side of the median nerve. When arising on the ulnar side, the motor branch is at extremely high risk in endoscopic techniques that do not provide adequate visualization.

Superficial palmar arch. The superficial palmar arch is located from 2 to 26 mm from the distal edge of the transverse carpal ligament. It is usually hidden by fatty tissue (see Fig. 15-12). Schwarz (1993) found that the blade of the Agee device (see p. 982) was less than 2 mm from the palmar arch in 4 of 13 cadaver specimens studied. This close proximity of the palmar arch to the carpal ligament is an important consideration in endoscopic release procedures.

Communicating branch between the median and ulnar nerves. In 80%–90% of cases the communicating branch is located near the distal ulnar edge of the transverse carpal ligament.

Fat pad. Between the transverse carpal ligament and palmar fascia is a fat pad that herniates into the carpal tunnel when the carpal ligament is divided and can prevent adequate visualization in endoscopic techniques.

Palmar cutaneous branch of the median nerve. Approximately 8 cm proximal to the wrist crease, the median nerve gives off a sensory branch that runs distally between the flexor carpi radialis and palmaris longus tendons. Because this branch takes a variable course at the wrist and also becomes very superficial, it is vulnerable to skin incisions. The incision for a carpal tunnel release should be placed ulnar to the palmaris longus tendon, therefore.

Operative Technique

The most widely used endoscopic techniques are described below, along with a minimally invasive technique that was developed by the authors.

1. Okutsu technique
2. Orr technique (Acufex)
3. Agee technique (3 M)
4. Chow technique (Smith and Nephew, Mansfield, USA)
5. Menon technique (Linvatec, Largo, FL, USA)
6. Preissler technique (Karl Storz, Tuttlingen, Germany)
7. Minimally invasive endoscopically controlled technique (Karl Storz, Tuttlingen, Germany)

The purely endoscopic techniques (see 1–6 above) start by creating a space over or beneath the transverse carpal ligament. In most cases a slotted cannula is introduced into this space and is used for inserting the endoscope and cutting instrument. The techniques differ in several aspects:

1. **Placement of the skin incision:**
   – Along the wrist crease
   – In the palm
2. **Number of skin incisions:**
   – Uniportal technique
   – Two-portal technique
3. **Direction of the cut:**
   – Proximal to distal
   – Distal to proximal

Okutsu Technique

A transverse incision of approximately 1 cm is made in the wrist crease on the ulnar side. The carpal tunnel is dilated with an obturator, and a clear plastic tube is advanced beneath the transverse carpal ligament. A retrograde hook knife is inserted parallel to the tube and drawn back to transect the ligament under endoscopic vision.

Orr Technique
(Fig. 15-2)

Instrumentation. The instrument set contains:
- Dilators
- Slotted cannula
- Retrograde knife
- Elevator
- Probe

All the components of this set are available as disposable items.

1. **Skin incision.** A transverse skin incision approximately 1.2–1.5 cm long is made about 1 cm proximal to the wrist crease on the ulnar side.

2. **Identifying the transverse carpal ligament.** The subcutaneous tissue is spread, and the forearm fascia is exposed and incised. A small elevator is introduced and advanced to the undersurface of the transverse carpal ligament. Adherent soft tissues are dissected from the ligament. All movements are directed along the axis of the ring finger ray while manual pressure is exerted on the carpal ligament.

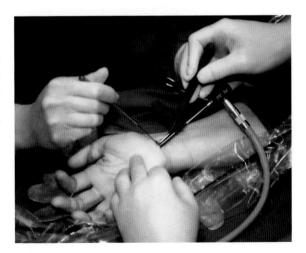

Fig. 15-2. The Orr technique. Endoscopic visualization is limited, because the light post prevents viewing the undersurface of the carpal ligament by rotating the scope

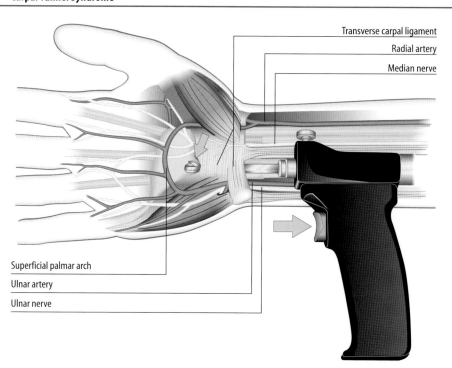

Transverse carpal ligament
Radial artery
Median nerve

Superficial palmar arch
Ulnar artery
Ulnar nerve

3. **Dilating the carpal tunnel.** A 6.5-mm dilator is inserted to develop a space beneath the transverse carpal ligament.

4. **Cutting the ligament.** A slotted cannula is introduced into the dilated space, and a 30° oblique endoscope is inserted into the cannula. A probe is inserted parallel to the scope to determine the distal extent of the carpal ligament. When the distal end has been located, a retrograde hook knife is inserted, the distal edge of the ligament is caught by the knife, and the knife is drawn back toward the skin incision (Fig. 15-2). After the ligament has been divided, fatty tissue appears within the cut. Finally the slotted cannula with the scope and the knife are withdrawn.

5. **Confirming a complete release.** A 10-mm dilator is inserted and advanced distally. According the manufacturer, free passage of the dilator indicates that the transverse carpal ligament has been completely divided. This technique does not permit visual confirmation of a complete release.

Agee Technique
(Fig. 15-3)

Instrumentation. The instrument set includes a pistol-grip handpiece with a disposable blade assembly. A window in the blade assembly permits viewing through a special endoscope that is coupled to the handpiece.

Fig. 15-3. The Agee technique. A pistol-grip handpiece with a trigger-actuated blade is inserted into the dilated carpal tunnel. The blade is elevated to divide the carpal ligament

1. **Skin incision.** A transverse skin incision is placed in the proximal wrist crease on the ulnar side.

2. **Identifying the transverse carpal ligament.** The forearm fascia is exposed by blunt dissection and opened with a distally based U-shaped incision.

3. **Dilating the carpal tunnel.** A special probe is inserted to enlarge the space beneath the transverse carpal ligament.

4. **Cutting the ligament.** The pistol-type grip with the blade assembly and endoscope is introduced, and the tip of the assembly is palpated just distal to the transverse carpal ligament. Under endoscopic vision, the blade is elevated and the release is initiated at the center of the ligament. When orientation has been sufficiently established, the release is continued from the distal edge. The disposable blade assembly consists of a retrograde knife in a slotted sheath. Pressing the trigger on the handpiece elevates the blade toward the undersurface of the ligament. As the device is pulled proximally to divide the ligament, the cutting process is monitored endoscopically. After the release is completed, the fatty tissue above the ligament appears within the cut.

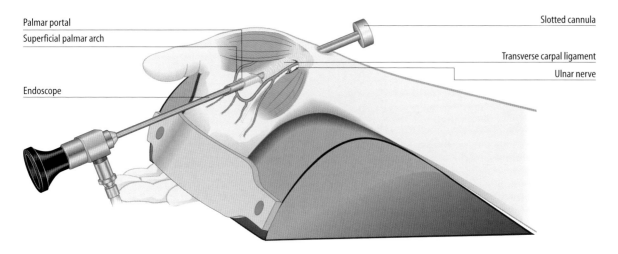

Palmar portal
Superficial palmar arch
Endoscope

Slotted cannula
Transverse carpal ligament
Ulnar nerve

Chow Technique
(Fig. 15-4)

Fig. 15-4. The Chow technique. The wrist is hyperextended over a special positioning wedge. The slotted cannula is introduced, and the endoscope is inserted from the distal side

Instrumentation. The complete instrument set includes a hand holder that fixes the wrist in hyperextension. Other components are a large-bore slotted cannula with a blunt obturator and three knives, which are available as disposable instruments.

Positioning. The wrist is hyperextended over a special hand holder that is part of the instrument set.

1. **Skin incision.** Before the skin is incised, the bony landmarks on the palmar surface (hook of the hamate, pisiform) are identified and marked. Reference lines and the endoscopic portals are also marked. Then a 1- to 1.5-cm transverse skin incision is made at the wrist.

2. **Identifying the transverse carpal ligament.** After blunt spreading of the subcutaneous tissue, the forearm fascia is exposed and a distally based U-shaped flap is raised with a scalpel. A curved dissector is used to dilate the carpal tunnel between the undersurface of the transverse carpal ligament and the tendon sheaths. A "washboard effect" is felt as the dissector is advanced across the transverse fibers of the ligament. The dissector is carefully advanced into the palm, and its tip is palpated beneath the skin.

3. **Distal skin incision.** Because this is a two-portal technique, a second skin incision is made in the surface of the palm. This is done by inserting a blunt trocar and slotted cannula beneath the carpal ligament into the carpal tunnel and carefully advancing the assembly toward the palm. The bony ulnar boundary of the carpal tunnel (the hook of the hamate) can be felt during the insertion.

▶ **Caution:** Advance the slotted cannula with blunt trocar along the axis of the ring finger ray. Do not deviate toward the radial side.
The tip of the trocar is palpated in the palm, and that site is marked and incised. The subcutaneous tissue and palmaris longus fascia are carefully spread open. If necessary, the distal palmar arch can be held distally with a special retractor.

4. **Cutting the ligament.** After the trocar is removed from the slotted cannula, a knife (antegrade or retrograde) is inserted from one side and the endoscope from the other. Before the carpal ligament is cut, the patient (under regional or local anesthesia) is told to slowly flex the fingers; this avoids interposition of the flexor tendons between the slotted cannula and carpal ligament. Then the ligament is divided under endoscopic control. Vision following the release is obscured by overlying fat herniating between the cut edges and into the slotted cannula.

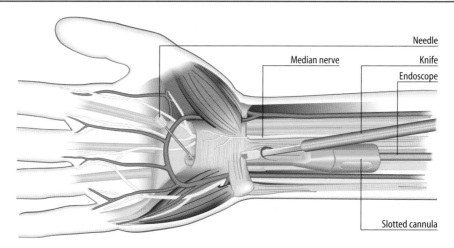

Needle
Knife
Endoscope
Median nerve
Slotted cannula

Menon Technique

Instrumentation. The instrument set includes the following components:
- Slotted cannula
- Matching trocar
- Dilators (5.5 and 7 mm)
- Antegrade knife

All the instruments are available in disposable form.

The operative technique is very similar to the Orr release (see above). The main difference is the somewhat different design of the slotted cannula. An antegrade knife similar to the Smillie knife is used (Fig. 15-5).

Preissler Technique

Instrumentation. This technique requires:
- 30° Forward oblique endoscope (diameter 2.7 mm, length 11 mm)
- Retractor with scope guide
- Smillie bayonet knife
- Dilators (4, 5, 6, and 7 mm)

1. **Skin incision.** A 1-cm skin incision is made over the distal edge of the transverse carpal ligament between the thenar and hypothenar eminences.

2. **Visualizing the transverse carpal ligament.** Because the carpal ligament is approached in a plane between the palmar fascia and ligament rather than between the median nerve and ligament, first the palmar aponeurosis is spread longitudinally in the direction of its fibers, and the middle fascial layer, distinguished by its oblique fiber course, is identified. Dilators are used to enlarge the space between the two layers to 7 mm. A special retractor with a scope guide (grooved

Fig. 15-5. The Menon technique. The slotted cannula is inserted beneath the transverse carpal ligament. The undersurface of the ligament is inspected with the endoscope and divided with an antegrade knife. The distal edge of the ligament is marked with a needle

retractor) is introduced into this space, and the transverse carpal ligament is visualized.

3. **Cutting the ligament.** The transverse carpal ligament is divided in several steps. It is easily identified by its transverse fibers. It is recommended that the cut be continued approximately 1–1.5 cm onto the forearm fascia. After the proximal part of the carpal ligament has been divided, the instruments are removed and the distal part of the ligament is cut under direct vision. This can be aided by inserting a small Langenbeck retractor, for example. The palmar arch, located somewhat distal to the palmar incision, can also be inspected and preserved.

Minimally Invasive Endoscopically Controlled Technique

Analysis of the known endoscopic techniques (see above) has shown that they are useful only for dividing the transverse carpal ligament. Little or no real "dissection" can be performed. This situation is comparable to the early days of knee arthroscopy, when both the arthroscope and the operating instruments were inserted through common sheath systems or working cannulas. "Arthroscopic surgery" in the true sense developed only when the instruments were inserted through a separate portal. This greatly increased the maneuverability of the instruments, enabling the surgeon to selectively palpate, dissect, resect, and divide anatomic structures with a high degree of precision. Because the purely

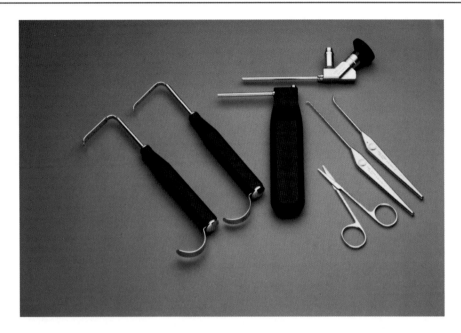

Fig. 15-6. Instrument set for *minimally invasive endoscopically assisted surgery*, consisting of an endoscope, scope holder, dissecting scissors, and retractor (Karl Storz, Tuttlingen, Germany)

endoscopic techniques lack this capability and do not satisfy the requirements of a minimally invasive procedure (see p. 979), we have developed our own minimally invasive endoscopically assisted technique for carpal tunnel release.

Instruments (Fig. 15-6). The instrument set consists of:
- 30° wide-angle endoscope (barrel length 11 mm, diameter 4.5 mm with angled eyepiece). The eyepiece is angled to provide more working space below the scope and keep the light post from getting in the way. Since a 4.5-mm scope is used, it provides excellent image quality that permits easily identification of anatomic structures.
- Scope holder
- Retractor with length markings
- Dissecting scissors
- Dissecting elevator
- Probe with a millimeter scale

1. Skin incision. A 1-cm skin incision is placed in the ulnar third of the wrist crease. A line from the ulnar border of the ring finger should bisect the skin incision at a right angle. Only the skin is incised.

2. Visualizing the transverse carpal ligament. The forearm fascia is exposed with a small, blunt dissecting scissors. The fascia is carefully incised, and the cut is extended distally while the subcutaneous tissue is elevated with a small Langenbeck retractor or the retractor from the instrument set (Fig. 15-7a). The first 5–10 mm is incised under direct vision or under endoscopic control (Fig. 15-7b). Then the retractor is inserted somewhat more deeply and angled (on its tip) to demonstrate the proximal edge of the transverse carpal ligament (Fig. 15-7b,c).

3. Cutting the ligament. The handpiece with scope inserted is advanced directly beneath the retractor. The undersurface of the carpal ligament is exposed with the elevator (Fig. 15-7c).

▶ **Tip:** Aim for the ulnar border of the ring finger. Do not deviate toward the radial side!
First the proximal edge of the transverse carpal ligament is incised with a small scissors (Fig. 15-7d). The median nerve and a portion of the flexor tendons are visible at this stage, so it should be possible to preserve them. If vision is obscured by herniating fat, the special retractor should be carefully advanced distally in line with the ring finger. The retractor can then be slightly angulated to regain a view of the carpal ligament so that the release can be continued in stepwise fashion (Fig. 15-8).
After the release has been completed, the probe is used to check for any remaining intact transverse structures that should also be divided (Fig. 15-9a,b).

4. Visualizing the motor branch. If necessary, the elevator or probe is used to carefully dissect toward the middle and radial thirds of the carpal ligament. The retractor should be angled to obtain adequate exposure of this area (Fig. 15-10). Generally the motor

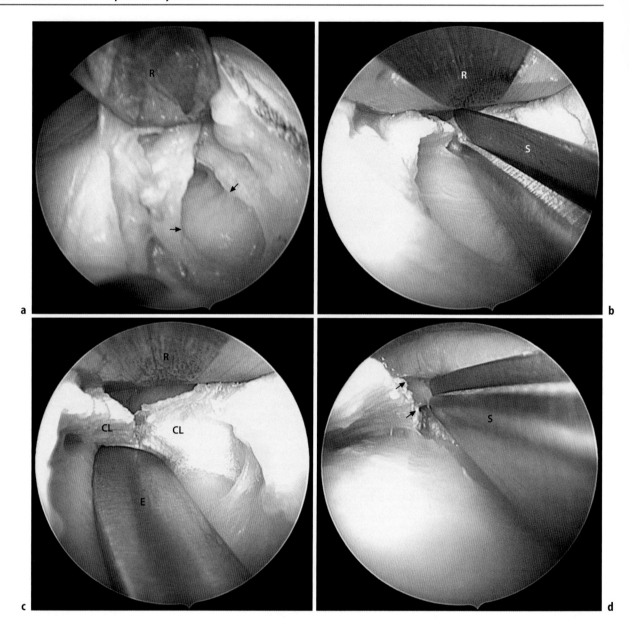

Fig. 15-7 a–d. Minimally invasive ECTR (left hand). **a** After the skin is incised, the retractor (*R*) is inserted and the forearm fascia (*arrows*) is opened. **b** A scissors (*S*) is used to continue the cut distally and carefully dissect beneath the transverse carpal ligament. **c** The undersurface of the carpal ligament (*CL*) is exposed with the elevator (*E*), and its proximal edge is incised. **d** The cut is continued with the scissors (*S*) (*arrows* cut edge of carpal ligament)

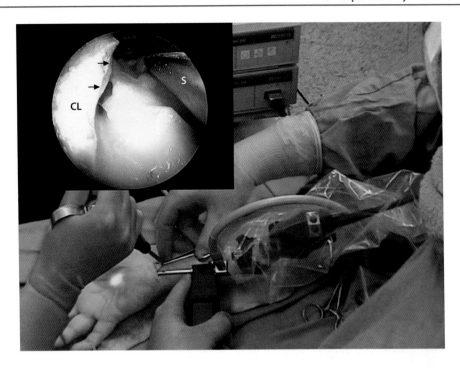

Fig. 15-8. Dividing the carpal ligament with a scissors. An assistant holds the retractor while the surgeon guides the endoscope holder and dissecting scissors. Endoscopic view (*upper left*). Division of the carpal ligament (*CL*) is continued with the scissors (*S*) (*arrows* cut edge)

branch of the median nerve can now be visualized. If thenar atrophy is present, the surgeon can proceed with endoscopically controlled dissection and neurolysis of the motor branch (Fig. 15-11). Numerous anatomic variants of the motor branch can be identified (Fig. 15-11 c–e).

Variable muscle fibers (e. g., of palmaris brevis) have also been observed. If the muscle is stretched tightly over the median nerve, it may have to be divided. This can be done endoscopically, and bleeding sites in the muscle can be selectively coagulated with electrocautery.

5. **Visualizing the palmar arch and the distal division of the median nerve.** If the transverse carpal ligament extends very far distally or if it is necessary to visualize the superficial palmar arch, the retractor and the holder/scope assembly are advanced farther distally. Because the arm has been exsanguinated, the palmar arch appears as a narrow, transverse, pinkish band (Fig. 15-12 b). Usually the median nerve has already split into its terminal branches at this level, but sometimes its point of division can be seen endoscopically.

6. **Confirming a complete release.** Before the operation is concluded, the retractor is reinserted to check the integrity of the median nerve and to exclude (or if necessary divide) any remaining intact transverse fibers of the carpal ligament (Fig. 15-12 a).

7. **Drainage and wound closure.** If it was necessary to divide a band of muscle tissue, a small drain (Ch 6 or 8) is inserted. This may be done under endoscopic control (Fig. 15-12 c). The skin incision is closed with simple interrupted sutures.

Postoperative Care

A well-padded elastic compression bandage is worn for five days after surgery. The wound drain is removed on the first postoperative day (without suction), and the sutures are removed on day 14. The patient should wear an elastic wrap on the operated wrist for four additional weeks. Patients engaged in heavy manual labor are advised to continue the elastic wrap for 6–8 weeks.

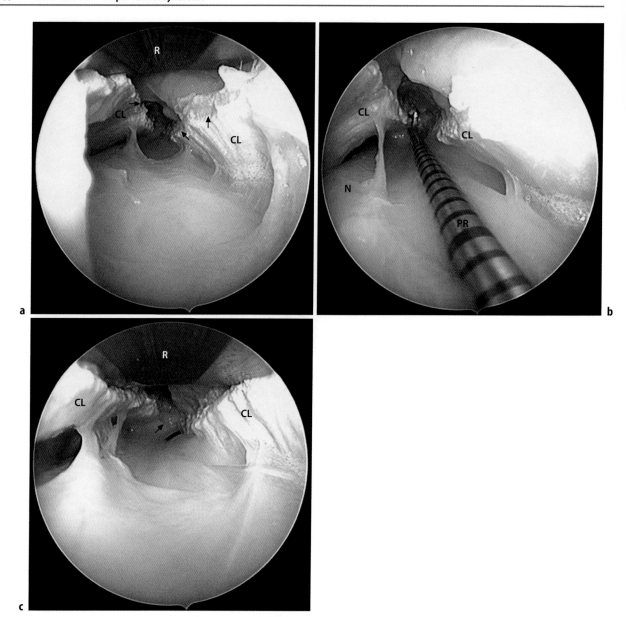

Fig. 15-9 a–c. Minimally invasive ECTR in the left hand (continued from Fig. 15-7). **a** With the retractor (*R*) in place, the cut edges (*arrows*) of the carpal ligament (*CL*) are visible following the release (*N* median nerve). **b** The probe (*PR*) is used to check for remaining intact fibers in the distal part of the ligament. **c** When the retractor is advanced farther distally and angled, it cannot be determined for certain whether residual fibers (*arrows*) are present, and careful probing is necessary to confirm a complete release

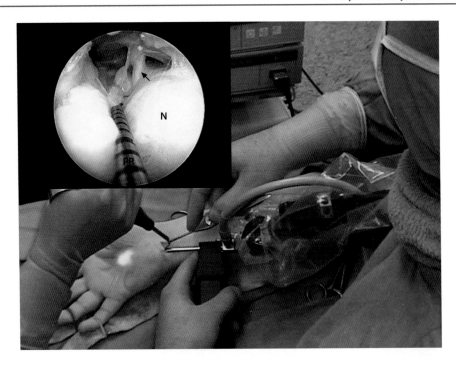

Fig. 15-10. Visualization of the motor branch (left hand). The median nerve (*N*) is pushed dorsalward with the probe (*PR*) until the motor branch of the median nerve (*arrow*) can be seen

Summary and Outlook

A comparison of the open, endoscopic, and minimally invasive endoscopically assisted techniques shows that carpal tunnel release can be performed through a small skin incision. The potential problems associated with purely endoscopic techniques have been discussed (see p. 976). The minimally invasive technique offers the following advantages:

1. **Positive identification of anatomic structures.**
2. **Visualization and neurolysis of the motor branch** (if required, see Figs. 15-10 and 15-11).
3. **Visualization of the median nerve.**
4. **Visualization of the superficial palmar arch** (if required, see Fig. 15-12 b).
5. **Small skin incision.**
6. **Ability to dissect tissues** in order to identify anatomic structures and divide the carpal ligament with adequate vision. This makes the minimally invasive technique more comparable to operating with a microscope or binocular loupe than the purely endoscopic techniques (see Fig. 15-12).
7. **No disposable instruments.**
8. **Instrument versatility.** The same instruments can be used for minimally invasive procedures in other regions (see Chap. 17).

To date, we have used this technique 122 patients with carpal tunnel syndrome (1995–1998). Motor branch neurolysis was performed in 21 patients, and a synovial biopsy was obtained in 8 patients. There were no instances of nerve or vascular injuries in any of the patients. Two patients had an indurated area in the palm due to excessive scarring, but this resolved in 6 and 11 months.

With its low morbidity, clear visualization (Figs. 15-7 to 15-12) and controlled dissection, this technique has become our procedure of first choice for carpal tunnel release. Long-term results are still needed, however.

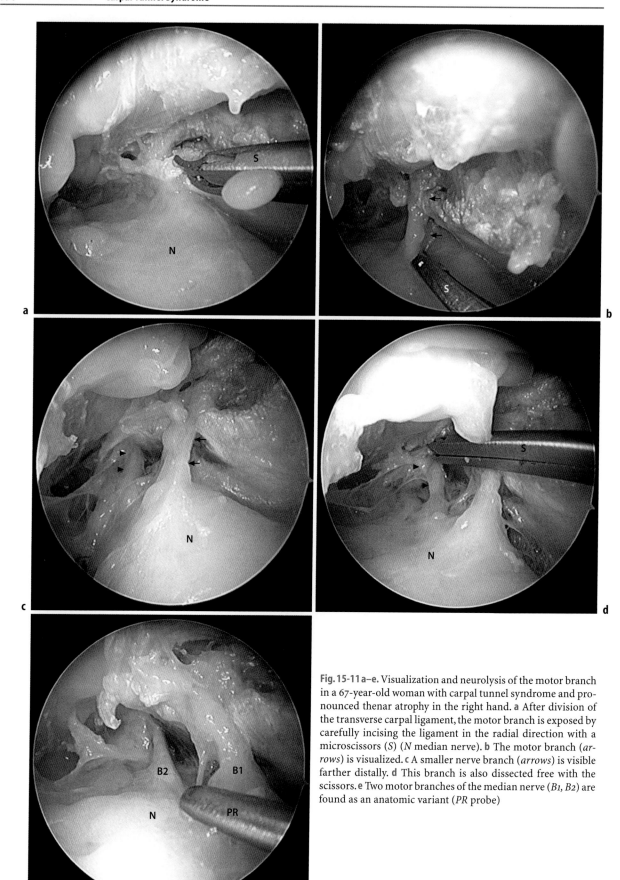

Fig. 15-11 a–e. Visualization and neurolysis of the motor branch in a 67-year-old woman with carpal tunnel syndrome and pronounced thenar atrophy in the right hand. **a** After division of the transverse carpal ligament, the motor branch is exposed by carefully incising the ligament in the radial direction with a microscissors (*S*) (*N* median nerve). **b** The motor branch (*arrows*) is visualized. **c** A smaller nerve branch (*arrows*) is visible farther distally. **d** This branch is also dissected free with the scissors. **e** Two motor branches of the median nerve (*B1, B2*) are found as an anatomic variant (*PR* probe)

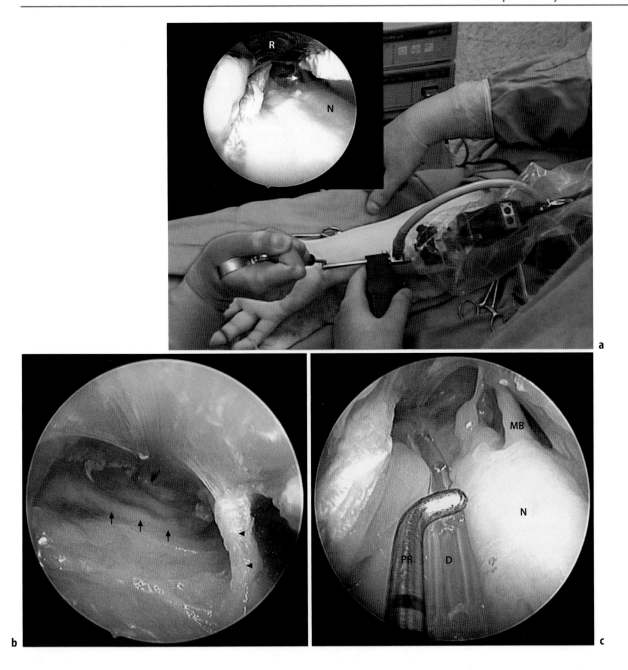

Fig. 15-12 a–c. Confirming a complete release (continued from Fig. 15-10). **a** The retractor (*R*) is advanced far distally and carefully angled. The median nerve (*N*) is visible and intact. The motor branch (*arrow*) is also visible. Residual carpal ligament fibers are excluded. **b** Visualization of the superficial palmar arch (*arrows*) after division of the carpal ligament (*arrowheads* cut edge of the distal ligament). **c** If desired, a drain (*D*) can be accurately placed with the probe under endoscopic control (*MB* motor branch)

Bursal Endoscopy

Given the ability of endoscopes to view the interior of anatomic cavities, it is logical to apply this capability to the prepatellar and olecranon bursae, i.e., distend the bursal cavity with fluid as a prelude to endoscopic inspection and excision.

16.1 Instrumentation

The instruments are the same as those used for knee and ankle arthroscopy. The small size of the bursae makes it advantageous to use a short-barreled scope (see Fig. 3.2-1).

16.2 Video System

The video setup is the same as in knee arthroscopy (see Sect. 1.3).

16.3 Probe

A short probing hook is necessary for palpating fibrotic bands.

16.4 Operating Instruments

The same operating instruments are used as in knee arthroscopy (see Sect. 1.6). Essential instruments are the motorized shaver (Rosenberg resector, meniscus cutter; see Fig. 1.6-6) and electrocautery (see Fig. 1.6-8).

16.5 Anesthesia

Several options are available: general anesthesia, spinal block, epidural anesthesia, or a brachial plexus block in the upper arm.

16.6 Positioning

For endoscopic surgery on the prepatellar bursa, the knee joint is placed in an extended position as for knee arthroscopy (see Sect. 1.8.1). For the endoscopic treatment of olecranon bursitis, the prone position is preferred (see Fig. 7.8-2).

16.7 Tourniquet

All operations are performed with a proximal tourniquet and exsanguinating wrap, because even slight bleeding can greatly obscure the field of view.

16.8 Draping

The limb is draped as for arthroscopy of the knee joint (see Sect. 1.10) or elbow joint (see Sect. 7.10).

16.9 Distention Medium

Because electrocautery instruments will be used, the bursa is distended with a nonelectrolytic solution.

16.10 Setup and Preparations for Endoscopy

The setup is the same as for knee arthroscopy (see Sect. 1.12) or elbow arthroscopy (see Sect. 7.12).

16.11 Portal Placement

One medial and one lateral portal are recommended. The exact placement site depends on the size of the bursa and its degree of distention.

16.11.1 Technique for Creating the Portals

A standard routine is recommended for establishing the portals:

1. **Needle insertion.** A needle is inserted into the bursa. The needle can be angled proximally and distally to confirm that it has entered the bursal cavity. This should present no problems in a fluid-filled bursa.

2. **Distention.** The bursa is tightly distended with fluid.

3. **Incision.** An incision 3–4 mm long is made through the skin and bursal tissue. The bursal walls may be

fibrotic, making it difficult to introduce the sheath and blunt obturator without incising the capsule. The obturator is withdrawn, the scope is inserted, and the bursa is inspected.

16.11.2 Instrument Portal

The instrument portal is established under endoscopic vision:

1. **Transillumination.** The external light spot from the endoscope marks the portion of the bursa that is located opposite the viewing portal.

2. **Needle insertion.** A needle is inserted at that site under endoscopic vision. There should be no difficulty in entering the bursa.

3. **Incising the skin and bursal wall.** The skin and bursal wall are incised with a scalpel. The incision should be no longer than 3–4 mm; a larger incision would allow considerable fluid extravasation that would hamper the rest of the procedure.

4. **Insertion of the probe and operating instruments.**

16.12 Complications

The only known complications are those generally associated with surgical operations: infection, thrombosis, effusion, skin injuries, reflex sympathetic dystrophy. Our only complication to date has been one effusion, which resolved after percutaneous aspiration.

16.13 Documentation

The documentation of endoscopic bursectomy must meet the same requirements as in arthroscopic procedures (see Sect. 1.16).

16.14 Outpatient Bursoscopy

All bursoscopies can be performed on an outpatient basis.

16.15 Indications

Endoscopic bursectomy is appropriate for refractory bursitis that is unresponsive to conservative treatment or to the single injection of a crystalloid cortisone solution.

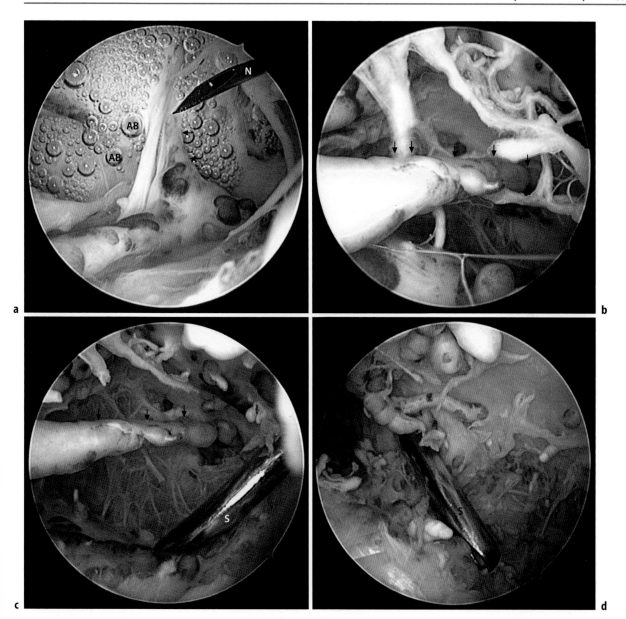

Fig. 16.17-1 a–d. Endoscopic bursectomy. a, b Inspection of the fluid-distended bursa reveals numerous air bubbles (*AB*) on the bursal wall. A percutaneous needle (*N*) is used to locate the site for the instrument portal. Numerous adhesions (*arrows*) are visible within the bursa. c, d Adhesions and inflammatory wall tissues are resected with a shaver (*S*)

16.16 Contraindications

Besides the general contraindications that apply to knee and elbow arthroscopy (see Sect. 1.19), bacterial bursitis is considered a relative contraindication. So far we have had no experience with the endoscopic treatment of bacterial bursitis, and no reports have been published in the literature.

16.17 Operative Technique

Endoscopic inspection reveals fibrotic adhesions in the bursa, which often are palpable and may be causing pain

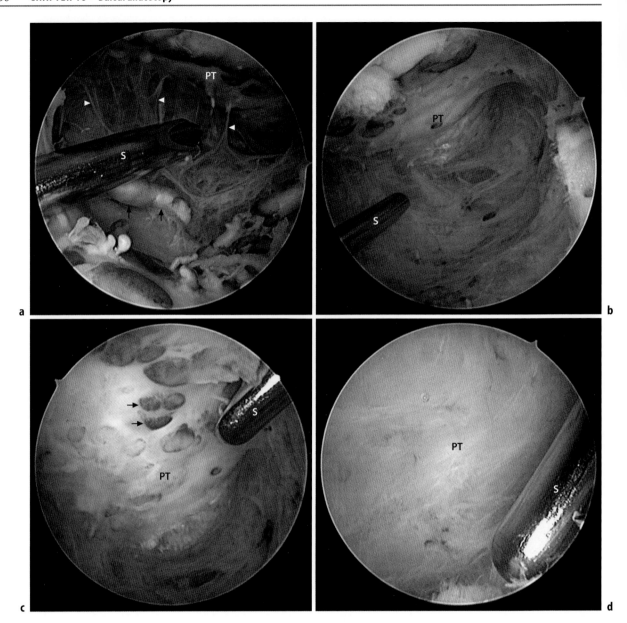

Fig. 16.17-2a–d. Endoscopic bursectomy (continued from Fig. 16.17-1). **a** The distal portion of the bursa also contains numerous adhesions (*arrowheads*) and thicker bands (*arrows*), which are removed (*S* shaver, *PT* anterior aspect of patellar tendon). **b** After the adhesions have been removed, the full distal extent of the bursa can be appreciated. **c, d** Inflammatory changes (*arrows*) on the patellar tendon are also removed

(Fig. 16.17-1). These bands are divided or excised with a basket forceps or shaver (Rosenberg resector or meniscus cutter). Since the bursal wall may be very fibrotic in chronic bursitis, it is first necessary to establish a starting point for the resection (Fig. 16.17-2). We recommend notching the bursal wall with an electrocautery knife or dividing the wall into multiple segments which can then be separately removed with the meniscus cutter or synovial resector. Larger segments that have been detached with the cautery knife can be extracted with a grasping forceps.

In a complete bursectomy, it is always necessary to interchange the viewing and instrumentation portals.

▶ **Note:** Suction should be carefully regulated when a power shaver is used. Since the bursa contains a very small amount of fluid, its walls can collapse relatively quickly.

When the bursectomy has been completed, the access portals are closed over a Ch 8 suction drain with simple interrupted sutures. The drain is removed on the first postoperative day.

16.18 Postoperative Care

The operated limb is immobilized in a removable splint for 7 to 10 days. Range of motion exercises and axial loading are permitted. Our single instance of effusion was probably due to premature mobilization, since vigorous exercises had been started in the immediate postoperative period.

16.19 Outlook and Personal Experience

In summary, it is evident that prepatellar and olecranon bursectomy can be performed endoscopically. It is reasonable to expect that the results will be comparable to those of "classic" open bursectomy. The main advantage of endoscopic bursectomy is a very inconspicuous scar. The main disadvantage is a longer operating time. Pässler (1996) states that the operating time is twice that of open surgery, and this is consistent with our own experience.

Nevertheless, endoscopic bursectomy should be considered in properly selected cases. It is advantageous for women or young patients who desire an optimum cosmetic result, and endoscopic prepatellar bursectomy will avoid prepatellar scars in patients whose occupation involves kneeling.

CHAPTER 17

Minimally Invasive Endoscopically Assisted Techniques

Endoscopic techniques are limited to articular spaces (arthroscopy) and other preexisting anatomic spaces (bursae, subacromial space, carpal tunnel). But by adding minimally invasive surgical techniques to endoscopic techniques, it is possible to visualize and treat areas that would not be accessible to endoscopy alone.

The desire to see an anatomic structure "with one's own eyes" or palpate it with the finger is not in itself a sufficient rationale for wide surgical exposure. It is only logical to facilitate inspection with a videoendoscope whose magnified view ($5\times$ to $30\times$) displays considerably more anatomic details than would be apparent to the unaided eye. Endoscopic surgery is comparable to operating with a binocular loupe or operating microscope, for even minute tissue changes can be visualized and documented.

Many of the practical aspects of minimally invasive endoscopic techniques have been worked out in cadaver studies, making it possible to apply these technique to the diagnosis and treatment of numerous disorders.

Instrumentation

Minimally invasive techniques employ a short, angled endoscope with an angled eyepiece (see Fig. 15-6). To facilitate handling, the scope is mounted in a holder before it is introduced into the dissected cavity. The holder is easy for surgeons to manipulate, regardless of handedness. The instrument set includes retractors of assorted lengths and widths, small blunt-ended scissors, a probe with a millimeter scale, and small dissector-elevators.

17.1 Stenosing Tenosynovitis

Cause

Stenosing tenosynovitis (de Quervain disease) is caused by overuse of the extensor tendons of the thumb. Females are predominantly affected. Acute, unaccustomed use of the wrist in flexion and ulnar deviation predisposes to the disorder.

Symptoms

The cardinal symptom is pain in the radial portion of the wrist and lateral distal forearm. The pain may radiate to the upper arm and toward the thumb.

Clinical Diagnosis

Physical examination elicits local tenderness over the first extensor compartment accompanied by a firm, localized swelling of variable degree. Patients typically have a positive Finkelstein test (severe pain on ulnar deviation of the wrist with the fingers closed over the thumb).

Therapeutic Management

Conservative treatment options include rest and immobilization, local nonsteroidal anti-inflammatory agents (in gel form), and activity modification. If conservative treatment is of no benefit, surgical release of the tendon compartment is indicated.

In the classic "open" operation, a 4- to 5-cm incision is used to expose the tendon compartment for the release. The classic procedure uses a palmar-convex skin incision that is not placed directly over the compartment that is to be released. It is necessary to identify and protect the superficial branch of the radial nerve. Many patients with large skin incisions complain of scar irritation, especially when wearing a bracelet or watch on the affected wrist. This problem can be avoided by using the minimally invasive technique described below.

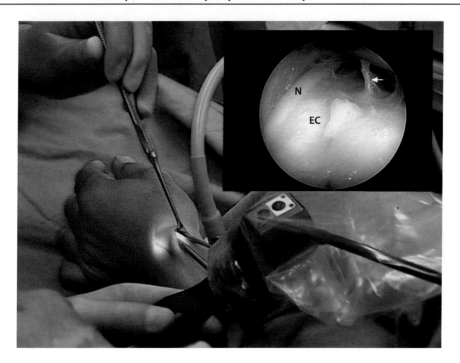

Fig. 17.1-1. Minimally invasive endoscopically assisted release of the first compartment for stenosing tenosynovitis. The angled arthroscope is introduced through a small skin incision (see Fig. 15.6). The first extensor compartment (*EC*) and an overlying nerve (*N*) are visualized (*arrow* small cutaneous nerve)

Operative Technique

1. **Skin incision.** An oblique skin incision about 1 cm long is placed 1.5 mm proximal to the extensor tendon compartment. The subcutaneous tissue is spread open with a fine scissors. Sometimes the superficial branch of the radial nerve can be located and held aside. Next a retractor is inserted, and the endoscope is introduced into the cavity that has been developed (Fig. 17.1-1).

2. **Exposing the extensor tendon compartment.** The tissue overlying the extensor compartment is bluntly spread open, creating a cavity that is held open with the retractor.

3. **Releasing the compartment.** The endoscope is placed into the cavity. The proximal expansions of the first compartment are incised first, exposing the extensor tendons (Fig. 17.1-2). The compartment is incised in the proximal-to-distal direction, exposing the course of the individual tendons. The extensor tendons are held aside with a fine probing hook to exclude accessory tendons (Fig. 17.1-3). It may be necessary to extend the compartment incision. The extensor tendons and floor of the compartment may show synovitic changes (Fig. 17.1-4).

The entire compartment and the tendons themselves are explored under visual control and evaluated for synovial changes. The scope can then be rotated to view the superficial branch of the radial nerve and assess its integrity. The magnified view enables the surgeon to identify and preserve small nerve branches that pass to the skin (see Fig. 17.1-1).

Experience to Date

So far we have performed minimally invasive release of the first compartment in 12 patients. There have been no instances of postoperative nerve irritation or wound healing problems, and we have not found it necessary to convert to an open release. The main advantages have been mild postoperative pain and an extremely favorable cosmetic result. The magnified view of the operative field on the monitor dispelled our original fears of inadequate visualization.

The case numbers to date are still too small to permit a definitive evaluation of this new technique. But the initial results have been very positive, and we are encouraged to continue the technique and develop it further.

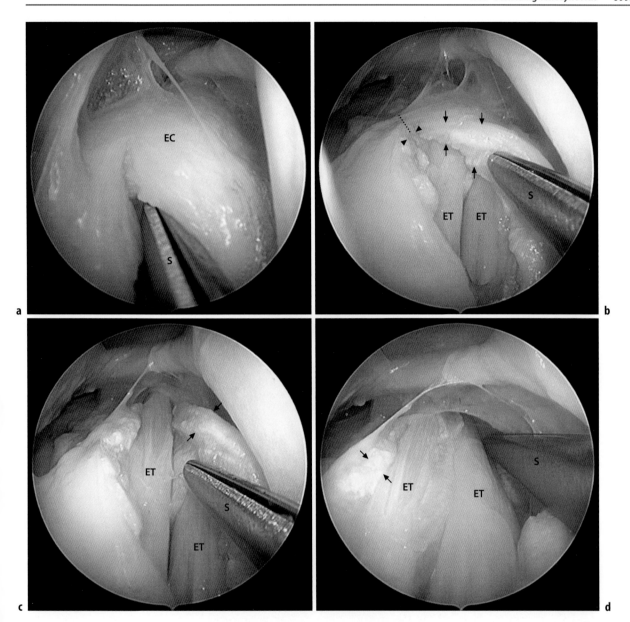

Fig. 17.1-2a–d. Minimally invasive endoscopically assisted release of the first compartment (continued from Fig. 17.1-1). **a** The compartment (*EC*) is opened with a scissors (*S*). **b** The compartment wall (*arrows*) shows considerable thickening over the two extensor tendons (*ET*) beneath it. Note that the compartment has not yet been completely divided (*dotted line, arrowheads*). **c, d** Appearance of the extensor tendons after completion of the release (*arrows* thickness of the extensor compartment)

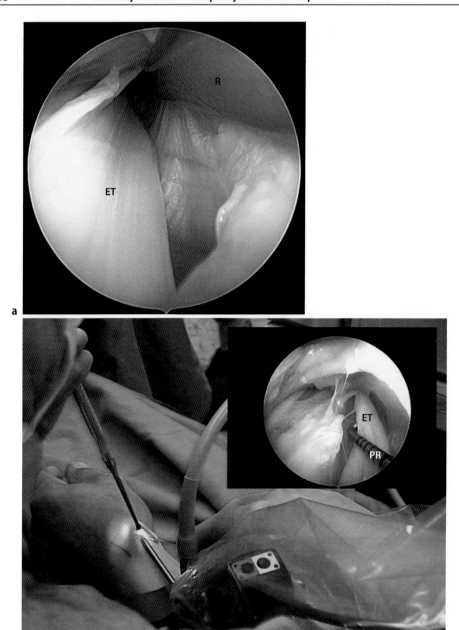

Fig. 17.1-3 a, b. Minimally invasive endoscopically assisted release of the first compartment (continued from Fig. 17.1-2). **a** Endoscopic view of the surface and course of the extensor tendon (*ET*) (*R* retractor). **b** The tendon is probed to exclude adhesions and synovial deposits (*PR* probe)

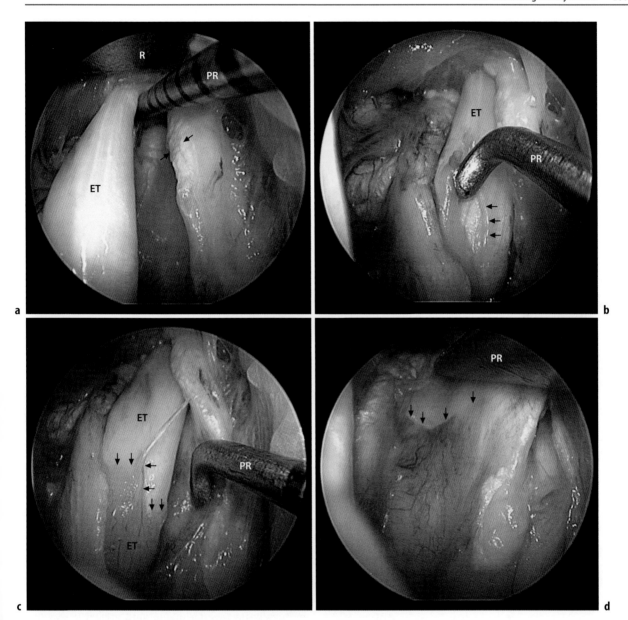

Fig. 17.1-4a–d. Minimally invasive endoscopically assisted release of the first compartment for stenosing tenosynovitis. **a** Endoscope demonstrates thickening of the extensor compartment (*arrows*) (*PR* probe, *ET* extensor tendon, *R* retractor)). **b** The tendon is covered by a thick synovial membrane (*arrows*), which has been endoscopically incised. **c** Proximal to the thickened compartment (site of narrowing) is an area of pronounced tendon degeneration (*arrows*) with synovial deposits. **d** Elevating the tendon from its bed reveals a marked synovial reaction (*arrows*) on the compartment floor. This reaction can be more clearly evaluated by endoscopy than by visual inspection during an open release

17.2 Retrocalcaneal Exostosis

Cause

The symptoms are precipitated by local pressure (e. g., from the back of a shoe) acting on an area of exostosis.

Symptoms

The hallmark is pain adjacent to the Achilles tendon insertion on the tuber calcanei.

Clinical Diagnosis

Physical examination gives the impression of a true exostosis. The skin is reddened and may even be inflamed. Bursitis may be present between the Achilles tendon and calcaneus.

Radiographs

Despite the clinical impression of a large exostosis, radiographs may show only a small spur on the tuber calcanei directed toward the Achilles tendon.

Therapeutic Management

If benefit is not derived from stretching of the lower leg muscles, local ointments, and shoe modification, surgical removal of the exostosis is recommended.

Treating the condition by open surgery requires a skin incision approximately 4–5 cm long. Again, a minimally invasive technique can be used to expose and remove the exostosis.

Operative Technique

1. **Skin incision.** A skin incision 10–15 mm long is made lateral to the Achilles tendon. The subcutaneous tissue is spread with a small scissors, and the tuber calcanei is approached by blunt dissection.

2. **Exposing the tuber calcanei.** A Langenbeck retractor is inserted to create a cavity bounded inferiorly by the exostosis on the tuber calcanei and posteriorly by the Achilles tendon. This space is visualized with the endoscope (Fig. 17.2-1, see also Fig. 15-6).

3. **Removing the exostosis.** First the exostosis is grossly removed with a small chisel (Fig. 17.2-1 d). The resection site is then smoothed with a round bur and bone curet (Fig. 17.2-2 a, b), and it is fine-smoothed with a file (Fig. 17.2-2 c). Finally it is cauterized with a ball-tipped electrode to minimize the postoperative bleeding risk (Fig. 17.2-2 d).

4. **Probing the Achilles tendon.** After the exostosis has been removed, indurated sites are found in the Achilles tendon. Marked thickening and induration are found proximal to the original site of the exostosis. The more distal portion of the tendon is thinner and shows no structural changes (Fig. 17.2-3).

5. **Skin closure.** The skin is closed with sutures over a suction drain (Fig. 17.2-3 b).

Experience to Date

We have used this technique in 14 patients. In all cases the pathologic changes were clearly visualized and could be evaluated with better precision than in the classic open procedure.

We cannot definitively assess the clinical value of this minimally invasive technique until greater case numbers have become available for analysis.

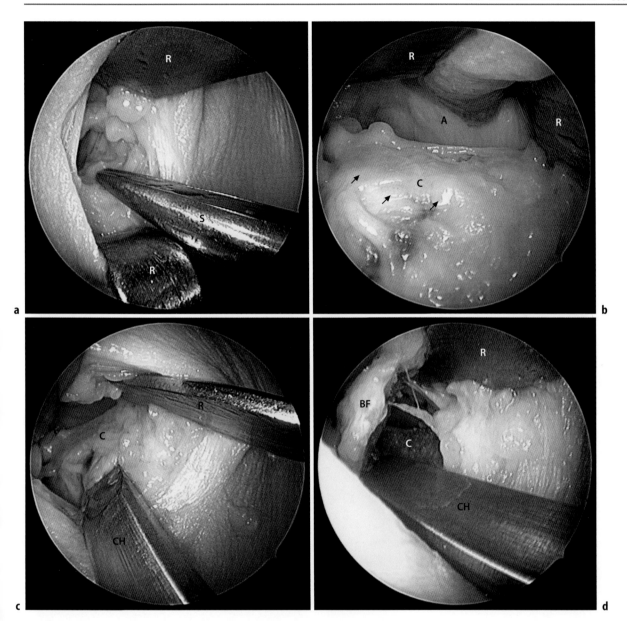

Fig. 17.2-1 a–d. Minimally invasive endoscopically assisted removal of retrocalcaneal exostosis. **a** The space over the exostosis is bluntly developed with a scissors (*S*). The wound is held open with two retractors (*R*). **b** The endoscope is inserted, revealing the bulge (*arrows*) on the calcaneus (*C*). **c** The exostosis is removed with a chisel (*CH*). **d** The detached bone fragment (*BF*) is removed

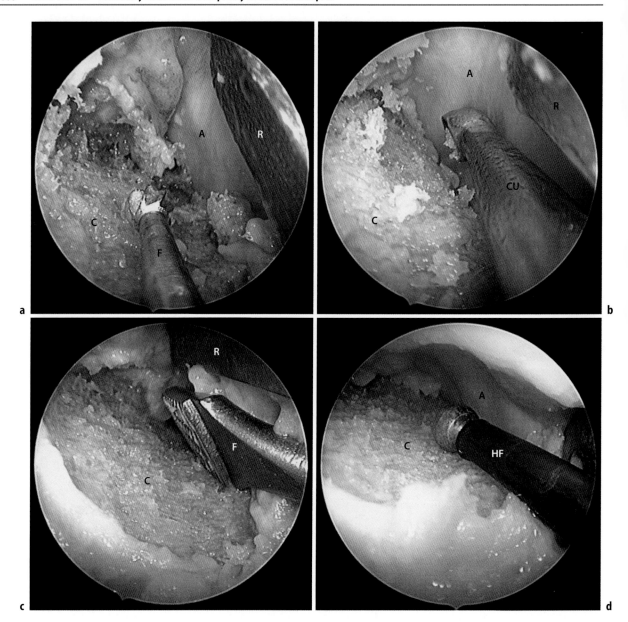

Fig. 17.2-2 a–d. Minimally invasive endoscopically assisted removal of retrocalcaneal exostosis (continued from Fig. 17.2-1). **a** The resection site is smoothed with a small round bur (*B*) (*A* Achilles tendon, *R* retractor, *C* calcaneus). **b** Final smoothing is done with a curet (*CU*), **c** a file (*F*), and **d** a ball-tipped electrode on the cautery probe (*HF*)

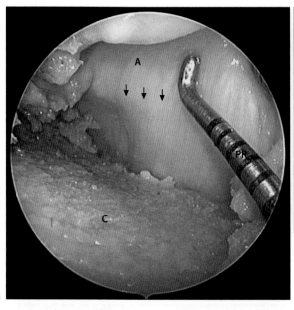

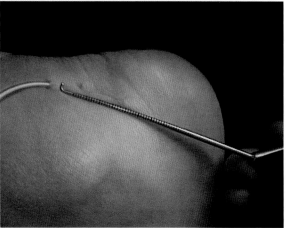

Fig. 17.2-3 a, b. Minimally invasive endoscopically assisted removal of retrocalcaneal exostosis (continued from Fig. 17.2-2). **a** The posterior surface of the Achilles tendon (*A*) bears a distinct indentation (*arrow*) caused by the distal exostosis. The resection site on the calcaneus (*C*) has been adequately smoothed (*PR* probe). **b** The skin incision is 1.4 cm long

17.3 Excessive Lateral Pressure Syndrome, Lateral Patellofemoral Osteoarthritis

Numerous changes in the patellofemoral joint can lead to lateralization of the patella and excessive lateral pressure. The causes, symptoms, clinical diagnosis, radiographic features, arthroscopic findings, and management of these conditions were discussed in an earlier chapter (see Sect. 1.5). If a lateral release is indicated, it remains to decide whether to use a purely arthroscopic technique (see Sect. 2.5, Figs. 2.5-4 to 2.5-6) or a minimally invasive endoscopically assisted technique.

▶ **Advantages:**
- **The synovial membrane remains intact.**
- **The surgeon can selectively dissect the blood vessels in the lateral retinaculum,** sparing or coagulating them as required.
- **There is no need for an extra skin incision.** The approach is made through the lateral arthroscope portal, which is extended by 1–2 mm.

Operative Technique

(Figs. 17.3-1 and 17.3-2)

1. **Skin incision.** The incision consists of a low anterolateral arthroscope portal 6 mm wide. It may be helpful to extend this portal by about 1–2 mm.

2. **Subcutaneous dissection.** A retractor is inserted into the portal, and the subcutaneous tissue is bluntly spread proximal to the capsular incision for the arthroscope portal to expose the surface of the lateral retinaculum.

3. **Dividing the retinaculum in layers.** First the superficial layer is divided with a scissors (Fig. 17.3-1b). It is not uncommon to encounter some fatty tissue beneath the superficial layer. Next the thicker layer (the "true" lateral retinaculum) is progressively divided from distal to proximal under endoscopic control (Fig. 17.3-1c). The surgery can be performed with or without a thigh tourniquet, and usually one or more blood vessels can be identified and preserved (Fig. 17.3-1). The release is continued to the distal border of the vastus lateralis muscle, which should not be incised. Bleeding points along the cut edges of the retinaculum are selectively cauterized (Fig. 17.3-1d).
The synovial membrane remains intact. The cut edges of the retinaculum are carefully separated from the synovial membrane, increasing the distance between them (Fig. 17.3-2b).
The integrity of the synovium is assessed by passing a probe through the medial instrument portal and palpating the synovium from inside the joint. The subsynovial position of the probe can be seen. An

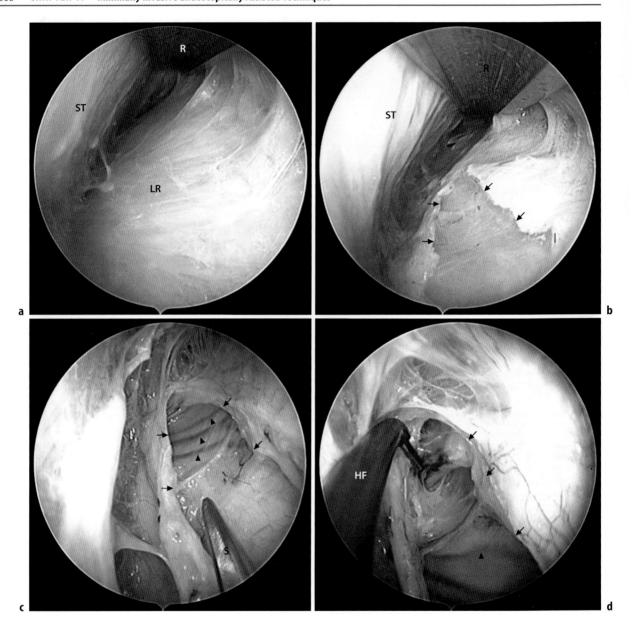

Fig. 17.3-1 a–d. Minimally invasive endoscopically assisted lateral release. **a** A subcutaneous space is developed over the lateral retinaculum (*LR*) (*ST* subcutaneous tissue, *R* retractor). **b** The superficial layers are divided (*arrows*). **c** The retinaculum proper is divided (*arrows*) with a scissors (*S*) while sparing the adjacent blood vessels (*arrowheads*). **d** Bleeding sites are controlled with electrocautery (*HF*)

identical technique is used in releasing the distal portions of the lateral retinaculum, i. e., working through the skin incision and progressively incising the retinaculum in the distal direction under vision.

4. **Hemostasis.** Bleeding points on the cut edges of the retinaculum are meticulously coagulated with the cautery probe (Fig. 17.3-2 b).

5. **Assessing patellar mobility.** After the release it should be easier to displace the patella medially, and the tilt test should be neutral. The arthroscope can be reinserted to evaluate patellar tracking.

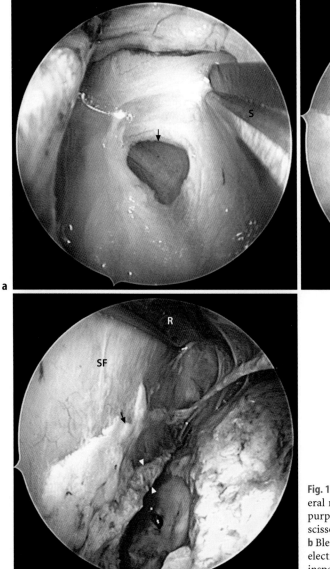

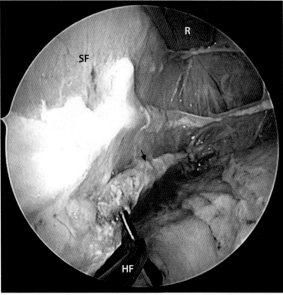

Fig. 17.3-2a–c. Minimally invasive endoscopically assisted lateral release (continued from Fig. 17.3-1). **a** For demonstration purposes, the synovial membrane has been incised with the scissors (*S*) so that the intraarticular space (*arrow*) can be seen. **b** Bleeding points on the cut edges (*arrows*) are controlled with electrocautery (*HF*) (*SF* subcutaneous fat, *R* retractor). **c** Final inspection after completion of the lateral release (*arrowheads* thickness of retinaculum, *arrow* superficial layer)

Postoperative Care

The postoperative protocol is the same as that following a purely arthroscopic release (see p. 274).

Experience to Date

We have performed our minimally invasive endoscopically controlled lateral release in 22 patients. We have found no significant differences between this procedure and a purely arthroscopic release with regard to bleeding risk or postoperative pain. A prospective study is now in preparation.

The minimally invasive release is particularly advantageous in very thin patients, who often have a palpable and sometimes visible gap in the lateral retinaculum following a purely arthroscopic release (which also divides the synovial membrane). Preservation of the synovial membrane in the minimally invasive procedure avoids this unpleasant effect in thin patients.

17.4 Screw Removal

Screws that have become displaced into soft tissues (e.g., the posterolateral capsule) can be removed using minimally invasive endoscopically assisted technique (see Sect. 2.14 and Fig. 2.14-18 for operative technique).

17.5 Division of Adhesions

If there is significant limitation of knee motion and the joint space is obliterated by scar tissue (e. g., following an infection), making it impossible to pass an arthroscope into the suprapatellar pouch, it is not helpful to establish a suprapatellar medial or lateral arthroscope portal in an effort to improve the situation. The minimally invasive, endoscopically controlled lysis of the adhesions offers an alternative to formal arthrotomy in these cases. The advantage of this technique is that after the adhesions have been divided, the arthroscopic procedure can be continued since only a minimal arthrotomy has been performed.

Operative Technique
(Fig. 17.5-1)

1. **Skin incision.** The skin is opened with a lateral or medial suprapatellar incision approximately 8–10 mm long.

2. **Dissection of the capsule.** The subcutaneous tissue is spread with a small, blunt scissors. A retractor is inserted into the skin incision and the developed subcutaneous tissue space in an effort to expose the capsule of the suprapatellar pouch.

3. **Lysis of adhesions.** Adhesive bands in the suprapatellar pouch are divided with a scissors. Progressive expansion of the joint space is noted as the adhesions are lysed (Fig. 17.5-1). The retropatellar cartilage provides a useful landmark for orientation.

4. **Further measures.** The rest of the procedure depends on the situation. The arthroscopic operation can be continued by inserting the sheath with blunt obturator into the anterolateral arthroscope portal. If this proves difficult, a concomitant minimally invasive release of the lateral retinaculum may be indicated to increase the mobility of the patella.

Postoperative Care

The postoperative regimen is the same as that following the arthroscopic lysis of adhesions (see Sect. 2.12).

Experience to Date

So far we have had experience with three cases. In none of these cases were we able to pass a sheath into the suprapatellar pouch. Two of the patients had extensive postinfectious joint adhesions. Further studies are needed on this operative technique.

17.6 Future Outlook

The minimally invasive technique has conceivable applications in other body regions. It must be possible to "elevate" the skin over the affected region and develop a subcutaneous cavity for insertion of the endoscope and operating instruments. The future outlook for these operative techniques is extremely promising.

Fig. 17.5-1 a–e. Minimally invasive endoscopically controlled ▶ lysis of adhesions in the suprapatellar pouch for postinfectious arthrofibrosis. The patient, a 53-year-old man, had a 0°–20°–45° range of knee motion after undergoing arthroscopic arthrolysis and manipulation under anesthesia on two previous occasions. When another arthroscopic release was attempted, the suprapatellar pouch could not be entered and therefore a minimally invasive technique was used. **a** A small lateral skin incision (*arrows*) is made just proximal to the patella (*R* retractor). **b** Intraarticular vision is obscured by numerous adhesive bands (*SC*) and dark synovitis (*arrows*). **c** The adhesions have been divided, creating a space that is separated from the patellofemoral joint by a sheet of scar tissue (*arrows*). **d** When the scar plaque is divided with a basket forceps (*PU*), the retropatellar cartilage (*P*) can be seen. **e** The sheath (*S*) can now be passed into the superior pouch through the anterolateral arthroscope portal, and the rest of the arthroscopic procedure can be continued

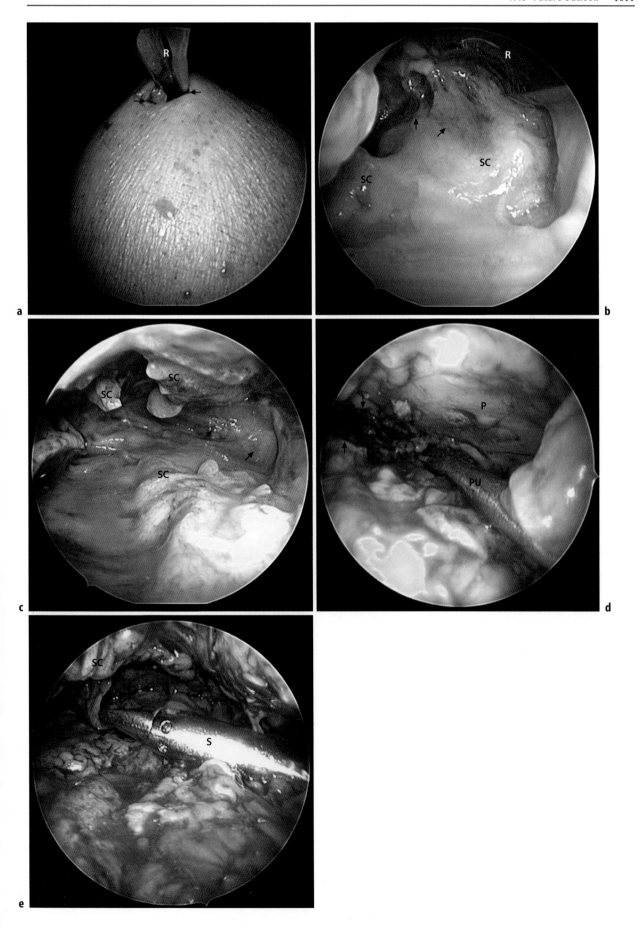

Ankle Joint

Aldrich MA, Arenson DJ (1985) Ankle joint evaluation – an overview of the arthroscopic techniques. J Foot Surg 24: 349–356

Alexander AH, Lichtman DM (1980) Surgical treatment of transchondral talar-dome fractures (osteochondritis dissecans). J Bone Joint Surg [Am] 62: 646–652

Amendola A, Petrik J, Webster Bogaert S (1996) Ankle arthroscopy: outcome in 79 consecutive patients. Arthroscopy 12: 565 573

Andrews JR, Previte WJ, Carson WG (1985) Arthroscopy of the ankle: technique and normal anatomy. Foot Ankle 6: 129–133

Arcomano JP, Kamhi E, Karas EH et al. (1987) Transchondral fracture and osteochondritis dissecans of talus. NY State J Med 78: 2183–2189

Baker CL, Andrews JR, Ryan JB (1986) Arthroscopic treatment of the transcondylar talar dome fractures. J Arthroscopy 2: 82–87

Barber FA, Britt BT, Ratliff HW, Sutker AN (1988) Arthroscopic surgery of the ankle. Orthop Rev 17: 446–451

Barber FA, Glick J, Britt BT (1990) Complications of ankle arthroscopy. Foot Ankle 10: 263–266

Bassett FH, Gates HS (1990) Talar impingement by the antero-inferior tibiofibular ligament. J Bone Joint Surg [Am] 72: 55–59

Benedetto KP, Glötzer W (1991) Indikation und Technik der Arthroskopie am oberen Sprunggelenk. Arthroskopie 4: 9– 14

Berndt AL, Harty M (1959) Transchondral fractures (osteochondritis dissecans) of the talus. J Bone Joint Surg [Am] 41: 988–1018

Berner W, Zwipp H, Lobenhoffer P, Südkamp N (1991) Vorteile der Distraktion bei der Arthroskopie des oberen Sprunggelenks. Arthroskopie 4: 32–36

Bühren V (1988) Arthroskopische Techniken am oberen Sprunggelenk. Unfallheilkunde 199: 168–173

Burmann MS (1931) Arthroscopy or direct visualization of joints: An experimental cadaver study. J Bone Joint Surg [Am] 13: 669–695

Campbell CJ, Renawat CS (1966) Osteochondritis dissecans: The question of etiology. J Trauma 6: 20–21

Canale ST, Belding RH (1980) Osteochondral lesions of the talus. J Bone Joint Surg [Am] 62: 97–107

Carrera CF, Guhl JF (1988) Radiological techniques. In: Guhl JF (ed) Ankle arthroscopy: pathology and surgical techniques. Slack, NJ, pp 25–37

Carson WG, Andrews JR (1987) Arthroscopy of the ankle. Clin Sports Med 6: 503–512

Casteleyn PP, Handelberg F (1995) Distraction for ankle arthroscopy. Arthroscopy 11: 633–634

Chen YC (1976) Clinical and cadaver studies of the ankle joint. Arthroscopy. J Jap Orthop Assoc 50: 631–651

Chen YC (1985) Arthroscopy of the ankle joint. In: Watanabe M (ed) Arthroscopy of small joints. Igaku-Shoin, Tokyo New York, pp 104–128

Cooper PS, Murray TF Jr (1996) Arthroscopy of the foot and ankle in the athlete. Clin Sports Med 15: 805–824

Corso SJ, Zimmer TJ (1995) Technique and clinical evaluation of arthroscopic ankle arthrodesis. Arthroscopy 11: 585–590

Crosby LA, Yee TC, Formanek TS, Fitzgibbons TC (1996) Complications following arthroscopic ankle arthrodesis. Foot Ankle Int 17: 340–342

Davidson AM, Steele HD, MacKenzie DA, Penny JA (1967) A review of twenty-one cases of transchondral fracture of the talus. J Trauma 7: 378–415

Dowdy PA, Watson BV, Amendola A, Brown JD (1996) Noninvasive ankle distraction: relationship between force, magnitude of distraction, and nerve conduction abnormalities. Arthroscopy 12: 64–69

Drez DJ, Guhl GF, Gollehon DL (1982) Ankle arthroscopy: Techniques and indications. Clin Sports Med 1: 35–45

Espejo Baena A, Lopez Arevalo R, Moro Robledo JA, Queipo de Llano A, Javier de Santos F (1997) Partial necrosis of the neck of the talus treated with arthroscopy. Arthroscopy 13: 245–224

Fallat LM (1987) Accuracy of diagnostic arthroscopy of the ankle joint. J Foot Surg 26: 26–32

Feiwell LA, Frey C (1994) Anatomic study of arthroscopic debridement of the ankle. Foot Ankle Int 15: 614–621

Ferkel RD, Fischer SP (1989) Progress in ankle arthroscopy. Clin Orthop 240: 210–220

Ferkel RD, Sgaglione NA (1993) Arthroscopic treatment of osteochondral lesions of the talus: long-term results. Orthop Trans 17: 1011

Ferkel RD, Heath DD, Guhl JF (1996) Neurological complications of ankle arthroscopy. Arthroscopy 12: 200–208

Ferkel RD (1996) Arthroscopic surgery. The foot and ankle. Lippincott, Philadelphia

Frank A, Cohen P, Beaufils P, Lamare J (1989) Arthroscopic treatment of the osteochondral lesions of the talar dome. Arthroscopy 5: 57–61

Freeman MAR (1965) Treatment of ruptures of the lateral ligament of the ankle. J Bone Joint Surg [Br] 47: 661

Friscia DA (1994) Pigmented villonodular synovitis of the ankle: a case report and review of the literature. Foot Ankle Int 15: 674–678

Gächter A (1989) Arthroskopische Spülung zur Behandlung infizierter Gelenke. Operat Orthop Traumatol 1: 196–199

Gächter A, Gerber BE (1991) Arthroskopie des oberen Sprunggelenks in Lokalanästhesie. Arthroskopie 4: 37–41

Gerber BE, Gächter A (1987) Arthroskopie des oberen Sprunggelenks – Indikation und Vorgehen, einsehbare Strukturen und Befunde. In: Gächter A (Hrsg) Fortschritte in der Arthroskopie, Bd 3. Enke, Stuttgart, S 92–98

Glasgow M, Jackson A, Jamieson AM (1980) Instability of the ankle after injury to the lateral ligament. J Bone Joint Surg [Br] 62: 196

Glick JM, Morgan CD, Myerson MS, Sampson TG, Mann JA (1996) Ankle arthrodesis using an arthroscopic method: long term follow up of 34 cases. Arthroscopy 12: 428–434

Glick JM, Ferkel RD (1996) Arthroscopic ankle arthrodesis. In: Ferkel RD (ed) Arthroscopic surgery. The foot and ankle. Lippincott, Philadelphia, pp 215–229

Gollehon DL, Drez DJ (1983) Ankle arthroscopy: Approaches and techniques. Orthopedics 6: 1150–1152

Gollehon DL, Drez DJ (1986) Arthroscopic evaluation of the ankle. In: Nicholas JAN, Hershman EB (ed) The lower extremity and spine in sport medicine. Mosby, St. Louis Toronto Princeton, pp 458–478

Guhl JF (1986) Arthroscopic advances: New techniques for arthroscopic surgery of the ankle joint: A preliminary report. Orthopedics 9: 261–269

Guhl JF (1988) Ankle arthroscopy: Pathology and surgical techniques. Slack, NJ

Guhl JF (1988) New concepts (distraction) in ankle arthroscopy. Arthroscopy 4: 160–167

Guman G (1987) Ankle arthroscopic portals and intraarticular anatomy. J Foot Surg 26: 13–21

Gumann G (1987) Ankle arthroscopic portals and techniques. Clin Podiatric Med Surg 4: 861–874

Gumann G (1987) Ankle arthroscopy. In: McClamry ED (ed) Comprehensive textbook of foot surgery. Williams & Wilkins, Baltimore, pp 821–832

Haas AF (1989) Operative ankle arthroscopy. Long-term follow-up. Am J Sports Med 17: 16–23

Hall RL, Shereff MJ, Stone J, Guhl JF (1995) Ankle arthroscopy in industrial injuries of the ankle. Arthroscopy 11: 127–133

Hamilton WG (1982) Sprained ankles in ballet dancers. Foot Ankle 3: 99–103

Hamilton WG (1988) Differential diagnosis of the ankle problems. In: Guhl JF (ed) Ankle arthroscopy: Pathology and surgical techniques. Slack, NJ, pp 69–79

Harty M (1988) Gross anatomy of the ankle joint. In: Guhl JF (ed) Ankle arthroscopy: Pathology and surgical techniques. Slack, NJ, pp 7–13

Hawkins RB (1987) Arthroscopic stapling repair for chronic lateral instability. Clin Podiatric Med Surg 4: 875–883

Hawkins RB (1988) Arthroscopic treatment of sports-related anterior osteophytes in the ankle. Foot Ankle 9: 87–90

Hawkins RB (1988) Stapling repair for chronic lateral ankle instability. In. Guhl JF (ed) Ankle arthroscopy. Slack, Thorofare, pp 123–133

Hawkins RB (1996) Arthroscopic approach to lateral ankle instability. In: Ferkel RD (ed) Arthroscopic surgery. The foot and ankle. Lippincott, Philadelphia, pp 201–213

Heller AJ, Vogler HW (1982) Ankle joint arthroscopy. J Foot Surg 21: 23–29

Huang T, Rodney RW, Bormadel R, Ray T (1979) Correlation of arthroscopy with other diagnostic modalities. Orthop Clin North Am 10: 523–534

Jaivin JS, Ferkel RD (1994) Arthroscopy of the foot and ankle. Clin Sports Med 13: 761 83

Jakubowski S (1973) Synovektomie des oberen Sprunggelenkes. Orthopädie 2: 79–80

Japour C, Vohra P, Giorgini R, Sobel E (1996) Ankle arthroscopy: follow up study of 33 ankles effect of physical therapy and obesity. J Foot Ankle Surg 35: 199–209

Jensen KU, Klein W (1989) Die arthroskopische Behandlung der septischen Gonitis. Arthroskopie 2: 104–111

Jensen KU, Klein W (1991) Die arthroskopische Chirurgie am oberen Sprunggelenk mit Gelenkdistraktion. Arthroskopie 4: 24–31

Jerosch J, Goetzen M, Reifenrath M (1991) Transarthroskopische Arthrodese des oberen Sprunggelenks Indikationen und operative Technik. Arthroskopie 4: 62–65

Jerosch J, Steinbeck J, Schroder M, Reer R (1996) Arthroscopically assisted arthrodesis of the ankle joint. Arch Orthop Trauma Surg 115: 182–189

Johnson EE, Markolf KL (1983) The contribution of the anterior talofibular ligament to ankle laxity. J Bone Joint Surg [Am] 65: 81

Josten C, Muhr G, Lies A (1990) Die arthroskopische Abrasionsarthroplastik am oberen Sprunggelenk. Langzeitergebnisse bei der Osteochondrosis dissecans. Unfallchirurgie 93: 110–114

Katchis SD, Smith RW (1997) A simple way to establish the posterolateral portal in ankle arthroscopy. Foot Ankle Int 18: 178–179

Kelikian H (1985) Disorders of the ankle. Saunders, Philadelphia

Kibler WB (1996) Arthroscopic findings in ankle ligament reconstruction. Clin Sports Med 15: 799–804

Kleiger B (1982) Anterior tibiotalar impingement syndromes in dancers. Foot Ankle 3: 69–73

Klein W, Jensen KU (1989) Technik und Probleme der arthroskopischen Synovektomie. Knie-, Schulter-, Ellbogen-, Sprunggelenk. Arthroskopie 2: 80–93

Kohn D (1991) Bisherige Erfahrungen bei der Arthroskopie des oberen Sprunggelenks. Arthroskopie 4: 15–19

Kristensen G, Lind T, Lavard P, Olsen PA (1990) Fracture stage 4 of the lateral talar dome treated arthroscopically using Biofix for fixation. Case Report. Arthroscopy 6: 242–244

Landgraf P (1990) Oberes Sprunggelenk. In: Hempfling H (Hrsg) Arthroskopie: Indikation, Bedeutung, Begutachtung. Fischer, Stuttgart, S 62–63

Landsiedl F (1991) Die Arthroskopie des oberen Sprunggelenks. Arthroskopie 4: 2–8

Lindholm TS, Osterman K, Vankka E (1980) Osteochondritis dissecans of elbow, ankle and hip: A comparison survey. Clin Orthop 148: 245–253

Liu SH, Nuccion SL, Finerman G (1997) Diagnosis of anterolateral ankle impingement. Comparison between magnetic resonance imaging and clinical examination. Am J Sports Med 25: 389–393

Lubell JD, Fallat LM (1986) Ankle joint arthroscopy. J Foot Surg 25: 128–132

Lundeen RO (1985) Arthroscopic anatomy of the anterior aspect of the ankle. J Am Podiatric Med Assoc 75: 367–371

Lundeen RO (1987) Arthroscopic treatment of intraarticular fractures of the ankle. Clin Podiatric Med Surg 4: 855–902

Lundeen RO (1987) Medial impingement lesions of the tibial plafond. J Foot Surg 26: 37–40

Lundeen RO (1987) Review of diagnostic arthroscopy of the foot and ankle. J Foot Surg 26: 33–36

Lundeen RO (1987) Techniques of ankle arthroscopy. J Foot Surg 26: 22–25

Lundeen RO (1989) Arthroscopic evaluation of traumatic injuries to the ankle and foot. Part I: Acute injuries. J Foot Surg 28: 499–511

Lundeen RO (1990) Arthroscopic evaluation of traumatic injuries to the ankle and foot. Part II: Chronic posttraumatic pain. J Foot Surg 29: 59–71

Lundeen RO (1992) Manual of ankle and foot arthroscopy. Churchill Livingstone, New York Edinburgh

Martin DF, Baker CL, Curl WW et al. (1989) Ankle arthroscopy: A method of distraction. Orthopedics 12: 1317–1320

Martin DF, Baker CL, Curl WW, Andrews JR, Robic DB, Haas AF (1989) Operative ankle arthroscopy: Long-term follow-up. Am J Sports Med 17: 16–23

Martin DF, Curl WW, Baker CL (1989) Arthroscopic treatment of chronic synovitis of the ankle. Arthroscopy 5: 110–114

McCullough CJ, Venugopal V (1979) Osteochondritis dissecans of the talus: The natural history. Clin Orthop 144: 264–268

Meislin RJ, Rose DJ, Parisien JS, Springer S (1993) Arthroscopic treatment of synovial impingement of the ankle. Am J Sports Med 21: 186–189

Miller MD (1997) Arthroscopically assisted reduction and fixation of an adult Tillaux fracture of the ankle. Arthroscopy 13: 1179

Morgan CD (1988) Arthroscopic tibiotalar arthrodesis. In: Guhl JF (ed) Ankle arthroscopy – Pathology and surgical techniques. Slack, New Jersey, pp 119–122

Myerson M, Allon SM (1989) Arthroscopic ankle arthrodesis. Contemp Orthop 19: 21

Naumetz VA, Schweigel JF (1980) Osteocartilaginous lesions of the talar dome. J Trauma 20: 924–927

Nitzschke E, Moraldo M, Aksu M, Blecker U (1992) Die arthroskopische Behandlung der Osteochondrosis dissecans am Knie – und Sprunggelenk. Arthroskopie 5: 24–32

O'Donoghue DH (1966) Chondral and osteochondral fractures. J Trauma 6: 469–481

O'Farrell TA, Costello BG (1982) Osteochondritis dissecans of the talus: The late results of surgical treatment. J Bone Joint Surg [Br] 64: 494–497

Ogilvie Harris DJ, Reed SC (1994) Disruption of the ankle syndesmosis: diagnosis and treatment by arthroscopic surgery. Arthroscopy 10: 561–568

Ogilvie Harris DJ, Sekyi Otu A (1995) Arthroscopic debridement for the osteoarthritic ankle. Arthroscopy 11: 433–436

Pappas AM (1981) Osteochondrosis dissecans. Clin Orthop 158: 59–69

Parisien JS (1983) Diagnostic and operative arthroscopy of the ankle – An experimental approach. Orthop Trans 7: 158

Parisien JS (1985) Diagnostic and operative arthroscopy of the ankle. Techniques and indications. Bull Hosp Joint Dis 45: 38–47

Parisien JS (1986) Arthroscopic treatment of osteochondral lesions of the talus. Am J Sports Med 14: 211–217

Parisien JS (1987) Ankle and subtalar joint arthroscopy – An update. Bull Hosp Joint Dis 47: 262–272

Parisien JS (1987) Arthroscopy of the subtalar joint. In: Slach (ed) Ankle arthroscopy: Pathology and surgical techniques. Thorofare, NJ, Slack, pp 133–142

Parisien JS (1988) Arthroscopic surgery of the ankle. In: Parisien JS (ed) Arthroscopic surgery. McGraw-Hill, New York, pp 259–282

Parisien JS (1988) Instumentation in arthroscopic surgery of the ankle. In: Guhl JF (ed) Ankle arthroscopy: pathology and surgical techniques. Slack, pp 37–49

Parisien JS, Shereff MJ (1981) The role of arthroscopy in the diagnosis and the treatment of disorders of the ankle. Foot Ankle 2: 144–149

Parisien JS, Vangsness T (1985) Operative arthroscopy of the ankle. Three years experience. Clin Orthop 199: 46–53

Parisien JS, Vangsness T, Feldman R (1987) Diagnostic and operative arthroscopy of the ankle. An experimental approach. Clin Orthop 224: 228–236

Patel D, Guhl JF (1988) Arthroscopic anatomy. In: Guhl JF (ed) Ankle arthroscopy: pathology and surgical techniques. Slack, NJ, pp 13–25

Patti JE, Mayo WE (1996) Arthroscopic synovectomy for recurrent hemarthrosis of the ankle in hemophilia. Arthroscopy 12(6): 652 6

Plank E, Burri C, Zeitler HP (1979) Die Technik der Arthroskopie des oberen Sprunggelenks, des Ellengelenks und des Handgelenks. In: Blauth W, Donner K (Hrsg) Arthroskopie des Kniegelenks. Thieme, Stuttgart, S 142–149

Plank E, Mutschler W (1978) Die Arthroskopie des oberen Sprunggelenkes. Unfallheilkunde 131: 245–251

Pritsch M, Horoshovski H, Farine I (1984) Ankle arthroscopy. Clin Orthop 184: 137–141

Pritsch M, Horoshovski H, Farine I (1986) Arthroscopic treatment of ostechondral lesions of the talus. J Bone Joint Surg [Am] 68: 862–865

Reagen BF, McInerny VK, Treadwell BV, Zarins B, Mankin HJ (1983) Irrigation solutions for arthroscopy: A metabolic study. J Bone Joint Surg [Am] 65: 629–631

Rehm KE, Kunze K, Ecke H (1985) Stellenwert der Arthroskopie des oberen Sprunggelenks. In: Hofer H (Hrsg) Fortschritte in der Arthroskopie. Enke, Stuttgart, S 111–116

Reichen A, Marti R (1974) Die frische fibulare Bandruptur. Diagnose, Therapie, Resultate. Arch Orthop Unfallchir 80: 211

Resnick RB, Jarolem KL, Sheskier SC, Desai P, Cisa J (1995) Arthroscopic removal of an osteoid osteoma of the talus: a case report. Foot Ankle Int 16: 212–215

Reynaert P, Gelen G, Geens G (1994) Arthroscopic treatment of anterior impingement of the ankle. Acta Orthop Belg 60: 384–348

Rixen D, Klein J, Ure BM, Tiling T (1991) Die Arthroskopie des oberen Sprunggelenks beim Sportler. Arthroskopie 4: 42–45

Roden S, Tillegaard P, Unander-Scharin L (1953) Osteochondritis dissecans and similar lesions of the talus. Acta Orthop Scand 23: 51–66

Saltzman CL, Marsh JL, Tearse DS (1994) Treatment of displaced talus fractures: an arthroscopically assisted approach. Foot Ankle Int 15: 630–633

Sartoretti C, Sartoretti Schefer S, Duff C, Buchmann P (1996) Angioplasty balloon catheters used for distraction of the ankle joint. Arthroscopy 12: 82–86

Schafer D, Hintermann B (1996) Arthroscopic assessment of the chronic unstable ankle joint. Knee Surg Sports Traumatol Arthrosc 4: 48–52

Scharling M (1978) Osteochondritis dissecans of the talus. Acta Orthop Scand 49: 89–94

Schießler W, Taruttis H, Stedtfeld HW (1991) Posttraumatische Veränderungen der Synovialmembran am oberen Sprunggelenk. Arthroskopische Diagnostik und Therapie. Arthroskopie 4: 51–57

Schonholtz GJ (ed) (1986) Complications of the arthroscopic surgery of the shoulder, elbow and ankle. In: Arthroscopic surgery of the shoulder, elbow and ankle. Thomas, Springfield, pp 73–78

Schonholtz GJ (1988) Indications and contraindications. In: Guhl JF (ed) Ankle arthroscopy: Pathology and surgical techniques. Slack, NJ, pp 63–69

Schultz W, Stinus H, Hess T (1991) Medialer Knorpelschaden am oberen Sprunggelenk nach Supinations-Inversions-Traumen. Arthroskopie 4: 58–61

Scranton PE, McDermott JE (1992) Anterior tibiotalar spurs: a comparison of open versus arthroscopic debridement. Foot Ankle 13: 125–132

Sefton GK, George J, Fitton JM (1979) Reconstruction of the anterior talofibular ligament for the treatment of the unstable ankle. J Bone Joint Surg [Br] 61: 352

Takahashi T, Yamamoto H (1997) Development and clinical application of a flexible arthroscopy system. Arthroscopy 13: 42–50

Trager S, Frederick LD, Seligeon D (1989) Ankle arthroscopy: A method of distraction. Orthopedics 12: 1317–1320

Turan I, Wredmark T, Fellander Tsai L (1995) Arthroscopic ankle arthrodesis in rheumatoid arthritis. Clin Orthop 320: 110–114

Van Buecken K, Barrack RL, Alexander AH, Ertl JP (1989) Arthroscopic treatment of the transchondral talar dome fractures. Am J Sports Med 17: 350–356

van Dijk CN, Scholte D (1997) Arthroscopy of the ankle joint. Arthroscopy 13: 90–96

van Duk CN, Verhagen RA, Tol JL (1997) Arthroscopy for problems after ankle fracture. J Bone Joint Surg [Br] 79: 280–284

Voto SJ, Ewing JW, Fleissner PR, Alfonso M, Kufel M (1989) Ankle arthroscopy: neurovascular and arthroscopic anatomy of standard and trans-achilles tendon portal placement. Arthroscopy 5: 41–46

Watanabe J (1971) Arthroscopy of small joint. J Jpn Orthop Assoc 45: 908

Wertheimer SJ, Weber CA, Loder BG, Calderone DR, Frascone ST (1995) The role of endoscopy in treatment of stenosing posterior tibial tenosynovitis. J Foot Ankle Surg 34: 15–22

Whipple TL (1991) Meniscoid lesions of the ankle. Clin Sport Med 10: 661–667

Wolin I, Glassman F, Sideman S (1950) Internal derangement of the talofibular component of the ankle. Surg Gynecol Obstet 91: 193–200

Wright G (1996) Technique tips. Skeletal traction for ankle arthroscopy. Foot Ankle Int 17: 119

Yao J, Weis E (1985) Osteochondritis dissecans. Orth Rev 14: 190–204

Yates CK, Grana WA (1983) A simple distraction technique for ankle arthroscopy. Arthroscopy 4: 103–105

Yvars MF (1976) Osteochondral fractures of the dome of the talus. Clin Orthop 114: 185–191

Wrist

Abrams RA, Petersen M, Botte MJ (1994) Arthroscopic portals of the wrist: an anatomic study. J Hand Surg Am 19: 940–944

Adolfsson L (1992) Arthroscopy for the diagnosis of post-traumatic wrist pain. J Hand Surg Br 17: 46–50

Adolfsson L (1994) Arthroscopic diagnosis of ligament lesions of the wrist. J Hand Surg Br 19: 505–512

Adolfsson L, Nylander G (1993) Arthroscopic synovectomy of the rheumatoid wrist. J Hand Surg Br 18: 92–96

Aghasi M, et al. (1981) Osteochondrosis dissecans des Scaphoids. J Hand Surg 6: 351

Ahmadi A, Kreutsch-Brinker R, Doll B, Münch W (1988) Die Aussagekraft der Arthroskopie bzw. der Arthrographie des Handgelenkes in der präoperativen Diagnostik. Orthop Praxis 7: 420–423

Ahmadi A, Pomsel Th (1990) Handgelenksarthroskopie bei unklaren posttraumatischen Beschwerden. Handchir Mikrochir Plast Chir 22: 71–73

Allende BT (1988) Osteoarthristis of the wrist secondary to non-union of the scaphoid. Int Orthop 12: 201–211

Ambrose L, Posner MA (1992) Lunate-triquetral and midcarpal joint instability. Hand Clin 8: 653–668

Bain GI, Roth JH (1995) The role of arthroscopy in arthritis: Ectomy procedures. Hand Clin North Am 11: 51–58

Bednar JM, Osterman AL (1994) The role of arthroscopy in the treatment of traumatic triangular fibrocartilage injuries. Hand Clin 10: 605–614

Bednar JM, Ostermann AL (1994) The role of arthroscopy in the treatment of traumatic triangular fibrocartilage injuries. Hand Clin North Am 10: 605–614

Bell MJ, Hill RJ, McMurtry YR (1981) Ulnar impingement syndrome. J Bone Surg [Br] 67: 126–129

Berger RA, Blair WF, El-Khoury GY (1983) Arthrotomography of the wrist. The triangular fibrocartilage complex. Clin Orthop 172: 257–264

Berghoff RA jr, Amadio PC (1993) Dorsales Handgelenksganglion: Ursache des dorsalen Handgelenkschmerzes. Orthopäde 22: 30–35

Bettinger PC, Cooney WP 3rd, Berger RA (1995) Arthroscopic anatomy of the wrist. Orthop Clin North Am 26: 707–19

Bittar ES, Dell PC (1990) Comparison of arthrography and arthroscopy of the wrist. Arthroscopy 2: 150

Bittar ES, Dell PC, Smith P (1988) Arthroscopic surgery of the wrist. Arthroscopy 4: 131

Bora FW, Osterman AL, Matin E, Bednar J (1986) The role of arthroscopy in treatment of disorders of the wrist. Contemp Orthop 12: 28–36

Botte MJ, Cooney WP, Linscheid RL (1989) Arthroscopy of the wrist: Anatomy and technique. J Hand Surg [Am] 14: 313–316

Brown DE, Lichtman DM (1984) The evaluation of chronic wrist pain. Orthop Clin North Am 15: 183–192

Broy SB, Stulberg AD, Schmid FR (1986) The role of arthroscopy in the diagnosis and management of the septic joint. Clin Rheum Dis 12: 489–500

Brüser P (1989) Arthroskopie des Handgelenks. Handchir Mikrochir Plast Chir 20: 49–53

Buck-Gramcko D (1985) Karpale Instabilitäten. Handchirurgie 17: 188

Buck-Gramcko D (1986) Instabilitäten der Handwurzel. Orthopäde 15: 88–94

Burman MS (1931) Arthroscopy or the direct visualization of joints. J Bone Joint Surg [Am] 13: 669–695

Buterbaugh GA (1994) Radiocarpal arthrosckopy portals and normal anatomy. Hand Clin North Am 10: 567–576

Cerofolini E, Luchetti R, Pederzini L, Soragni O, Colombini R, D'Alimonte P, Romagnoli R (1990) MR evaluation of triangular fibrocartilage complex tears in the wrist: comparison with arthrography and arthroscopy. J Comput Assist Tomogr 14: 963–967

Chen YC (1979) Arthroscopy of the wrist and finger joints. Orthop Clin North Am 10: 723–733

Chen YC (1985) Arthroscopy of the wrist joint. In: Watanabe M (ed) Arthroscopy of small joints. Igaku Shoin, Tokyo New York, pp 85–90

Christian L Jantea, Balzer A, Ruther W (1995) Arthrocopic repair of radial-sided lesions of the triangular fibrocartilage complex. Hand Clin North Am 11: 31–36

Chung KC, Zimmerman NB, Travis MT (1996) Wrist arthrography versus arthroscopy: a comparative study of 150 cases. J Hand Surg Am 21: 591–594

Coleman HM (1960) Injuries of the articular disk at the wrist. J Bone Joint Surg [Br] 42: 522–529

Conney WP, Dobyns JH, Linscheid RL (1990) Arthroscopy of the wirst. Anatomy and classification of carpal instability. Arthroscopy 6: 133–140

Cooney WP (1993) Evaluation of chronic wrist pain by arthrography, arthroscopy, and arthrotomy. J Hand Surg Am 18: 815–822

Cooney WP (1995) The future of arthroscopic surgery in the hand and wrist. Hand Clin 11: 97–99

Cooney WP, Berger RA (1993) Treatment of complex fractures of the distal radius. Combined use of internal and external fixation and arthroscopic reduction. Hand Clin 9: 603–612

Cooney WP, Linscheid RL, Dobyns JH (1994) Triangular fibro-cartilage tears. J Hand Surg Am 19: 143–154

Corso SJ, Savoie FH, Geissler WB, Whipple TL, Jiminez W, Jenkins N (1997) Arthroscopic repair of peripheral avulsions of the triangular fibrocartilage complex of the wrist: a multicenter study. Arthroscopy 13: 78–84

Craig SM (1987) Wrist arthroscopy. Clin Sports Med 6: 551–556

Culp RW, Osterman AL (1995) Arthroscopic reduction and internal fixation of distal radius fractures. Orthop Clin North Am 26: 739–748

Dautel G, Goudot B, Merle M (1993) Arthroscopic diagnosis of scapho-lunate instability in the absence of X-ray abnormalities. J Hand Surg Br 18: 213–218

Dautel G, Merle M (1997) Chondral lesions of the midcarpal joint. Arthroscopy 13: 97–102

de Araujo W, Poehling GG, Kuzma GR (1996) New Tuohy needle technique for triangular fibrocartilage complex repair: preliminary studies. Arthroscopy 12: 699–703

De Smet L, Dauwe D, Fortems Y, Zachee B, Fabry G (1996) The value of wrist arthroscopy. An evaluation of 129 cases. J Hand Surg Br 21: 210–212

Drewniany JJ, Palmer AK (1986) Injuries to the distal radioulnar joint. Orthop Clin North Am 17: 451–459

Drobner WS, Hausman MR (1992) The distal radioulnar joint. Hand Clin 8: 631–644

Dvorak J (1993) Neurologische Ursachen für einen Handgelenksschmerz. Orthopäde 22: 25–29

Ekman EF, Poehling GG (1994) Principles of arthroscopy and wrist arthroscopy equipment. Hand Clin 10: 557–566

Feldkamp G, Whipple TL (1992) Stellenwert der Arthroskopie für die Handchirurgie heute. Handchir Mikrochir Plast Chir 24: 296–303

Fellinger M, Peicha G, Seibert FJ, Grechenig W (1997) Radial avulsion of the triangular fibrocartilage complex in acute wrist trauma: a new technique for arthroscopic repair. Arthroscopy 13: 370–374

Fisk GR (1970) Carpal instability and the fractured scaphoid. Ann R Coll Surg Engl 46: 63–76

Fortems Y, Mawhinney I, Lawrence T, Stanley JK (1994) Traction radiographs in the diagnosis of chronic wrist pain. J Hand Surg Br 19: 334–337

Fortems Y, Mawhinney I, Lawrence T, Trial IA, Stanley JK (1995) Late rupture of extensor pollicis longus after wrist arthroscopy. Arthroscopy 11: 322–323

Fowler JL, Wicks MH (1990) Osteochondritis dissecans of the lunate. J Hand Surg [Am] 15: 571–572

Gan BS, Richards RS, Roth JH (1995) Arthroscopic treatment of triangular fibrocartilage tears. Orthop Clin North Am 26: 721–729

Geisl H, Spritzendorfer E (1981) Der Riß des Discus articularis als Ursache des posttraumatischen Handgelenkschmerzes. Unfallheilkunde 84: 55–59

Geissler WB (1995) Arthroscically assisted reduction of intraarticular fractures of the distal radius. Hand Clin North Am 11: 19–30

Geissler WB, Fernandez DL, Lamey DM (1996) Distal radioulnar joint injuries associated with fractures of the distal radius. Clin Orthop 327: 135–146

Geissler WB, Freeland AE (1996) Arthroscopically assisted reduction of intraarticular distal radial fractures. Clin Orthop 327: 125–134

Gekeler-Steinle B, Hempfling H (1990) Die Arthroskopie aller Gelenke. Ein Leitfaden für das OP-Personal. Fischer, Stuttgart

Green DP (1988) Operative hand surgery. Churchill Livingstone, New York

Haage H (1966) Die Arthrographie des Handgelenkes. I. Das normale Gelenk und seine Variationen. Radiologe 6: 50–57

Haage H, Cornelius H (1966) Die Arthographie des Handgelenkes. II. Der pathologische Discus articularis. Radiologe 6: 58–63

Hanker GJ (1991) Diagnostic and operative arthroscopy of the wrist. Clin Orthop 263: 165–174

Hempfling H (1986) Die arthroskopische Untersuchung des Schultergelenkes und des Ellenbogengelenkes, des oberen Sprunggelenkes, des Hand – und Hüftgelenkes. Orthop Praxis 22: 97–102

Hempfling H (1988) Arthroskopie des Handgelenkes. In: Feldmeier C (Hrsg) Sporttraumatologie 1: Verletzungen und Schäden der Hand. Zuckerschwerdt, München, S 26–33

Hempfling H (1992) Die Arthroskopie am Handgelenk. Wissenschaftliche Verlagsgesellschaft, Stuttgart

Hempfling H (1995) Farbatlas der Arthroskopie großer Gelenke, 2. Aufl. Fischer, Stuttgart

Hodgson SP, Royle SG, Stanley JK (1995) An approach to the diagnosis of chronic wrist pain. J R Coll Surg Edinb 40: 407–410

Hulsizer D, Weiss AP, Akelman E (1997) Ulna-shortening osteotomy after failed arthroscopic debridement of the triangular fibrocartilage complex. J Hand Surg Am 22: 694–698

Jantea CL, Baltzer A, Ruther W (1995) Arthroscopic repair of radial-sided lesions of the triangular fibrocartilage complex. Hand Clin 11: 31–36

Johnson LL (1981) Diagnostic and surgical arthroscopy: 1. wrist joint. In: Arthroscopic surgery: Principles and practice. Mosby, St. Louis

Johnson RP, Carrera GF (1986) Chronic capitoulnate instability. J Bone Joint Surg [Am] 68: 1164–1176

Jones KJ (1996) Arthroscopy in hand surgery. Clin Plast Surg 23: 463–476

Jones WA, Lovell ME (1996) The role of arthroscopy in the investigation of wrist disorders. J Hand Surg Br 21: 442–445

Kaempffe F, Peimer CA (1990) Distraction for wrist arthroscopy. J Hand Surg Am 15: 520–521

Kauer JMG (1975) The articular disc of the hand. Acta Anat 93: 590–605

Kelly EP, Stanley JK (1990) Arthroscopy of the wrist. J Hand Surg [Br] 15: 236–242

Kessler I, Silberman Z (1961) An experimental study of the radiocarpal joint by arthrography. Surg Gynec Obstet 112: 33–40

Kirschenbaum D, Coyle MP, Leddy JP (1993) Chronic lunotriquetral instability: diagnosis and treatment. J Hand Surg Am 18: 1107–1112

Knopp W, Neumann K (1988) Handgelenksarthroskopie. Hefte Unfallheilkd 199: 155–167

Knopp W, Neumann K, Muhr G, Hinrichsen K (1988) Die Arthroskopie des proximalen Handgelenkes. indikation, Technik und klinische Ergebnisse. Unfallchirurg 91: 22–28

Knopp W, Neumann K, Muhr G, Josten Ch (1987) Arthroskopische Diagnostik des Handgelenkes. Handchir Mikrochir Plast Chir 19: 295–298

Koebke J, Brade A (1980) Zur Läsion des Discus articularis des Handgelenkes. Z Orthop 118: 616

Koman LA, Mooney, JF, Poehling GG (1990) Fractures and ligamentous injuries of the wrist. Hand Clin 6: 477–491

Koman LA, Poehling GG, Toby EB, Kamire G (1990) Chronic wrist pain: Indications for wrist arthroscopy. Arthroscopy 6: 116–119

Kuschner SH, Lane CS (1997) Evaluation of the painful wrist. Am J Orthop 26: 95–102

Lanz U (1986) Der Ulnavorschub nach distaler Radiusfraktur. In: Nigst H (Hrsg) Handverletzungen, Hippokrates, Stuttgart

LaStayo P, Howell J (1995) Clinical provocative tests used in evaluating wrist pain: a descriptive study. J Hand Ther 8: 10–17

Leibovic SJ, Bowers WH (1995) Arthroscopy of the distal radioulnar joint. Orthop Clin North Am 26: 755–757

Leibovic SJ, Geissler WB (1994) Treatment of complex intra-articular distal radius fractures. Orthop Clin North Am 25: 685–706

Lester B, Halbrecht J, Levy IM, Gaudinez R (1995) „Press test" for office diagnosis of triangular fibrocartilage complex tears of the wrist. Ann Plast Surg 35: 41–45

Levin LS, Rehnke R, Eubanks S (1995) Endoscopic surgery of the upper extremity. Hand Clin North Am 11: 59–70

Levinsohn EM, Palmer AK (1983) Arthrography of the traumatized wrist. Radiology 146: 647–651

Levy HJ, Gardner RD, Lemak LJ (1991) Bilateral osteochondral flaps of the wrist. Arthroscopy 7: 118–119

Levy HJ, Glickel SZ (1993) Arthroscopic assisted internal fixation of volar intraarticular wrist fractures. Arthroscopy 9: 122–124

Lichtman DM, Schneider JR, Swafford AR, Mack GR (1981) Ulnar midcarpal instability – Clinical and laboratory analysis. J Hand Surg 6: 515–523

Lindblad S, Hedfors E, Malmborg A (1985) Rifamycin SV in local treatment of synovitis – A clinical, arthroscopic and pharmacologic evaluation. J Rheumatol 12(5): 900–903

Linscheid RL, Dobyns JH (1992) Treatment of scapholunate dissociation. Rotatory subluxation of the scaphoid. Hand Clin 8: 645–652

Linscheid RL, Dobyns JH (1993) Karpale Instabilitäten. Orthopäde 22: 72–78

Martinek H (1977) Traumatologie des Discus articularis des Handgelenkes: Teil I/II. Arch Orthop Unfallchir 87: 285, 299

Mayfield JK (1984) Wrist ligamentous anatomy and pathogeneses of carpal instability. Orthop Clin North Am 15: 209–216

Mayfield JK (1988) Pathogenesis of wrist ligament instability. In: Lichtman DM (ed) The wrist and its disorders. Saunders, Philadelphia, pp 61–63

Mayfield JK, Johnson RP, Kilcoyne KRK (1980) Carpal dislocation. Pathomechanics and progressive perilunar instability. J Hand Surg 5: 226–241

Mayfield JK, Johnson RP, Kilcoyne RF (1976) The ligaments of the human wrist and their functional significance. Anat Rec 186: 417–428

Menon J (1996) Arthroscopic management of trapeziometacarpal joint arthritis of the thumb. Arthroscopy 12: 581–587

Menon J, Wood VE, Shoene HR, Frykman GK, Hohl JC, Bestard EA (1984) Isolated tears of the triangular fibrocartilage of the wrist: Results of partial excision. J Hand Surg [Am] 9: 527–530

Mikic ZD (1978) Age changes in the triangular fibrocartilage of the wrist joint. J Anat 126: 367–384

Mikic ZD (1984) Arthrography of the wrist joint. J Bone Joint Surg [Am] 66: 371–378

Minami A, Ishikawa J, Suenaga N, Kasashima T (1996) Clinical results of treatment of triangular fibrocartilage complex tears by arthroscopic debridement. J Hand Surg Am 21: 406–411

Mital MA, Karlin LI (1980) Diagnostic arthroscopy in sport injuries. Orthop Clin North Am 11: 771–784

Mizuseki T, Watari S, Ishida O, Ikuta Y (1986) A case report of isolated traumatic tear of the triangular fibrocartilage. Hiroshima J Med Sci 35: 63–66

Mollenhoff G, Walz M, Knopp W, Muhr G (1996) Arthroscopic diagnosis of posttraumatic disorders of the wrist. Arch Orthop Trauma Surg 115: 351–356

Mooney JF, Poehling GG (1991) Disruption of the ulnolunate ligament as a cause of chronic ulnar wrist pain. J Hand Surg Am 16: 347–349

Mossing N (1975) Isolated lesions of the radio-ulnar disk treated with excision. Scand. J Plast Reconstr Surg 9: 231–233

Nagle DJ (1994) Arthroscopic treatment of degenerative tears of the triangulare fibrocartilage. Hand Clin North Am 10: 615–624

Nagle DJ, Benson LS (1992) Wrist arthroscopy: Indications and results. Arthroscopy 8: 198–203

Nakamura R, Imaeda T, Tsuge S, Watanabe K (1991) Scaphoid non-union with D.I.S.I. deformity. A survey of clinical cases with special reference to ligamentous injury. J Hand Surg Br 16: 156–161

Nakao E, Nakamura R, Tsunoda K (1996) Triquetrohamate impaction syndrome: a case report. J Hand Surg Br 21: 778–780

Nichols CD (1989) Wrist arthroscopy. AORN J 49: 759–771

North ER, Meyer S (1990) Wrist injuries: correlation of clinical and arthroscopic findings. J Hand Surg Am 15: 915–920

North ER, Thomas S (1988) An anatomic guide for arthroscopic visualization of the wrist capsula ligaments. J Hand Surg [Am] 13 A: 815–822

Oneson SR, Timins ME, Scales LM, Erickson SJ, Chamoy L (1997) MR imaging diagnosis of triangular fibrocartilage pathology with arthroscopic correlation. AJR 168: 1513–1518

Osterman AL (1990) Arthroscopic debridement of triangular fibrocartilage complex tears. Arthroscopy 6: 120–124

Osterman AL, Mikulics M (1988) Scaphoid nonunion. Hand Clin 4: 437–455

Osterman AL, Raphael J (1995) Arthroscopic resection of dorsal ganglion of the wrist. Hand Clin North Am 11: 7–12

Osterman AL, Seidman GD (1995) The role of arthroscopy in the treatment of lunatotriquetral ligament injuries. Hand Clin 11: 41–50

Osterman AL, Terrill RG (1991) Arthroscopic treatment of TFCC lesions. Hand Clin 7: 277–281

Palmer AK (1989) Triangular fibrocartilage complex lesions: A classification. J Hand Surg [Am] 14: 594–606

Palmer AK (1990) Triangular fibrocartilage disorders: Injury pattern and treatment. Arthroscopy 6: 125–132

Palmer AK, Glisson RR, Werner FW Mech ME (1984) Relationship between ulnar variance and triangular fibrocartilage complex thickness. J Hand Surg [Am] 9: 681–683

Palmer AK, Skahen JR, Werner FW, Glisson R (1985) The extensor retinaculum of the wrist: Anatomical and biomechanical study. J Hand Surg [Br] 10: 11–16

Palmer AK, Werner FW (1981) The triangular fibrocartilage complex of the wrist – Anatomy and function. J Hand Surg [Br] 6: 153–162

Palmer AK, Werner FW, Glisson RR, Murphy DJ (1988) Partial excision of the triangular fibrocartilage complex: An experimental study. J Hand Surg [Am] 13: 391–394

Pederzini L, Luchetti R, Soragni O et al. (1992) Evaluation of the triangular fibrocartilage complex tears by arthroscopy, arthrography, and magnetic resonance imaging. Arthroscopy 8: 191–197

Peicha G, Seibert FJ, Fellinger M, Grechenig W, Schippinger G (1997) Lesions of the scapholunate ligaments in acute wrist trauma-arthroscopic diagnosis and minimally invasive treatment. Knee Surg Sports Traumatol Arthrosc 5: 176–183

Pianka G (1992) Wrist arthroscopy. Hand Clin 8: 621–630

Plank E, Burri C, Zeitler HP (1979) Die Technik der Arthroskopie des oberen Sprunggelenks, des Ellenbogengelenks und des Handgelenks. In: Blauth W, Donner K (Hrsg) Arthroskopie des Kniegelenks – Symposion Kiel 1978. Thieme, Stuttgart, S 142–149

Pomsel T, Kreusch-Brinker R, Ahmadi A (1989) Die arthroskopische Diagnostik der Handgelenks-Discusverletzung. Z Orthop 127: 331–335

Rettig ME, Amadio PC (1994) Wrist arthroscopy. Indications and clinical applications. J Hand Surg Br 19: 774–777

Rominger MB, Bernreuter WK, Kenney PJ, Lee DH (1993) MR imaging of anatomy and tears of wrist ligaments. Radiographics 13: 1233–1246, discussion 1247–1248

Rosenthal A (1949) Die Verletzungen des Discus articularis bei der typischen Radiusfraktur. Langenbecks Arch Dtsch Z Chir 262: 390–403

Roth JH (1988) Wrist Arthroscopy – Radiocarpal arthroscopy. Orthopaedics 11: 1309–1312

Roth JH (1990) Arthroscopic „-ectomy" surgery of the wrist. Arthroscopy 6: 141–147

Roth JH, Haddad RG (1986) Radiocarpal arthroscopy and arthrography in the diagnosis of ulnar wrist pain. Arthroscopy 2: 234–243

Roth JH, Poehling GG (1990) Arthroscopic „-ectomy" surgery of the wrist. Arthroscopy 6: 141–147

Roth JH, Poehling GG, Whipple TL (1988) Arthroscopic surgery of the wrist. Instruct Course Lect 37: 183–194

Roth JH, Poehling GG, Whipple TL (1988) Hand instrumentation for small joint arthroscopy. Arthroscopy 4: 126–128

Ruch DS, Poehling GG (1996) Arthroscopic management of partial scapholunate and lunotriquetral injuries of the wrist. J Hand Surg Am 21: 412–417

Ruch DS, Siegel D, Chabon SJ, Koman LA, Poehling GG (1993) Arthroscopic categorization of intercarpal ligamentous injuries of the wrist. Orthopedics 16: 1051–1056

Sagerman SD, Short W (1996) Arthroscopic repair of radial-sided triangular fibrocartilage complex tears. Arthroscopy 12: 339–342

Savoie F (1995) The role of arthroscopy in the diagnosis and management of cartilagous lesions of the wrist. Hand Clin North Am 11: 1–6

Savoie FH 3rd (1995) The role of arthroscopy in the diagnosis and management of cartilaginous lesions of the wrist. Hand Clin 11: 1–5

Savoie FH 3rd, Grondel RJ (1995) Arthroscopy for carpal instability. Orthop Clin North Am 26: 731–738

Savoie FH 3rd, Whipple TL (1996) The role of arthroscopy in athletic injuries of the wrist. Clin Sports Med 15: 219–233

Scheck RJ, Kubitzek C, Hierner R, Szeimies U, Pfluger T, Wilhelm K, Hahn K (1997) The scapholunate interosseous ligament in MR arthrography of the wrist: correlation with non-enhanced MRI and wrist arthroscopy. Skeletal Radiol 26: 263–271

Schers TJ, van-Heusden HA (1995) Evaluation of chronic wrist pain. Arthroscopy superior to arthrography: comparison in 39 patients. Acta Orthop Scand 66: 540–542

Sennwald G (1987) Das Handgelenk. Springer, Berlin Heidelberg New York Tokyo

Sennwald GR, Zdravkovic V (1997) Wrist arthroscopy: a prospective analysis of 53 post-traumatic carpal injuries. Scand J Plast Reconstr Surg Hand Surg 31: 261–266

Sennwald W, Kern HP, Jacob HAC (1993) Die Arthrose des Handgelenks als Folge der karpalen Instabilität: Therapeutische Alternativen. Orthopäde 22: 65–71

Stanley J, Saffar P (1994) Handgelenkarthroskopie. Chapman & Hall, London Glasgow

Staehlin P (1993) Die Handgelenksarthroskopie. Orthopäde 22: 19–24

Taleisnik J (1976) The ligaments of the wrist. J Hand Surg 1: 110–118

Taleisnik J (1985) The wrist. Churchill Livingstone, New York

Taleisnik J (1988) Current concepts review: Carpal instability. J Bone Joint Surg [Am] 70: 1262–1268

Taleisnik J (1988) Scapholunate ligament excision. J Hand Surg Am 13: 790–792

Taleisnik J, Gelbermann RH, Miller BW, Szabo RM (1984) The extensor retinaculum of the wrist. J Hand Surg [Am] 9: 495–501

Tehranzadeh J, Labosky DA, Gabriele OF (1983) Ganglion cysts and tear of triangular fibrocartilages of both wrists in a cheerleader. Am J Sports Med 11: 357–359

Terrill RQ (1994) Use of arthroscopy in the evaluation and treatment of chronic wrist pain. Hand Clin 10: 593–603

Terrill RQ (1994) Use of arthroscopy in the evaluation and treatment of chronic wrist pain. Hand Clin North Am 10: 593–604

Thiru-Pathi RG. (1986) Arterial anatomy of the triangular fibrocartilage of the wrist and its surgical significance. J Hand Surg 11 A: 258–263

Totterman SM, Miller RJ, McCance SE, Meyers SP (1996) Lesions of the triangular fibrocartilage complex: MR findings with a three-dimensional gradient-recalled-echo sequence. Radiology 199: 227–232

Trumble TE, Gilbert M, Vedder N (1996) Arthroscopic repair of the triangular fibrocartilage complex. Arthroscopy 12: 588–597

Trumble TE, Gilbert M, Vedder N (1997) Isolated tears of the triangular fibrocartilage: management by early arthroscopic repair. J Hand Surg Am 22 A: 57–65

Van Heest AE (1995) Wrist arthroscopy. Scand J Med Sci Sports 5: 2–6

Vanden Eynde S, De Smet L, Fabry G (1994) Diagnostic value of arthrography and arthroscopy of the radiocarpal joint. Arthroscopy 10: 50–3

Vesely DG (1967) The distal radio-ulnar joint. Clin Orthop 51: 75–91

Viegas S (1994) Medicarpal arthroscopy: Anatomy and portals. Hand Clin North Am 10: 577–588

Viegas SF (1986) Intraarticular ganglion of the dorsal interosseous scapholunate ligament: A case for arthroscopy. Arthroscopy 2: 93–95

Viegas SF (1988) Arthroscopic treatment of osteochondritis dissecans of the scaphoid. Arthroscopy 4(4): 278–281

Viegas SF (1990) The lunatohamate articulation of the midcarpal joint. Arthroscopy 6: 5–10

Viegas SF (1992) Midcarpal arthroscopy: anatomy and technique. Arthroscopy 8: 385–390

Viegas SF (1994) Midcarpal arthroscopy: anatomy and portals. Hand Clin 10: 577–587

Viegas SF (1995) Arthroscopic assessment of carpal instabilities and ligament injuries. Instr Course Lect 44: 151–154

Viegas SF, Ballantyne G (1987) Attritional lesions of the wrist joint. J Hand Surg [Am] 12: 1025–1029

Viegas SF, Calhoun JH (1987) Osteochondritis dissecans of the lunate. J Hand Surg [Am] 12: 130–133

Warhold LG, Ruth RM (1995) Complications of arthrocopy and how to prevent them. Hand Clin North Am 11: 81–90

Warhold LG, Ruth RM (1995) Complications of wrist arthroscopy and how to prevent them. Hand Clin 11: 81–89

Watanabe K, Nakamura R, Imaeda T (1995) Arthroscopic assessment of Kienbock's disease. Arthroscopy 11: 257–262

Watanabe M (1971) Arthroscopy of small joint. J Jpn Orthop Assoc 45: 908

Watanabe M (1976) Recent advances in arthroscopy. Rheumatologie 33: 29–33

Watanabe M (1985) Arthroscopy of small joints: 6. Arthroscopy of the wrist joint. Igaku-Shoin, Tokyo New York, pp 85–90

Watanabe M, Ito K, Fujii S (1985) Equipments and procedures of small joint arthroscopy. In: Watanabe M (ed) Arthroscopy of small joints. Igaku Shoin, Tokyo New York, pp 3–30

Watanabe M, Takeda S, Ikeuchi H (1979) Atlas of arthroscopy, 3nd edn. Igaku-Shoin, Tokyo New York

Weber ER (1988) Wrist mechanics and its a association with ligamentous instability. In: Lichtman DM (ed) The wrist and its disorders. Saunders, Philadelphia

Wehbe MA, Parisien JS (1988) Arthroscopy of the wrist. In: Parisien JS (ed) Arthroscopic surgery. Mc Graw-Hill, New York, pp 293–299

Weigl K, Spira E (1969) The triangular fibrocartilage of the wrist joint. Reconstr Surg Traumatol 11: 139–153

Weiss AP, Akelman E (1995) Diagnostic imaging and arthroscopy for chronic wrist pain. Orthop Clin North Am 26: 759–767

Weiss AP, Akelman E, Lambiase R (1996) Comparison of the findings of triple-injection cinearthrography of the wrist with those of arthroscopy. J Bone Joint Surg [Am] 78: 348–356

Weiss AP, Sachar K, Glowacki KA (1997) Arthroscopic debridement alone for intercarpal ligament tears. J Hand Surg Am 22: 344–349

Werner FW, Glisson RR, Murphy DJ, Palmer AK (1986) Force transmission through the distal radioulnar carpal joint: Effect of ulnar lengthening and shortening. Handchir Mikrochir Plast Chir 18: 304–308

Whipple TL (1986) Clinical applications of wrist arthroscopy. Arthroscopy 2: 116–117

Whipple TL (1988) Powered instruments for wrist arthroscopy. Arthroscopy 4: 290–294

Whipple TL (1990) Precautions for arthroscopy of the wrist. Arthroscopy 6: 3–4

Whipple TL (1991) Arthroscopy of the wrist: Introduction and indications. In: McGinty IB et al. (eds) Operative arthroscopy. Raven, New York

Whipple TL (1992) Arthroscopic surgery: The wrist. Lippincott, Philadelphia

Whipple TL (1992) The role of arthroscopy in the treatment of wrist injuries in the athlete. Clin Sports Med 11: 227–238

Whipple TL (1994) Arthroscopy of the distal radioulnar joint: Indications, portals and Anatomy. Hand Clin North Am 10: 589–592

Whipple TL (1995) The role of arthroscopy in the treatment of intra-articular wrist fractures. Hand Clin 11: 13–18

Whipple TL (1995) The role of arthroscopy in the treatment of scapholunate Instability. Hand Clin North Am 11: 37–40

Whipple TL, Geissler WB (1993) Arthroscopic management of wrist triangular fibrocartilage complex injuries in the athlete. Orthopedics 16: 1061–1067

Whipple TL, Marotta JJ, Powell JH (1986) Techniques of wrist arthroscopy. Arthroscopy 2: 244–252

Williams CS, Jupiter JB (1993) Das schmerzhafte Ulnokarpalgelenk: Diagnostik und Therapie. Orthopäde 22: 36–45

Wnorowski DC, Palmer AK, Werner FW, Fortino MD (1992) Anatomic and biomechanical analysis of the arthroscopic wafer procedure. Arthroscopy 8: 204–212

Wolfe SW, Easterling KJ, Yoo HH (1995) Arthroscopic-assisted reduction of distal radius fractures. Arthroscopy 11: 706–714

Xu JS (1988) Wrist arthroscopy in clinical applications. Chung Hua Wai Ko Tsa Chih 26: 598–600, 637

Yung Ch (1979) Arthroscopy of the wrist and finger joints. Orthop Clin North Am 10: 723

Zachee B, De Smet L, Fabry G (1993) Arthroscopic suturing of TFCC lesions. Arthroscopy 9: 242–243

Zachee B, De Smet L, Fabry G (1994) Frayed ulno-triquetral and ulno-lunate ligaments as an arthroscopic sign of longstanding triquetro-lunate ligament rupture. J Hand Surg Br 19: 570–571

Zachee B, DeSmet L, Fabry G (1993) A snapping wrist due to a loose body. Arthroscopic diagnosis and treatment. Arthroscopy 9: 117–118

Elbow Joint

Andrews JR, Carson WG (1985) Arthroscopy of the elbow. Arthroscopy 1: 97–107

Andrews JR, Craven WM (1991) Lesions of the posterior compartment of the elbow. Clin Sports Med 10: 637–652

Andrews JR, McKenzie PJ (1991) Arthroscopic surgical treatment of elbow pathology. In: McGinty JB (ed) Operative arthroscopy. Raven, New York, p 595

Andrews JR, Pierre RK, Carson WG (1986) Arthroscopy of the elbow. Clin Sports Med 5: 653–662

Andrews JR, Wilson FD (1985) Valgus extension overload in the pitching elbow. In: Zarins B, Andrews JR, Carson WG (eds) Injuries to the throwing arm. Saunders, Philadelphia

Andrews JR, Soffer SR (1994) Elbow arthroscopy. Mosby, St. Louis Baltimore

Andrews JR, Baumgarten TE (1995) Arthroscopic anatomy of the elbow. Orthop Clin North Am 26: 671–677

Baker CL, Shalvoy RM (1991) The prone position for elbow arthroscopy. Clin Sports Med 10: 623–628

Baker CL, Brooks AA (1996) Arthroscopy of the elbow. Clin Sports Med 15: 261–281

Barthel T, Jäger A, Würstle R (1994) Ergebnisse der arthroskopischen Chirurgie des Ellenbogengelenks. Arthroskopie 7: 34

Berner W (1988) Arthroskopische Operationstechnik am Ellenbogengelenk. Hefte Unfallheilkd 199: 149–155

Berner W, Hendrich Ch (1994) Arthroskopie des Ellenbogengelenks nach traumatischer Luxation. Arthroskopie 7: 40

Boe S (1986) Arthroscopy of the elbow. Diagnosis and extraction of loose bodies. Acta Orthop Scand 57: 52–53

Burman MS (1932) Arthroscopy of the elbow joint:A cadaver study. J Bone Joint Surg [Am] 14: 349–350

Byrd JW (1994) Elbow arthroscopy for arthrofibrosis after type I radial head fractures. Arthroscopy 10: 162–165

Cameron SE, Travis MT, Kruse RW (1993) Foreign body arthroscopically retrieved from the elbow. Arthroscopy 9: 220–221

Carson WG (1988) Arthroscopy of the elbow. In: Torg J, Welsh RP (eds) Current therapy in sports medicine. Decker, Philadelphia

Carson WG, Andrews JR (1985) Arthroscopy of the elbow. In Zarins B, Andrews JR, Carson WG (eds) Injuries to the throwing arm. Saunders, Philadelphia, pp 221–227

Carson WG, Meyers JF (1991) Diagnostic arthroscopy of the elbow:Surgical technique and arthroscopic and portal anatomy. In: McGinty JB (ed) Operative arthroscopy. Raven, New York, pp 583–594

Carson WG:Complications of elbow arthroscopy (1988) In Minkoff J, Sherman O (eds) Arthroscopic surgery. Williams & Wilkins, Baltimore, pp 166–179

Casscells SW (1987) Editor's comment:Neurovascular anatomy and elbow arthroscopy: Inherent risks. Arthroscopy 2: 190

Clarke RP (1988) Symptomatic, lateral synovial fringe (plica) of the elbow joint. Arthroscopy 4: 112–116

Cohen B, Constant CR (1992) Extension-supination sign in prearthroscopic elbow distension. Arthroscopy 8: 189–190

Commandre FA, Taillan B, Benezis C, Follacci FM, Hammou JC (1988) Plica synovialis (synovial fold) of the elbow. Report on one case. J Sports Med Phys Fitness 28: 209–210

Day B (1996) Elbow arthroscopy in the athlete. Clin Sports Med 15: 785–797

Ekman EF, Cory JW, Poehling GG (1997) Pigmented villonodular synovitis and synovial chondromatosis arthroscopically diagnosed and treated in the same elbow. Arthroscopy 13: 114–116

Ekman EF, Poehling GG (1994) Arthroscopy of the elbow. Hand Clin 10: 453–460

Esch JC, Baker JI (1993) Surgical arthroscopy: The shoulder and elbow. Lippincott, Philadelphia

Faulkner JR, Jackson RW (1980) Arthroscopy of the elbow. J Bone Joint Surg [Br] 62: 130

Field LD, Altchek DW (1996) Evaluation of the arthroscopic valgus instability test of the elbow. Am J Sports Med 24: 177–181

Field LD, Altchek DW, Warren RF, O'Brien SJ, Skyhar MJ, Wickiewicz TL (1994) Arthroscopic anatomy of the lateral elbow: a comparison of three portals. Arthroscopy 10: 602–607

Field LD, Callaway GH, O'Brien SJ, Altchek DW (1995) Arthroscopic assessment of the medial collateral ligament complex of the elbow. Am J Sports Med 23: 396–400

Figgie MP, Inglis AE, Mow CS, Figgie HE (1989) Total elbow arthroplasty for complete ankylosis of the elbow. J Bone Joint Surg [Am] 71: 513–519

Gallay SH, Richards RR, O'Driscoll SW (1993) Intraarticular capacity and compliance of stiff and normal elbows. Arthroscopy 9: 9–13

Glötzer W, Künzel KH (1990) Ellbogen und Handgelenk. In: Hempfling H (Hrsg) Arthroskopie. Fischer, Stuttgart New York

Greis PE, Halbrecht J, Plancher KD (1995) Arthroscopic removal of loose bodies of the elbow. Orthop Clin North Am 26: 679–689

Gruber J, Schießler W, Stedtfeld HW, Dittrich V (1994) Technik und Komplikationen der Ellenbogenarthroskopie. Arthroskopie 7: 1 8–23

Guhl JF (1985) Arthroscopy and arthroscopic surgery of the elbow. Orthopedics 8: 1290–1296

Hempfling H (1983) Die endoskopische Untersuchung des Ellbogengelenkes vom dorsoradialen Zugang. Z Orthop 121: 331–332

Hempfling H (1984) Die Arthroskopie des Ellbogengelenkes – Indikation und Ergebnisse. Z Orthop 122: 750–753

Hempfling H (Hrsg) (1994) Die Arthroskopie des Ellenbogengelenkes. In: Farbatlas der Arthroskopie großer Gelenke, 2 Aufl. Fischer, Stuttgart New York

Husband JB, Hastings H (1990) The lateral approach for operative release of posttraumatic contracture of the elbow. J Bone Joint Surg [Am] 72: 1353

Ito K (1979) The arthroscopic anatomy of the elbow joint. Arthroscopy 4: 2–9

Ito K (1981) Arthroscopy of the elbow joint. Arthroscopy 6: 14–24

Ito K (1985) Arthroscopy of the elbow joint. In: Watanabe M (ed) Arthroscopy of small joints. Igaku Shoin, Tokyo New York pp 57–84

Jackson DW, Silvino N, Reiman P (1989) Osteochondritis in the femal gymnast's elbow. Arthroscopy 5: 129–136

Janarv PM, Hesser U, Hirsch G (1997) Osteochondral lesions in the radiocapitellar joint in the skeletally immature: radiographic, MRI, and arthroscopic findings in 13 consecutive cases. J Pediatr Orthop 17: 311–314

Jerosch J, Castro WHM, Assheuer J (1992) Arthroskopie des Ellenbogengelenks, Langzeitergebnisse, Komplikationen und Indikationen. Unfallchirurg 95: 405–411

Jerosch J, Drescher H, Steinbeck J, Schröder M (1994) Arthroskopie des Ellenbogengelenkes. Indikationen, Ursachen von neurologischen Komplikationen, Prävention. Arthroskopie 7: 25

Johnson LL (1981) Elbow Joint. In: Johnson LL (ed) Diagnostic and surgical arthroscopy. Mosby, St. Louis, pp 390–399

Jones GS, Savoie FH 3d (1993) Arthroscopic capsular release of flexion contractures (arthrofibrosis) of the elbow. Arthroscopy 9: 277–283

Josefsson PO, Johnell O, Gentz CF (1984) Long-term sequelae of simple dislocation of the elbow. J Bone Joint Surg [Am] 66: 927–930

Kathrein A, Inderster A, Benedetto KP, Künzel KH (1994) Einfluß der Kapselfüllung auf die Lagebeziehung der neurovaskulären Strukturen am Ellenbogengelenk. Eine experimentelle Studie. Arthroskopie 7: 6

Kerschbaumer F, Koydl G, Herresthal J (1997) Arthroskopische Synovektomie des rheumatischen Ellbogens Arthroskopie 10: 27–30

Kim SJ, Kim HK, Lee JW (1995) Arthroscopy for limitation of motion of the elbow. Arthroscopy 11: 680–683

Knopp W, Neumann K (1993) Indikation zur diagnostischen und therapeutischen Arthroskopie kleiner Gelenke. Chirurg 64: 163–169

Lee BP, Morrey BF (1997) Arthroscopic synovectomy of the elbow for rheumatoid arthritis. A prospective study. J Bone Joint Surg [Br] 79: 770–772

Lindenfeld TN (1989) The medial approach for elbow arthroscopy. Arthroscopy 5: 159

Lindenfeld TN (1990) Medial approach in elbow arthroscopy. Am J Sports Med 18: 413–417

Lo IK, King GJ (1994) Arthroscopic radial head excision. Arthroscopy 10: 689–692

Lokietek JC, De Cloedt, F Legaye J et al. (1988) Extraction of a foreign body from the elbow using arthroscopy. Rev Chir Orthop 74: 93–98

Lutz M, Konzett Ch, Benedetto KP, Künzel KH (1994) Makroskopische und arthroskopische Anatomie des Ellenbogengelenks. Arthroskopie 7: 2–9

Lynch GJ, Meyers JF, Whipple TL, Caspari RB (1986) Neurovascular anatomy and elbow arthroscopy:Inherent risks. Arthroscopy 2 : 190–197

Marshall PD, Fairclough JA, Johnson SR, Evans EJ (1993) Avoiding nerve damage during elbow arthroscopy. J Bone Joint Surg [Br] 75: 129–131

Miller CD, Jobe CM, Wright MH (1995) Neuroanatomy in elbow arthroscopy. J Shoulder Elbow Surg 4: 168–174

Mital MA (1980) Diagnostic arthroscopy in sports injuries. Elbow joint. Orthop Clin North Am 11: 771–785

Morrey BF (1985) Arthroscopy of the elbow. In: Morrey BF (ed) The elbow and its disorders. Saunders, Philadelphia, pp 7–24

Nowicki KD, Shall LM (1992) Arthroscopic release of a posttraumatic flexion contracture in the elbow: a case report and review of the literature. Arthroscopy 8: 544–547

O'Driscoll SW (1992) Elbow arthroscopy for loose bodies. Orthopedics 15: 855–859

O'Driscoll SW (1995) Arthroscopic treatment for osteoarthritis of the elbow. Orthop Clin North Am 26: 691–706

O'Driscoll SW, Morrey BF (1992) Arthroscopy of the elbow: Diagnostic and therapeutic benefits and hazards. J Bone Joint Surg [Am] 74: 84–94

O'Driscoll SW, Morrey BF, An KN (1990) Intraartiular pressure and capacity of the elbow. Arthroscopy 6: 100–103

Ogilvie Harris DJ, Gordon R, MacKay M (1995) Arthroscopic treatment for posterior impingement in degenerative arthritis of the elbow. Arthroscopy 11: 437–443

Ogilvie Harris DJ, Schemitsch E (1993) Arthroscopy of the elbow for removal of loose bodies. Arthroscopy 9: 5–8

Oretorp N (1984) Arthroscopy of joints other than the knee – Elbow. Technique of examination. In: Casscells SW (ed) Arthroscopy – Diagnostic and surgical practice. Lea & Febiger, Philadelphia, pp 77–78

Papilion JD, Neff RS, Shall LM (1988) Compression neuropathy of the radial nerve as a compliation of elbow arthroscopy: A case report and review of the literature. Arthroscopy 4: 284–286

Parisien JS (1988) Arthroscopic surgery of the elbow. Bull Hosp Joint Dis Orthop Inst 48: 149–158

Poehling GG (1989) Elbow arthroscopy. A new technique. Arthroscopy 5: 222–224

Poehling GG, Sisco L, Whipple T (1989) Elbow arthroscopy: A new technique. Arthroscopy 5: 153–154

Poeling GG, Whipple T, Sisco L, Goldmann B (1989) Elbow arthroscopy: A new technique. Arthroscopy 5: 222–224

Poehling GG, Koman LA, Pope TL, Siegel DB (1994) Arthroscopy of the wrist and elbow. Raven, New York

Poehling GG, Ekman EF (1995) Arthroscopy of the elbow. Instr Course Lect 44: 217–223

Quinn SF, Haberman JJ, Fitzgerald SW, Traughber PD, Belkin RI, Murray WT (1994) Evaluation of loose bodies in the elbow with MR imaging. J Magn Reson Imaging 4: 169–172

Redden JF, Stanley D (1993) Arthroscopic fenestration of the olecranon fossa in the treatment of osteoarthritis of the elbow. Arthroscopy 9: 14–16

Robla J, Hechtman KS, Uribe JW, Phillipon MS (1996) Chondromalacia of the trochlear notch in athletes who throw. J Shoulder Elbow Surg 5: 69–72

Ruch DS, Poehling GG (1991) Arthroscopic treatment of Panner's disease. Clin Sports Med 10: 629–636

Rupp S, Tempelhof S (1995) Arthroscopic surgery of the elbow. Therapeutic benefits and hazards. Clin Orthop 313: 140–145

Ruth RM, Groves RJ (1996) Synovial osteochondromatosis of the elbow presenting with ulnar nerve neuropathy. Am J Orthop 25: 843–844

Schmidt K, Miehlke RH (1994) Arthroscopic synovectomy of shoulder – and elbow. Orthop Traumatol 3: 11–28

Schmidt K, Miehlke RK (1994) Die arthroskopische Synovektomie des Ellbogengelenkes. Aktuel Rheumatol 19: 50–44

Schneider T, Hoffstetter I, Fink B, Jerosch J (1994) Long-term results of elbow arthroscopy in 67 patients. Acta Orthop Belg 60: 378–383

Schonholtz GJ (ed) (1986) Arthroscopic surgery of the elbow joint. In: Arthroscopic surgery of the shoulder, elbow and ankle. Thomas, Springfield, III, pp 49–57, 73–78

Shaffer B, Parisien JS (1989) Elbow arthroscopy. Surg Rounds Orthop 3: 113–117

Sheppard JE, Marion JD, Hurst DI (1991) Arthroscopic elbow surgery five year experience and observations in 48 cases. Am J Arthroscopy 1: 13–19

Sojbjerg JO (1996) The stiff elbow. Acta Orthop Scand 67: 626–631

Stothers K, Day B, Regan WR (1995) Arthroscopy of the elbow: anatomy, portal sites, and a description of the proximal lateral portal. Arthroscopy 11: 449–457

Tedder JL, Andrews JR (1992) Elbow arthroscopy. Orthop Rev 21: 1047–1053

Thomas MA, Fast A, Shapiro D (1987) Radial nerve damage as a complication of elbow arthroscopy. Clin Orthop 215: 130–131

Timmerman LA, Andrews JR (1994) Histology and arthroscopic anatomy of the ulnar collateral ligament of the elbow. Am J Sports Med 22: 667–673

Timmerman-LA, Andrews JR (1994) Arthroscopic treatment of posttraumatic elbow pain and stiffness. Am J Sports Med 22: 230–235

Verhaar J, van Mameren H, Brandsma A (1991) Risks of neurovascular injury in elbow arthroscopy: starting anteromedially or anterolaterally? Arthroscopy 7: 287–290

Ward WG, Anderson TE (1993) Elbow arthroscopy in a mostly athletic population. J Hand Surg Am 18: 220–224

Ward WG, Belhobek GH, Anderson TE (1992) Arthroscopic elbow findings: correlation with preoperative radiographic studies. Arthroscopy 8: 498–502

Watanabe M (1985) Arthroscopy of small joints. Igaku Shoin, Tokyo New York

Wilson FD, Andrews JA, Blackburn TA, Mc Cluskey G (1983) Valgus extension overload in the pitching elbow. Am J Sports Med 11: 83

Woods WG (1987) Elbow arthroscopy. Clin Sports Med 6: 557–564

Shoulder Joint

Adolfsson L, Lysholm J (1991) Arthroscopy for the diagnosis of shoulder pain. Int Orthop 15: 275–278

Altchek DW (1995) Arthroscopy of the shoulder. Scand J Med Sci Sports 5: 71–75

Altchek DW, Warren RF, Wickiewicz TL, Skyhar MJ, Ortiz G, Schwartz E (1990) Arthroscopic acromioplasty. Technique and results J Bone Joint Surg [Am] 72: 1198–1207

Andrews JR, Broussard TS, Carson WG (1985) Arthroscopy of the shoulder in the management of partial tears of the rotator cuff: a preliminary report. Arthroscopy 1: 117–122

Andrews JR, Carson WG (1983) Shoulder joint arthroscopy. Orthopaedics 6: 1157–1162

Andrews JR, Carson WG, McLeod WD (1985) Glenoid labrum tears related to long head of biceps. Am J Sports Med 13: 337

Andrews JR, Carson WG, Ortega K (1984) Arthroscopy of the shoulder. Technique and normal antamoy. Am J Sport Med 12: 1–7

Andrews JR, Kupferman SP, Dillman CJ (1991) Labral tears in throwing and racquet sports. Clin Sports Med 10: 901–911

Arcioro RA, Taylor DC, Snyder RJ, Uhorchak JM (1995) Arthroscopic biosorbale tack stabilization of initial anterior shoulder dislocation: a preliminary report. Arthroscopy 11: 410–417

Ark JW, Block TJ, Flatow EL, Bigliani LU (1992) Arthrocopic treatment of calcific tendinitis of the shoulder. Arthroscopy 8: 183–188

Bach BR Jr (1990) Arthroscopic removal of painful Bristow hardware. Arthroscopy 6: 324–326

Baker CL, Uribe JW, Whitman C (1990) Arthroscopic evaluation of acute initial anterior shoulder dislocations. Am J Sports Med 18: 25–28

Barber FA, Herbert FA, Click JN (1995) The ultimate strength of suture anchors. Arthroscopy 11: 21–28

Beer CH, Foster CR (1980) Inferior capsular shift for involuntary inferior and multdirectional instability of the shoulder. J Bone Joint Surg [Am] 62: 897–908

Benedetto KP, Glötzer W (1987) Die arthroskopische Limbusrefixation. Hefte Unfallheilkd 186: 137–140

Benedetto KP, Glötzer W (1988) Die arthroskopische Bankart-Operation mittels Nahttechnik – Indikation, Technik und Ergebnisse. Arthroskopie 1: 185–189

Benedetto KP, Glötzer W (1992) Arthroscopic Bankart procedure by suture technique: indications, technique ans resulsts. Arthroscopy 8: 111–115

Berg EB, Ellison AE (1990) The inside-out Bankart procedure. Am J Sports Med 18: 129–133

Biedert R, Kentsch A (1989) Arthroskopische Revision des subakromialen Raumes bei Impingement-Syndrom. Unfallchirurgie 92: 500–504

Bigliani LU, Dalsey RM, McCann PD, April EW (1990) An anatomical study of the suprascapular nerve. Arthroscopy 6: 301–305

Bigliani LU, Flatow EL, Deliz ED (1991) Complications of shoulder arthroscopy. Orthop Rev 20: 743–751

Boszotta H, Helperstorfer W (1996) Ruptur der langen Bizepssehne. Arthroskopischer Befund, morphologische Einteilung und therapeutische Konsequenzen. Arthroskopie 9: 44–48

Boszotta H, Helperstorfer W (1997) Indikation, Technik und Ergebnisse der arthroskopischen Naht der Rotatorenmanschette. Arthroskopie 175–180

Brown AR, Weiss R, Greenberg C, Flatow EL, Bigliani LU (1993) Interscalene block for shoulder arthroscopy: comparison with general anesthesia. Arthroscopy 9: 295–300

Brunner U, Weidemann E, Trupka A, Habermeyer P (1995) Langzeitergebnisse nach arthroskopischer Bankart-Naht bei vorderen Schulterinstabilitäten (modifizierte Morgan-Technik). Arthroskopie 8: 168–172

Bunker T, Wallace WA (1991) Shoulder arthroscopy. Dunitz, London

Burkhart SS (1990) Deep venous thrombosis after shoulder arthroscopy. Arthroscopy 6: 61–63

Burkhart SS (1991) Arthroscopic treatment of massive rotator cuff tears. Clinical results and biomechanical rationale. Clin Orthop 45–56

Burkhart SS (1996) Shoulder arthroscopy. New concepts. Clin Sports Med 15: 635–653

Burkhart SS, Fox DL (1992) SLAP-lesions in association with complete tears of the long head of the biceps tendon. A report of two cases. Arthroscopy 8: 31–35

Buuck DA, Davidson MR (1996) Rehabilitation of the athlete after shoulder arthroscopy. Clin Sports Med 15: 655–672

Cameron SE (1996) Venous pseudoaneurysm as a complication of shoulder arthroscopy. J Shoulder Elbow Surg 5: 404–406

Canniggia M, Maniscalco P, Pagliantini L, Bocchi L (1995) Titanium anchors for the repair of rotator cuff tears: preliminary report of a surgical technique. J Orthop Trauma 9: 312–317

Carson WG Jr (1992) Arthroscopy of the shoulder: anatomy and technique. Orthop Rev 21: 143–153

Cash JD (1991) Recent advances and perspectives on arthroscopic stabilization of the shoulder. Clin Sports Med 10: 871–886

Caspari RB (1982) Shoulder arthroscopy: a review of the present state of the art. Contemp Orthop 4: 523–531

Cofield RH (1983) Arthroscopy of the shoulder. Mayo Clin Proc 58: 501–508

Coughlin L, Rubinovich M, Johansson J, White B, Greenspoon J (1992). Arthroscopic staple capsulorrhaphy for anterior shoulder instability. Am J Sports Med 20: 253–256

Craft DV, Moseley JB, Cawley PW, Noble PC (1996) Fixation strength of rotator cuff repairs with suture anchors and the transosseous technique. J Shoulder Elbow Surg 15: 32–40

Craig EV (1996) Shoulder arthroscopy in the throwing athlete. Clin Sports Med 15: 673–700

Davidson PA, Tibone JE (1995) Anterior-inferior (5 o'clock) portal for shoulder arthroscopy. Arthroscopy 11: 519–525

Denti M, Monteleone M, Trevisan C, De-Romedis B, Barmettler F (1995) Magnetic resonance imaging versus arthroscopy for the investigation of the osteochondral humeral defect in anterior shoulder instability. A double-blind prospective study. Knee Surg Sports Traumatol Arthrosc 3: 184–186

Dietzel DP, Ciullo JV (1996) Spontaneous pneumothorax after shoulder arthroscopy: a report of four cases. Arthroscopy 12: 99–102

Ellmann H (1987) Arthroscopic subacromial decompression: analysis of one to three year results. Arthroscopy 3: 173–181

Ellman H (1990) Diagnosis and treatment of incomplete rotator cuff tears. Clin Orthop 254: 64–74

Ellman H, Kay SP (1991) Arthroscopic subacromial decompression for chronic impingement. Two – to five-year results. J Bone Joint Surg Br 73: 395–398

Ellmann H, Kay SP, Wirth M (1993) Arthroscopic treatment of full-thickness rotator cuff tears: two to seven year follow up study. Arthroscopy 9: 195–200

Ellmann MH, Hankes G, Bayer M (1986) Repair of the rotator cuff. J Bone Joint Surg [Am] 68: 158–167

Esch JC, Ozerkin LR, Helgager JA, Kane N, Lilliott N (1988) Arthroscopic subacromial decompression: results according to the degree of rotator cuff tear. Arthroscopy 4: 241–249

Esch JC, Baker CL (1993) Arthroscopic surgery. The shoulder and elbow. Lippincott, Philadelphia

Gächter A, Seelig W (1988) Schulterarthroskopie. Arthroskopie 1: 162–170

Gächter A, Seelig W (1992) Arthroscopy of the shoulder joint. Arthroscopy 8: 89–97

Gartsmann GA (1996) Arthrocopic assessment of rotator cuff tear reparability. Arthroscopy 12: 546–549

Gartsmann GM (1990) Arthroscopic acromioplasty for leasion of the rotator cuff. J Bone Joint Surg [Am] 72: 169–180

Gerber C, Schneeberger AG, Beck M et al. (1994) Mechanical strength of repairs of the rotator cuff. J Bone Joint Surg [Br] 76: 371–380

Goldberg BJ, Nirschl RP, Mc Connell JP, Petrone FA (1993) Arthroscopic transglenoid suture capsulolabral repair: Preliminary results. Am J Sports Med 21: 656–665

Grana WA, Buchlea PD, Yates CK (1993) Arthroscopic Bankart suture repair. Am J Sports Med 1: 276–284

Gross ML, Seeger LL, Smith JB, Mandelbaum BR, Finerman GA (1990) Magnetic resonance imaging of the glenoid labrum. Am J Sports Med 18: 229–234

Gross RM (1989) Arthorscopic shoulder capsulorrhaohy: does it work ? Am J Sports Med 17: 495–500

Gross RM, Fritzgibbons TC (1985) Shoulder arthroscopy: a modified approach. Arthroscopy 1: 156–159

Habermeyer P (1989) Sehnenruptur im Schulterbereich. Orthopädie 18: 257–267

Habermeyer P, Kaiser E, Knappes M, Kremser T, Wiedemann E (1987) Zur funktionellen Anatomie und Biomechanik der langen Bizepssehne. Unfallchirurgie 90: 319–329

Habermeyer P, Schuller U (1990) Die Bedeutung des Labrum glenoidale für die Stabilität des Glenohumeralgelenkes. Unfallchirurgie 93: 19–26

Habermeyer P, Schweiberger L (1996) Schulterchirurgie, 2. Aufl. Urban & Schwarzenberg, München

Habermeyer P, Wiedemann E (1989) Rationelle Therapie der Schulterinstabilität beim Sportler. Chirurg 60: 765–773

Hawkins RB (1989) Arthroscopic stapling repair for shoulder instability: a retrospective study of 50 cases. Arthroscopy 5: 122–128

Hawkins RJ, Misamare GW, Hobeika PE (1985) Surgery for full thickness rotator cuff tears. J Bone Joint Surg [Am] 67: 1349–1355

Hedtmann A, Fett H (1989) Die sogenannte Periarthopathia humeroscapularis. Z Orthop 127:643–649

Hedtmann A, Fett H (1991) Atlas und Lehrbuch der Schultersonografie. Enke, Stuttgart

Hedtmann A, Fett H (1995) Schultersonographie bei Subakromialsyndromen mit Erkrankungen und Verletzungen der Rotatorenmanschette. Orthopäde 24:498–508

Helpertorfer W, Boszotta H (1994) Eine selten Ursache für das Impingementsyndrom: intraartikuläre Ruptur der Bizepssehne. Arthroskopische Therapie. Arthroskopie 7: 235–238

Hempfling H (1989) Komplikationen bei der Schulterarthroskopie. Arthroskopie 2: 53–57

Henderson AA, Haines JF (1993) An early sign to confirm intraarticular injection of fluid in shoulder arthroscopy. Arthroscopy 9: 334–335

Hennrikus WL, Mapes RC, Bratton MW, Lapoint JM (1995) Lateral traction during shoulder arthroscopy: its effect on tissue perfusion measured by pulse oximetry. Am J Sports Med 23: 444–446

Hoffmann F, Reif G, Schiller M (1997. Arthroskopische Rotatorenmanschettenrekonstruktion mit Minischrauben oder Knochenankern. Arthroskopie 184

Hsu SY, Chan KM (1991) Arthroscopic distension in the management of frozen shoulder. Int Orthop 15: 79–83

Hurley JA, Anderson TE (1990) Shoulder arthroscopy: its role in evaluating shoulder disorders in the athlete. Am J Sports Med 18: 480–483

Jakobs RP, Johner R (1983) Indikation und Technik der Schulterarthroskopie. Hefte Unfallheilkd 165: 162–164

Jerosch J (1990) Einfluß der Gelenkmobilität auf die Ergebnisse der transarthroskopischen subakromialen Dekompression. Arthroskopie 3: 146–152

Jerosch J (1991) Arthroskopische Resektion des lateralen Klavikulanedes:, anatomisch-pathologische Grundlagen, operative Technik. Arthroskopie 4: 147–153

Jobe FW, Fobe CM (1983) Painful athletic injuries of the shoulder. Clin Orthop 173: 117–124

Johnson LL (1980) Arthroscopy of the shoulder. Orthop Clin North Am 2: 174–204

Klein W (1990) Die arthroskopische Bankart-Operation bei habitueller vorderer Schultergelenksluxation in Caspari-Technik. Arthroskopie 3: 153–158

Klein W, Gassen A (1992) Nachuntersuchungsergebnisse nach arthroskopischer Bankart Operation in Caspari-Technik. Arthroskopie 5: 229–234

Kölbel R (1989) Biomechanik und Pathobiomechanik des Schultergelenkes. In: Hedtmann A (Hrsg) Degenerative Schultererkrankungen. Enke, Stuttgart

Landsiedl F (1992) Arthroscopic therapy of recurrent anterior luxation of the shoulder by capsular repair. Arthroscopy 8: 296–305

Landsiedl F (1995) Arthroskopische Behandlungsmöglichkeiten an der Rotatorenmanschette. Orthopäde 24: 529–540

Landsiedl F, Leitner M (1997) Langzeitverlauf der arthroskopischen Therapie von Verkalkungen der Rotatorenmanschette. Arthroskopie 190

Lau KY (1993) Pneumomediastinum caused by subcutaneous emphysema in the shoulder. A rare complication of arthroscopy. Chest 103: 1606–1607

Laurencin CT, Deutsch A, O'Brien SJ, Altchek DW (1994) The superolateral portal for arthroscopy of the shoulder. Arthroscopy 10: 255–258

Legan JM, Burkhard TK, Goff WB 2d et al. (1991) Tears of the glenoid labrum: MR imaging of 88 arthroscopically confirmed cases. Radiology 179: 241–246

Levy AS, Kelly B, Lintner S, Speer K (1997) Penetration of cryotherapy in treatment after shoulder arthroscopy. Arthroscopy 13: 461–464

Levy HJ, Gardner RD, Lemak LJ (1991) Arthroscopic subacromial decompression in the treatment of full-thickness rotator cuff tears. Arthroscopy 7: 8–13

Levy HJ, Uribe JW, Delaney LG (1990) Arthroscopic assisted rotator cuff repair: preliminary results. Arthroscopy 6: 55–60

Lilleby H (1984) Shoulder arthroscopy. Acta Orthop Scand 55: 561–566

Macnab I (1981) Die pathologische Grundlage der sogenannten Rotatorenmanschetten-Tendinitis. Orthopädie 10: 1991–195

Mc Glynn FJ, Carpari RB (1984) Arthroscopic findings in the subluxating shoulder. Clin Orthop 183: 173–178

Mohtadi NG (1991) Advances in the understanding of anterior instability of the shoulder. Clin Sports Med 10: 863–870

Mok DW, Fogg AJ, Hokan R, Bayley JI (1990) The diagnostic value of arthroscopy in glenohumeral instability. J Bone Joint Surg [Br] 72: 698–700

Montgomery TJ, Yerger B, Savoie III FH (1994) Management of rotator cuff tears: a comparison of arthroscopic debridement ans surgical repair. J Shoulder Elbow Surg 3: 70–78

Moran MC, Warren RF (1989) Development of a synovial cyst after arthroscopy of the shoulder. J Bone Joint Surg [Am] 71: 127–129

Morgan CD (1991) Arthroscopic transglenoid suture repair. Operat Tech Orthop 2: 171–179

Morgan CD, Bodenstab AB (1987) Arthroscopic Bankart suture repair, technique and early results. Arthroscopy 3: 111–122

Mullins RC, Drez D Jr, Cooper J (1992) Hypoglossal nerve palsy after arthroscopy of the shoulder and open operation with the patient in the beach-chair position. A case report. J Bone Joint Surg [Am] 74: 137–139

Neer CS II (1983) Impingement lesions. Clin Orthop 173: 77–79

Neer CS II, Graig EV, Fukuda H (1983) Cuff-tear arthropathy. J Bone Joint Surg [Am] 65: 1232–1244

Neer CS II, Marberry TA (1981) One the disadvantages of radical acromioectomy. J Bone Joint Surg [Am] 63: 416

Neumann CH, Petersen SA, Jahnke AH (1991) MR imaging of the labral-capsular complex: normal variations. AJR 157: 1015–1021

Neviaser TJ (1980) The role of the biceps tendon in the impingement syndrom. Orthop Clin North Am 11: 343–348

Neviaser TJ (1993) The anterior labroligamentous periosteal sleeve avulsion: A cause of anteriore instability of the shoulder. Arthroscopy 9: 17–21

Neviaster TF (1987) Arthroscopy of the shoulder. Orthop Clin North Am 18: 361–372

Norlin R (1989) Arthroscopic subacromial Decompression vesus open acromioplasty. Arthroscopy 4: 321–323

O'Brien SJ, Neves MC, Arnoczyki SP et al. (1990) The anatomy and histology of the inferior glenohumeral ligament compley of the shoulder. Am J Sports Med 18: 449–456

Ogilvie Harris DJ, Boynton E (1990) Arthroscopic acromioplasty: extravasation of fluid into the deltoid muscle. Arthroscopy 6: 52–54

Ogilvie Harris DJ, D'Angelo G (1990) Arthroscopic surgery of the shoulder. Sports Med 9: 120–128

Ogilvie Harris DJ, Wiley AM, Sattarian J (1990) Failed acromioplasty for impingement syndrome. J Bone Joint Surg [Br] 72: 1070–1072

Ogilvie-Harris DJ, Demaziere A (1993) Arthroscopic debridement versus open repair for rotator cuff tears. J Bone Joint Surg [Br] 75: 416–420

Oglivie-Harris DJ, Biggs DJ, Fitsialos DP, Mc Day M (1995) The resistant frozen shoulder. Clin Orthop 319: 238–248

Paletta GA, Warner JP, Altchek DW, Wieckiewicz TL, O'Brien SJ, Warren RF (1993) Arthroscopic assisted rotator cuff repair: evaluation of results and comparison of techniques. Orthop Trans 17: 139

Pattee GA, Snyder SF (1988) Sonographic evaluation of the rotator cuff: correlation with arthroscopy. Arthroscopy 4: 15–20

Paulos LE, Franklin JL (1990) Arthroscopic shoulder decompression development and application. A five year experience. Am J Sports Med 18: 235–244

Pieper HF, Radas C, Blank M (1997) Häufigkeit der Rotatorenmanschettenruptur im höheren Lebensalter. Autoptische Untersuchung. Arthroskopie 175

Pollock RG, Duralde XA, Flatow EL, Bigliani LU (1994) The use of arthroscopy in the treatment of resistant frozen shoulder. Clin Orthop 304: 30–36

Resch H (1991) Neuere Aspekte in der arthroskopischen Behandlung der Schulterinstabilität. Orthopädie 20: 273–281

Resch H, Beck E (1991) Arthroskopie der Schulter. Springer, Wien New York

Resch H, Benedetto KP, Kadletz R, Oberhammer J (1985) Die Indikation zur Bankart'schen Operation. Akt Traumatol 15: 122–126

Resch H, Golser K, Sperner G, Thöni H (1992) Die arthroskopische extraartikuläre Limbusverschraubung bei unidirektionaler vorderer Schulterinstabilität. Arthroskopie 5: 79–86

Resch H, Golser K, Sperner G, Thöni H (1992) Die arthroskopische Labrumfixation mit resorbierbaren Staples. Arthroskopie 5: 89–95

Resch H, Kathrein A, Gosler K, Sperner G (1992) Arthroskopische und perkutane Verschraubungstechniken mit einem neuen Verschraubungssystem. Unfallchirurg 95: 91–98

Resch H, Sperner G, Gosler K. Thöni H, Kathrein A (1992) Die arthroskopische extraartikuläre Limbusverschraubung bei unidirektionaler vorderer Schulterinstabilität. Arthroskopie 5: 79–86

Richman JD, Rose DJ (1990) The role of arthroscopy in the management of synovial chondromatosis of the shoulder. A case report. Clin Orthop 257: 91–93

Richmond JC, Donaldson WR, Fu FH (1991) Modification of the Bankart reconstruction with a suture anchor. Report of a new technique. Am J Sports Med 19: 343–346

Rowe CR (1988) The shoulder. Churchill Livingston, New York

Sampson TG, Nisbet JK, Glick JM (1991) Precision acromioplasty in arthroscopic subacromial decompression of the shoulder. Arthroscopy 7: 301–307

Scarpinato DF, Bramhall JP, Andrews JR (1991) Arthroscopic management of the throwing athlete's shoulder: indications, techniques, and results. Clin Sports Med 10: 913–927

Seiler H (1988) Operative Schultergelenksathroskopie. Hefte Unfallheilkd 199: 13–17

Shaffer B, Tibone JE, Kerlan RK (1992) Frozen shoulder. A long-term follow up. J Bone Joint Surg [Am] 74: 738–746

Shea KP, Lovallo JLL (1991) Scapulothoracis penetration of a beath pin: An unusual complication of arthroscopic Bankart suture repair. Arthroscopy 7: 115–117

Shea KP, O'Keefe RM Jr, Fulkerson JP (1992) Comparison of initial pull-out strength of arthroscopic suture and staple Bankart repair techniques. Arthroscopy 8: 179–182

Shiley AM (1988) Arthroscopy for shoulder instability and a technique for arthroscopic repair. Arthroscopy 4: 25–30

Skyhar MR, Altchek DW, Warren RF (1988) Shoulder arthroscopy with the patient in the beach-chair position. Arthroscopy 4: 256–259

Snyder SJ (1991) Rotator cuff lesions. Acute and chronic. Clin Sports Med 10: 595–614

Snyder SJ, Brachner EJ (1993) Arthroscopic fixation of rotator cuff tears: a preliminary report. Arthroscopy 9: 342

Snyder SJ, Karzel RP, Del Pisso W, Ferkel RD (1990) SLAP lesions of the shoulder. Arthroscopy 6: 274–279

Snyder SJ, Karzel RP, Del Pizzo W, Ferkel RD, Friedman MJ (1990) SLAP lesions of the shoulder. Arthroscopy 6: 274–279

Snyder SJ, Pachelli AF, Del Pizzo W, Friedmann MJ, Ferkel RD, Pattee G (1991) Partial thickness rotator cuff tears: results of arthroscopic treatment. Arthroscopy 7: 1–7

Souryal TO, Baker CL (1990) Anatomy of the supraclavicular fossa portal in shoulder arthroscopy. Arthroscopy 6: 297–300

Speer KP, Lohnes J, Garrett WE Jr (1991) Arthroscopic subacromial decompression: results in advanced impingement syndrome. Arthroscopy 7: 291–296

Sperner G, Resch H, Golser K, Thöni H (1992) Arthorskopisches Management bei Tendinosus calcarea. Arthroskopie 5: 74–78

Stanish WD, Peterson DC (1995) Shoulder arthroscopy and nerve injury: pitfalls and prevention. Arthroscopy 11: 458–466

Strafford BB, Del Pizzo W (1993) A historical review of shoulder arthroscopy. Orthop Clin North Am 24: 1–4

Suder PA, Frich LH, Hougaard K, Lundorf E, Wulff-Jakobsen B (1995) Magnetic resonance imaging evaluation of capsulolabral tears after traumatic primary anterior shoulder dislocation. A prospective comparison with arthroscopy of 25 cases. J Shoulder Elbow Surg 4: 419–428

Tibone JE, Jobe FW, Kerlan RK, Carter VS, Shields CL, Lombardo SJ, Yocum LA (1985) Shoulder impingement syndrom in athletes treated by anterior acromioplasty. Clin Orthop 198: 134–140

Tsutsui H (1981) Arthroscopic approach to shoulder disorders. Arthroscopy 7: 9–12

Uhthoff HK, Sarkar K, Löhr J (1988) Die Pathologie der Rotatorenmanschette. Hefte Unfallheilkd 195: 125–131

Uitvlugt G, Detricac DA, Johnson LL, Austin MD, Johnson C (1993) Arthroscopic obvervations before and after manipulation of frozen shoulder. Arthroscopy 9: 181–185

Warner JJP, Miller MD, Marks P, Fu FH (1995) Arthroscopic Bankart repair with the Suretac Device. Arthroscopy 11: 2–13

Warner JJP, Warren RF (1991) Arthroscopic Bankart repair using a cannulated absorbable fixation device. Operative technique. Orthopaedics 1: 192–1998

Wasilewski SA, Frankl U (1991) Rotator cuff pathology. Arthroscopic assessment and treatment. Clin Orthop 267: 65–70

Weiner DS, Macnab I (1970) Superior migration of the humeral head. A radiological aid in the diagnosis of the rotator cuff. J Bone Joint Surg [Am] 52: 524–527

Wheeler JH, Rayn JB, Arciero RA, Molinari RN (1989) Arthroscopic versus monoperative treatment of acute shoulder dislocation in young athletes. Arthroscopy 5: 213–217

Wiley AM (1982) Arthroscopic examination of the shoulder. In: Bayley I, Kessel L (eds) Shoulder surgery. Springer, Berlin Heidelberg New York, pp 113–118

Wiley AM (1988) Arthroscopy for shoulder instability and a technique for arthroscopic repair. Arthroscopy 4: 25–30

Wiley AM (1991) Arthroscopic appearance of frozen shoulder. Arthroscopy 7: 138–143

Wiley AM, Older MWJ (1980) Shoulder arthroscopy. Investigation with a fibrooptic instrument. Am J Sport Med 8: 31–38

Yoneda M, Hirooka A, Saito S, Yamamoto T, Ochi T, Shino K (1991) Arthroscopic stapling for detached superior glenoid labrum. J Bone Joint Surg [Br] 73: 746–750

Zuckermann JD, Kummer FJ, Cuomo F, Simon J, Rosenblum S (1992) The influence of coracoacromial arch anatomy on rotator cuff tears. J Shoulder Elbow Surg 1: 4–14

Zuckermann JD, Matsen FA (1984) Complications about the glenohumeral joint related to the use of screws and staples. J Bone Joint Surg [Am] 66: 175–180

Zvjiac J, Leva HJ, Lemak LJ (1995) Athroskopic subacromial decompression in the treatment of full thickness rotator cuff tears: a 3- to 6-year follow up. Adv Orthop Surg 19: 117–119

Subtalar Joint

Bohay DR, Manoli A 2d (1996) Occult fractures following subtalar joint injuries. Foot Ankle Int 17 : 164–169

Buratti RA, Johnson JD, Buratti D (1994) Concurrent ankle and subtalar joint arthrodesis. J Foot Ankle Surg 33: 278–282

Drayer Verhagen F (1993) Arthritis of the subtalar joint associated with sustentaculum tali facet configuration. J Anat 183 631–634

Ferkel RD (ed) (1996) Subtalar arthroscopy. In: Arthroscopic surgery. The foot and ankle. Lippincott, Philadelphia, pp 231–254

Frey C, Gasser S, Feder K (1994) Arthroscopy of the subtalar joint. Foot Ankle Int 15: 424–428

Kato T (1995) The diagnosis and treatment of instability of the subtalar joint. J Bone Joint Surg [Br] 77: 400–406

Lundeen RO (1994) Arthroscopic fusion of the ankle and subtalar joint. Clin Podiatr Med Surg 11: 395–406

Lundeen RO (1987) Review of diagnostic arthroscopy of the foot and ankle. J Foot Surg 26: 33–36

Mekhail AO, Heck BE, Ebraheim NA, Jackson WT (1995) Arthroscopy of the subtalar joint: establishing a medial portal. Foot Ankle Int 16: 427–432

Parisien JS (1987) Arthroscopy of the subtalar joint. In: Slach (ed) Ankle arthroscopy: Pathology and surgical techniques. Thorofare, NJ, Slack, pp 133–142

Parisien JS, Vangsness T (1985) Arthroscopy of the subtalar joint: an experimental approach. Arthroscopy 1: 53–57

Parisien JS, Vangsness T (1986) Arthroscopy of the subtalar joint: A preliminary report. Foot Ankle 6: 219–224

Pisani G (1996) Chronic laxity of the subtalar joint. Orthopedics 19: 431–437

Rockar PA Jr (1995) The subtalar joint: anatomy and joint motion. J Orthop Sports Phys Ther 21: 361–372

Rollo VJ, Wapner KL (1993) Pigmented villonodular synovitis of the subtalar joint: a case report. Foot Ankle 14: 471–475

Villani C, Tucci G, Di Mille M, Di Gennaro S, Corsi A (1996) Extra-articular localized nodular synovitis (giant cell tumor of tendon sheath origin) attached to the subtalar joint. Foot Ankle Int 17: 413–41 6

Joints of the Toes

Alvarez R, Haddad RJ, Gould N, Trevino S (1984) The simple bunion: anatomy at the metatarsophalangeal joint oft the great toe. Foot Ankle 4: 229

Bartlett DH (1988) Arthroscopic management of osteochondritis dissecans of the first metatarsal head. Arthroscopy 4: 51–54

Clanton TO, Butler JE, Aggert A (1986). Injuries to the metatarsophalangeal joints in athletes. Foot Ankle 7: 162

Ferkel RD, Van Buecken K(1991) Great toe arthroscopy: Indications, technique and results. Presented at Arthroscopy Association of North America, San Diego

Ferkel RD (ed) (1996) Great toe arthroscopy. In: Arthroscopic surgery. The foot and ankle. Lippincott, Philadelphia, pp 255–272

Lundeen RO (1987). Arthroscopic approaches to the joints of the foot. J Am Podiatr Med Assoc 77: 451

Lundeen RO (1992) Manual of Ankle and foot arthroscopy. Churchill Livingstone, New York Edinburgh

Joints of the Fingers

Adolfsson L, Nylander G (1993) Arthrocopic synovectomy of the rheumatoid wrist. J Hand Surg Br 18: 92

Chen YC (1979) Arthrocopy of the wrist and finger joints. Orthop Clin North Am 10: 723

Chen YC (1985) Arthroscopy of the finger joints. In: Watanabe M (ed) Arthroscopy of small joints. Igaku Shoin, Tokyo New York, pp 91–96

Menon J (1996) Arthroscopic management of trapeziometacarpal joint arthritis of the thumb. Arthroscopy 12: 581–587

Wilkes LL (1987) Arthroscopic synovectomy in the rheumatoid metacarpophalangeal joint. J Med Assoc Ca 76: 638–639

Hip Joint

Blitzer CM (1993) Arthroscopic management of septic arthritis of the hip. Arthroscopy 9: 414–416

Bould M, Edwards D, Villar RN (1993) Arthroscopic diagnosis and treatment of septic arthritis of the hip joint. Arthroscopy 9: 707–708

Byrd JW (1994) Hip arthroscopy utilizing the supine position. Arthroscopy 10: 275–280

Byrd JW (1996) Hip arthroscopy for posttraumatic loose fragments in the young active adult: three case reports. Clin J Sport Med 6: 129–133

Byrd JW (1996) Labral lesions: an elusive source of hip pain case reports and literature review. Arthroscopy 12: 603–612

Byrd JW, Pappas JN, Pedley MJ (1995) Hip arthroscopy: an anatomic study of portal placement and relationship to the extra articular structures. Arthroscopy 11: 418–423

Chung WK, Slater GL, Bates EH (1993) Treatment of septic arthritis of the hip by arthroscopic lavage. J Pediatr Orthop 13: 444–446

DiStefano VJ, Kalman VR, O'Malley JS (1996) Femoral nerve palsy after arthroscopic surgery with an infusion pump irrigation system. A report of three cases. Am J Orthop 25: 145–148

Dvorak M, Duncan CP, Day B (1990) Arthroscopic anatomy of the hip. Arthroscopy 6: 264–273

Edwards DJ, Lomas D, Villar RN (1995) Diagnosis of the painful hip by magnetic resonance imaging and arthroscopy. J Bone Joint Surg Br 77: 374–376

Funke EL, Munzinger U (1996) Complications in hip arthroscopy. Arthroscopy 12: 156–159

Futami T, Kasahara Y, Suzuki S, Seto Y, Ushikubo S (1992) Arthroscopy for slipped capital femoral epiphysis. J Pediatr Orthop 12: 592–597

Grontvedt T, Engebretsen L (1995) Arthroscopy of the hip. Scand J Med Sci Sports 5: 7–9

Gross RH (1977) Arthroscopy in hip disorders in children. Orthop Rev 6: 43–49

Hogersson S, Brattstrom H, Mogensen B, Lindren L (1981) Arthroscopy of the hip in juvenile chronic arthritis. J Pediatr Orthop 1: 273–278

Hunter DM, Ruch DS (1996) Hip arthroscopy. J South Orthop Assoc 5: 243–250

Ide T, Akamatsu N, Nakajima I (1991) Arthroscopic surgery of the hip joint. Arthroscopy 7: 204–211

Ikeuchi H (1985) Arthroscopy of the hip joint. In: Watanabe M (ed) Arthroscopy of small joints. Igaku Shoin, Tokyo New York, pp 97–103

Keene GS, Villar RN (1994) Arthroscopic anatomy of the hip: an in vivo study. Arthroscopy 10: 392–399

Keene GS, Villar RN (1994) Arthroscopic loose body retrieval following traumatic hip dislocation. Injury 25: 507–510

Lage LA, Patel JV, Villar RN (1996) The acetabular labral tear: an arthroscopic classification. Arthroscopy 12: 269–272

Mah ET, Bradley CM (1992) Arthroscopic removal of acrylic cement from unreduced hip prosthesis. Aust N Z J Surg 62: 508–510

McCarthy JC, Busconi B (1995) The role of hip arthroscopy in the diagnosis and treatment of hip disease. Orthopedics 18: 753–756

Nordt W, Giangarra CE, Levy I, Habermann ET (1987) Arthroscopic removal of entrapped debris following dislocation of a total hip arthroplasty. Arthroscopy 3: 196–198

Norman Taylor FH, Villar RN (1994) Arthroscopic surgery of the hip: current status. Knee Surg Sports Traumatol Arthrosc 2: 255–258

Parisien SJ (1983) Arthroscopy of the hip present status. Bull Hops Joint Dis Orthop Inst 45: 127–132

Schindler A, Lechevallier JJ, Rao NS, Bowen JR (1995) Diagnostic and therapeutic arthroscopy of the hip in children and adolescents: evaluation of results. J Pediatr Orthop 15: 317–321

Skaggs DL, Grelsamer RP (1993) Use of a sheathed knife in hip arthroscopy. Orthop Rev 22: 1171–1172

Suzuki S, Kasahara Y, Seto Y, Futami T, Furukawa K, Nishino Y (1994) Arthroscopy in 19 children with Perthes' disease. Pathologic changes of the synovium and the joint surface. Acta Orthop Scand 65: 581–584

Takahashi T, Yamamoto H (1997) Development and clinical application of a flexible arthroscopy system. Arthroscopy 13: 42–50

Ueo T, Suzuki S, Iwasaki R, Yosikawa J (1990) Rupture of the labra acetabularis as a cause of hip pain detected arthroscopically, and partial limbectomy for successful pain relief. Arthroscopy 6: 48–51

Vakili F, Salvati EA, Warren RF (1980) Entrapped foreign body within the acetabular cup in total hip replacement. Clin Orthop Relat Res 150: 159–169

Villar RN (1992) Hip arthroscopy. Br J Hosp Med 2: 47: 763–766

Villar RN (1992) Hip arthrosopy. Butterworth Heinemann, Oxford London

Villar RN (1995) Hip arthroscopy [editorial]. J Bone Joint Surg [Br] 77: 517–518

Williams MS, Hutcheson RL, Miller AR (1997) A new technique for removal of intraarticular bullet fragments from the femoral head. Bull Hosp Joint Dis 56: 107–110

Carpal Tunnel Syndrome

Ablove RH, Peimer CA, Diao E, Oliverio R, Kuhn JP (1994) Morphologic changes following endoscopic and two-portal subcutaneous carpal tunnel release. J Hand Surg Am 19: 821–826

Agee JM, McCarroll HR Jr, Tortosa RD, Berry DA, Szabo RM, Peimer CA (1992) Endoscopic release of the carpal tunnel: a randomized prospective multicenter study. J Hand Surg Am 17: 987–995

Agee JM, Peimer CA, Pyrek JD, Walsh WE (1995) Endoscopic carpal tunnel release: a prospective study of complications and surgical experience. J Hand Surg Am 20: 165–171

Agee M, Peimer CA, Pyrek JD (1995) Endoscopic carpal tunnel relaese. A propective study of complications and surgical experience. J Hand Surg Am 20: 165–171

Akelman E, Weiss AP (1995) Carpal tunnel syndrome. Etiology and endoscopic treatment. Orthop Clin North Am 26: 769–778

Arner M, Hagberg L, Rosen B (1994) Sensory disturbances after two-portal endoscopic carpal tunnel release: a preliminary report. J Hand Surg Am 19: 548–551

Atroshi I, Johnsson R, Ornstein E (1997) Endoscopic carpal tunnel release: prospective assessment of 255 consecutive cases. J Hand Surg Br 22: 42–47

Bensimon RH, Murphy RX Jr (1996) Midpalmar approach to the carpal tunnel: an alternative to endoscopic release. Ann Plast Surg 36: 462–465

Berger RA (1994) Endoscopic carpal tunnel release. A current perspective. Hand Clin 10: 625–636

Biyani A, Downes EM (1993) An open twin incision technique of carpal tunnel decompression with reduced incidence of scar tenderness. J Hand Surg Br 18: 331–334

Born T, Mahoney J (1995) Cutaneous distribution of the ulnar nerve in the palm: does it cross the incision used in carpal tunnel release? Ann Plast Surg 35: 23–25

Bozentka DJ, Ostermann L (1995) Complications of endoscopic carpal tunnel release. Hand Clin North Am 11: 91–96

Bromley GS (1994) Minimal-incision open carpal tunnel decompression. J Hand Surg Am 19: 119–120

Brown MG, Keyser B, Rothenberg ES (1992) Endoscopic carpal tunnel release. J Hand Surg Am 17: 1009–1011

Brown RA, Gelberman RH, Seiler JG 3rd et al. (1993) Carpal tunnel release. A prospective, randomized assessment of open and endoscopic methods. J Bone Joint Surg [Am] 75: 1265–1275

Brown RA, Gelbermann RH, Seiler JGR (1993) Carpal tunnel release. A prospective, randomized assessment of open and endoscopic methods. J Bone Joint Surg [Am] 75: 1265–1275

Brug E (1995) Karpaltunnelsyndrom. In: Brug E, Rieger H, Strobel M (Hrsg) Ambulante Chirurgie. Deutscher Ärzteverlag, Köln, S 155–159

Brug E (1996) Die endokopische Operation des Karpaltunnels -[Editorial]. Chir Praxis 51: 171–172

Chow JC (1989) Endoscopic release of the carpal ligament: A new technique for carpal tunnel syndrome. Arthroscopy 5: 679–683

Chow JC (1990) Endoscopic release of the carpal ligament for carpal tunnel syndrome: 22-month clinical result. Arthroscopy 6: 288–296

Chow JC (1993) The Chow technique of endoscopic release of the carpal ligament for carpal tunnel syndrome: four years of clinical results. Arthroscopy 9: 301–314

Chow JC (1994) Endoscopic carpal tunnel release. Two-portal technique. Hand Clin 10: 637–646

Citron ND, Bendall SP (1997) Local symptoms after open carpal tunnel release. A randomized prospective trial of two incisions. J Hand Surg Br 22: 317–321

Cobb TK, Carmichael SW, Cooney WP (1994) The ulnar neurovascular bundle at the wrist. A technical note on endoscopic carpal tunnel release. J Hand Surg Br 19: 24–26

Cobb TK, Cooney WP (1994) Significance of incomplete release of the distal portion of the flexor retinaculum. Implications for endoscopic carpal tunnel surgery. J Hand Surg Br 19: 283–285

Cobb TK, Cooney WP, An KN (1994) Clinical location of hook

of hamate: a technical note for endoscopic carpal tunnel release. J Hand Surg Am 19: 516–518

Cobb TK, Knudson GA, Cooney WP (1995) The use of topographical landmarks to improve the outcome of Agee endoscopic carpal tunnel release. Arthroscopy 11: 165–172

De Smet L, Fabry G (1994) The results of carpal tunnel release: open versus endoscopic technique. J Hand Surg Br 19: 14–17

De Smet L, Fabry G (1995) Transection of the motor branch of the ulnar nerve as a complication of two portal endoscopic carpal tunnel release – a case report. J Hand Surg Am 20: 18–19

Del Pinal F, Cruz Camara A, Jado E (1997) Total ulnar nerve transection during endoscopic carpal tunnel release. Arthroscopy 13: 235–237

Deune EG, Mackinnon SE (1996) Endoscopic carpal tunnel release. The voice of polite dissent. Clin Plast Surg 23: 487–505

Dumontier C, Sokolow C, Leclercq C, Chauvin P (1995) Early results of conventional versus two-portal endoscopic carpal tunnel release. A prospective study. J Hand Surg Br 20: 658–662

Erdmann MW (1994) Endoscopic carpal tunnel decompression J Hand Surg Br 19: 5–13

Feinstein PA (1993) Endoscopic carpal tunnel release in a community based series. J Hand Surg Am 18: 451–454

Fischer TJ, Hastings H 2nd (1996) Endoscopic carpal tunnel release. Chow technique. Hand Clin 12: 285–297

Gibbs KE, Rand W, Ruby LK (1996) Open vs endoscopic carpal tunnel release. Orthopedics 19: 1025–1028

Hunt TR, Ostermann AL (1994) Complications of the treatment of carpal tunnel syndrome. Hand Clin 10: 63–71

Jacobsen MB, Rahme H (1996) A prospective, randomized study with an independent observer comparing open carpal tunnel release with endoscopic carpal tunnel release. J Hand Surg Br 21: 202–204

Jebson PJ, Agee JM (1996) Carpal tunnel syndrome: unusual contraindications to endoscopic release. Arthroscopy 12: 749–751

Karlsson-MK, Lindau-T, Hagberg-L (1997) Ligament lengthening compared with simple division of the transverse carpal ligament in the open treatment of carpal tunnel syndrome. Scand J Plast Reconstr Surg Hand Surg 31: 65–69

Katz JN, Gelberman RH, Wright EA, Abrahamsson SO, Lew RA (1994) A preliminary scoring system for assessing the outcome of carpal tunnel release. J Hand Surg Am 19: 531–538

Kelly CP, Pulisetti D, Jamieson AM (1994) Early experience with endoscopic carpal tunnel release J Hand Surg Br 19: 18–21

Kerr CD, Gittins ME, Sybert DR (1994) Endoscopic versus open carpal tunnel release: clinical results. Arthroscopy 10: 266–269

Kiritsis PG, Kline SC (1995) Biomechanical changes after carpal tunnel release: a cadaveric model for comparing open, endoscopic, and step-cut lengthening techniques. J Hand Surg Am 20: 173–180

Lanz UL (1977) Anatomical variations of the median nerve in the carpal tunnel. J Hand Surg [Am] 2: 44–53

Lee DH, Masear VR, Meyer RD, Stevens DM, Colgin S (1992) Endoscopic carpal tunnel release: a cadaveric study. J Hand Surg Am 17: 1003–1008

Lee H, Jackson TA (1996) Carpal tunnel release through a limited skin incision under direct visualization using a new instrument, the carposcope. Plast Reconstr Surg 98: 313–319, discussion 320

Lee WP, Plancher KD, Strickland JW (1996) Carpal tunnel release with a small palmar incision. Hand Clin 12: 271–284

Levy HJ, Soifer TB, Kleinbart FA, Lemak LJ, Bryk E (1993) Endoscopic carpal tunnel release: an anatomic study. Arthroscopy 9: 1–4

Lewicky RT (1994) Endoscopic carpal tunnel release: the guide tube technique. Arthroscopy 10: 39–49

Luallin SR, Toby EB (1993) Incidental Guyon's canal release during attempted endoscopic carpal tunnel release: an anatomical study and report of two cases. Arthroscopy 9: 382–326

Menon J (1991) Endoscopic release of carpal ligaments. Arthroscopy 7: 413–414

Menon J (1994) Endoscopic carpal tunnel release: Preliminary report. Arthroscopy 10: 31–38

Mirza MA, King ET (1996) Newer techniques of carpal tunnel release. Orthop Clin North Am 27: 355–371

Mirza MA, King ET Jr, Tanveer S (1995) Palmar uniportal extrabursal endoscopic carpal tunnel release. Arthroscopy 11: 82–90

Murphy RXJ, Jennings JF, Wukich DK (1994) Major neurovascular complications of endoscopic carpal tunnel release. J Hand Surg Am 19: 114–118

Nagle D, Harris G. Foley M (1994) Prospective review of 278 endoscopic carpal tunnel releases using the modified Chow technique. Arthroscopy 10: 259–265

Nagle DJ (1996) Endoscopic carpal tunnel release. In favor. Clin Plast Surg 23: 477–486

Nagle DJ, Fischer TJ, Harris GD et al. (1996) A multicenter prospective review of 640 endoscopic carpal tunnel releases using the transbursal and extrabursal chow techniques. Arthroscopy 12: 139–143

Nath RK, Mackinnon SE, Weeks PM (1993) Ulnar nerve transection as a complication of two-portal endoscopic carpal tunnel release: a case report. J Hand Surg Am 18: 896–898

Okutsu I, Ninomiya S, Natsuyama M (1987) Subcutaneous operation and examination under universal endoscopic. J Jpn Orthop Assoc 61: 491–498

Okutsu I, Ninomiya S, Takatori Y (1989) Endoscopic management of carpal tunnel syndrome. Arthroscopy 5: 11

Palmer AK, Toivonen DA (1995) Complications of endoscopic and open carpal tunnel release. Presented at the 50th Annual Meeting of the ASSH, San Francisco

Palmer DH, Paulson JC, Lane Larsen CL, Peulen VK, Olson JD (1993) Endoscopic carpal tunnel release: a comparison of two techniques with open release. Arthroscopy 9: 498–508

Palmer DH, Paulson JC, Lane-Larsen CL (1993) Endoscopic carpal tunnel release: A comparison of two techniques with open release. Arthroscopy 9: 498–508

Pennino R, Tavin E (1996) Endoscopic-assisted carpal tunnel release: a coupling of endoscopic and open techniques. Ann Plast Surg 36: 458–461

Preißler P (1996) Die palmar-dorsale endoskopische Karpalbandspaltung. Arthroskopie 9: 11–16

Rieger H, Grünert J, Brug E (1996) A severe infection following endoscopic carpal tunnel release. J Hand Surg Br 21: 672–674

Roth JH, Richards RS, MacLeod MD (1994) Endoscopic carpal tunnel release. Can J Surg 37: 189–193

Rotman MB, Manske PR (1993) Anatomic relationships of an endoscopic carpal tunnel device to surrounding structures. J Hand Surg Am 18: 442–450

Rowland EB, Kleinert JM (1994) Endoscopic carpal-tunnel release in cadavera. An investigation of the results of twelve surgeons with this training model. J Bone Joint Surg [Am] 76: 266–268

Schwartz JT, Waters PM, Simmons BP (1993) Endoscopic carpal tunnel release: a cadaveric study. Arthroscopy 9: 209–213

Scoggin JF, Whipple TL (1992) A potential complication of endoscopic carpal tunnel release. Arthroscopy 8: 363–365

Seiler JG 3d, Barnes K, Gelberman RH, Chalidapong P (1992) Endoscopic carpal tunnel release: an anatomic study of the two-incision method in human cadavers. J Hand Surg Am 17: 996–1002

Sellers DS (1995) Endoscopic carpal tunnel release. Clin Plast Surg 22: 775–780

Serra JM, Benito JR, Monner J (1997) Carpal tunnel release with short incision. Plast Reconstr Surg 99: 129–135

Shinya K, Lanzetta M, Conolly WB (1995) Risk and complications in endoscopic carpal tunnel release. J Hand Surg Br 20: 222–227

Stark RH (1994) Ulnar nerve transection as a complication of two-portal endoscopic carpal tunnel release. J Hand Surg Am 19: 522

Tsai TM, Tsuruta T, Syed SA, Kimura H (1995) A new technique for endoscopic carpal tunnel decompression. J Hand Surg Br 20: 465–469

Urbaniak JR, Desai SS (1996) Complications of nonoperative and operative treatment of carpal tunnel syndrome. Hand Clin 12: 325–335

Van Heest A, WatersP, Simmons B, Schwartz JT (1995) A cadaveric study of the single-portal endoscopic carpal tunnel release. J Hand Surg Am 20: 363–6

Viegas SF, Pollard A, Kaminksi K (1992) Carpal arch alteration and related clinical status after endoscopic carpal tunnel release. J Hand Surg Am 17: 1012–1016

Wheatley MJ (1996) A simple technique for identification of the distal extent of the transverse carpal ligament during single-portal endoscopic carpal tunnel release. J Hand Surg Am 21: 1109–1110

Wilson KM (1994) Double-incision open technique for carpal tunnel release: An alternative to endoscopic release. J Hand Surg Am 19: 907–912

Worseg AP, Kuzbari R, Korak K, Hocker K, Wiederer C, Tschabitscher M, Holle J (1996) Endoscopic carpal tunnel release using a single-portal system. Br J Plast Surg 49: 1–10

Zimmermann JA, Nitzsche T, Steen M (1997) Light at the beginning of the carpal tunnel? Plast Reconstr Surg 99: 2101–2102

Bursal Endoscopy

Kerr DR (1993) Prepatellar and olecranon arthroscopic bursectomy. Clin Sports Med 12: 137–142

Pässler HH (1996) Bursaendoskopie. Arthroskopie 9: 22–25

J

Y

Z